The Essential
SUDHIR KAKAR

'Sudhir Kakar, a great intellectual, psychoanalyst and anthropologist, is one of the principal figures in contemporary Indian thought, and on top of all that, a novelist of repute.'

—*Le Monde*, Paris

'[Sudhir Kakar is] by common consent, our foremost psychoanalyst, who will remain indispensable to our understanding of Indian men and women.'

—*The Hindu*

'[Kakar's] books have laid bare the Indian psyche, and shown how Indian culture, society and family structure condition our behaviour as adults.'

—*Indian Express*

'In the history of India's cultural awakening in the twentieth century … some books will stand out as seminal. Among these Sudhir Kakar's will certainly find a place.'

—*Indian Book Chronicle*

'To read Sudhir Kakar's books is always a great joy. The mix of knowledge, humour and wisdom is as uncommon as is the combination of literary and psychoanalytic approaches to the world.

—*Die Tageszeitung*, Berlin

The Essential
SUDHIR KAKAR

OXFORD
UNIVERSITY PRESS

OXFORD
UNIVERSITY PRESS

Oxford University Press is a department of the University of Oxford. It furthers the University's objective of excellence in research, scholarship, and education by publishing worldwide. Oxford is a registered trademark of Oxford University Press in the UK and in certain other countries.

Published in India by
Oxford University Press
22 Workspace, 2nd Floor, 1/22 Asaf Ali Road, New Delhi 110002, India

First Edition published in 2011
Oxford India Paperbacks 2021

ISBN 13: 978-0-19-012915-6
ISBN 10: 0-19-012915-8

Typeset in Adobe Garamond Pro 10.5/12.5
by BeSpoke Integrate Solutions, Puducherry, India 605 008
Printed in India by Rakmo Press, New Delhi 110 020

Contents

Preface[†]

THERE ARE SOME PARTS of the world that, no matter how many times you visit, always give you a new sense of reality. For me, India is such a place. Not only because multiple and contradictory views and forms of life co-exist here, but also because this is the home of great souls and strong characters. As Emerson says, 'Character is higher than intellect. A great soul will be strong [enough] to live as well as think.'

Sudhir Kakar is such a man; his peculiar moral strength and integrity of character has had, after seventy years of courageous effort, an ever-growing effect on fellow Indians and other people around the world. I had the privilege of conversing with Kakar and have now developed a deep and abiding friendship with him. He is neither a holy man living on top of a mountain nor a pretentious scholar not willing to listen to and learn from others; he is a remarkable human being and a passionate analyst of the Indian cultural imagination, who has studied the explicit link between modernity and tradition in India for more than forty years. Today, Kakar is a well-known name in Indian psychoanalysis and is an influential figure in the international intellectual arena. He has been described by the French magazine *Le Nouvel Observateur* as one of the twenty-five major thinkers of the world. He is the author of novels such

[†] First published as 'Capturing the Indian Psyche', in *India Analysed: Sudhir Kakar in Conversation with Ramin Jahanbegloo* (OUP 2009).

as *The Ascetic of Desire*, based on the life of Vatsyayana, and *Ecstasy*, which is an exploration of the relationship between guru and disciple as is seen in the mutual admiration of Miraben and the revered father of the Indian nation, Mahatma Gandhi.

While analysing sexuality as practised in ancient India, Kakar remains a severe critic of the conservative and puritanical sexual mores of contemporary India. As such, his new and fresh translation of the *Kamasutra*, done jointly with Wendy Doniger, appears to be an effort to critique modern Indian sexual behaviours through the presentation of this classical erotic text. *Kamasutra*, which many tourists who visit India wrongly regard as a textbook about sexual positions, is actually one of the oldest Hindu texts about the art of living. The book provides a fascinating glimpse into the society of ancient India along with much advice on cultivating knowledge of the arts, good manners, and grooming. Kakar's translation and study of the *Kamasutra* recovers and reconstructs the ancient text's insistence on the indispensable balance between the erotic and the spiritual. For Kakar, Indian spirituality is intended to be an intensely practical affair concerned with the alchemy of the libido. Here morality and sexuality are fused together, and it is true that individualism, in its Western form, is foreign to the traditional Indian sexual and spiritual consciousness and experience. For Kakar there are hidden images of individuality incorporated into Indian culture, and mystical experiences in India illustrate this fact. But the question which remains at the centre of Kakar's work is: to what extent is psychoanalytic theory that has originated primarily in the Western canon valid and meaningful when applied to the Indian context? Can the psychological make sense of the cultural in all human experience? The only way to understand Kakar's methodology is to recognize the fact that he has a measure of the modern as well as of the traditional.

Kakar invites his readers to participate in open debates about the universalistic pretensions of psychoanalytic theory when he applies them to Indian culture. A psychological analysis of the Hindu world image by Kakar makes sense because it provides readers with an analysis of the distinctive features of the Indian social and spiritual structures based on notions such as dharma, moksha, and karma. Realizing that these three coordinates are typical traits of Indian individuality/sociality that are different from Western traits, Kakar contextualizes them in his psychological analysis of India as forms of relational existence.

'The idea that every individual's svadharma is unique,' writes Kakar in his book *The Inner World*, 'enhances a deeply held belief in a pervasive equality at a personal level, among all human beings … It is more a belief that each individual has a dignified, rightful place and function in the society, a belief which transcends the formal patterns of deference to caste, class, and family hierarchies, but does not hold the promise of an egalitarian society.' In other words, the Hindu mind has a strong inclination to subjectivize timeless mythical events as if they were personal material. 'In India,' affirms Kakar, 'historical events have little immediacy in the lives of individuals; they seem to recede almost instantly into a distant past, to become immemorial legend … On the other hand, mythical figures like Rama or Hanuman are as actual and as psychologically real (if not more so) as recent historical characters such as Ramakrishna or Shivaji.' This is the reason why, for Kakar, the Oedipus complex is inverted in the Indian context. Kakar chooses the myth of Ganesha to show how the father envies the son for his possessions, including his mother. Kakar's emphasis is also on the goddess as mother and especially as mother of the sons, Ganesha and Skanda, who psychologically represent the two childhood positions of the Indian son. According to Kakar, Skanda and Ganesha personify the two opposing wishes of the older child on the eve of the Oedipus complex: a powerful push for independence and an equally strong pull towards surrender to the maternal from which he has just emerged. Thus, in Hindu culture Ganesha's surrender is considered to be superior to Skanda's wish for independence. Therefore, Kakar suggests that unlike the conflicted male of Western thought, the Indian man is at one with the mother's wish to not separate her son from herself.

In his 1986 publication, *Tales of Love, Sex and Danger*, written with the New York based psychoanalyst, John M. Ross, Kakar analyses the 'paradigmatic love story of Hindu India'—the story of the milkmaid Radha and her union with the god Krishna. For Kakar, the Radha–Krishna relation amounts to a 'depersonalized voluptuous state' recalling the earliest attachment of the infant to his mother. What the legendary Radha–Krishna love story illustrates is that in the protected childhood of Indian men there is an absence of social pressure 'to give up non-logical modes of thinking and communication'. An Indian child, thus, in contrast to a Western child, 'is encouraged to continue to live in a mythical, magical world for a long time'. It is interesting to examine Kakar's methodology by understanding the ways in which he presents the Indian cultural viewpoint before applying psychoanalysis to it. Kakar's research on the Indian psyche and sexual behaviours relies profoundly on Indian classical texts, Indian popular culture such as Hindi movies and folktales, and on primary source material such as biographies and letters. Kakar's art lies in the fact that he is a gifted story-teller and a brilliant analyst. Finally, Kakar's contribution to cultural psychology is his technique of interplaying the universalist theoretical approach and the cultural relativist view. As he underlines in his book *Intimate Relations*, 'Indian myths constitute a cultural idiom that aids the individual in the construction and integration of his inner world.'

However, not all Indians agree fully with Kakar's critical analysis of everyday Indian psychological behaviours. Many Indians feel that Kakar's psycho-biographic work on Indian spiritual figures is of a reductionist nature: it fails to appreciate the true essence of Indian mystic traditions correctly. Kakar's response to all these misconceptions and misunderstandings has been: '… mysticism is a kind of individualized religious experience that is limited to very few people; it can be expressed in a society that respects that, and India very much respects mystics. It is comparable to Gandhi: I will not be an ascetic like Gandhi, but I nevertheless respect Gandhi. This means India allows Gandhis to live their lives as it allows mystics to flourish and not put them into any kind of asylum.' What Kakar seems to be reminding us of here is that the ecstatic state of mysticism cannot be achieved without an ascetic state of being. As such, 'Shades of both "infinity" and "personality" will exist in every mystic.' As Kakar shows in his book *The Analyst and the Mystic*, the mystic blends the quest for the divine with the search for a higher self. In this context, the sense of individual identity is used to progress along the spiritual path. As Kakar points out clearly in *The Analyst and the Mystic*, 'Even the passions—lust, anger, greed, inordinate attachment, pride, egoism—which have been traditionally held as obstacles to spiritual progress, do not need to be vanquished in devotional mysticism.' Therefore, for Kakar, the mystical goal is not only to fuse with the Cosmic Being, but also to reach out for a relation with the mother through the 'recovery of a childlike innocence'. Quoting Ramakrishna, Kakar illustrates this relationship of the mystic with the cosmos as one that suggests the child's point of view: 'To my Mother I prayed only for pure devotion … Mother, here is your virtue, here is your vice. Take them both and grant me only pure love for you. Here is your purity and here is your impurity. Take them both Mother and grant me only pure devotion for you. Here is your dharma and here is your adharma. Take them both Mother and grant me only pure devotion for you.' In the course of his analysis of Ramakrishna's private space of passion and desire, Kakar surveys the psychotherapeutic function of the guru as a healer of emotional suffering. The guru is formulated as 'the culturally sanctioned addressee of a collective request for the transforming experience'. Thus in Kakar's formulation, the core of the guru–disciple relationship is 'an increasing surrender to the self-object experience of the merging kind'. In addition to this 'surrender', Kakar says that we can find 'an idealizing transference' in this relationship which touches the deeper layers of the human psyche. What becomes evident here is the expectation of immediate healing by a spiritual teacher rather than a religious promise of gaining a lost paradise. Therefore, while reading Kakar, it becomes clear that for him the two notions of 'spiritual' and 'religious' are not identical.

Looking back at Kakar's life and work, one can easily understand his interest in both religion and spirituality as a form of interplay between the individual and society. According to Kakar, 'It is the core of religion that is important for religious people, and that is spiritual rather than sectarian.' What Kakar calls 'sectarianism' or 'communalism', when viewed psychologically, is a change from the idea of community to that of communalism. Kakar observes that 'religious community is the interactive aspect of religious identity' and what is considered to be dangerous to this identity gives birth to 'communalism and the potential of social violence'. That is to say, religion has a greater emotional intensity and a deeper motivational thrust than ethnic pride or national identity. Taking into account one of Kakar's famous works, *The Colors of Violence*, one should remember that he grew up in a district town in west Punjab where he directly experienced the Partition and the religious confrontation between Hindus and Muslims. It would be wrong, however, to consider Kakar's cultural and psychological writings as the work of a 'Hindu' or a simple analysis of 'Hindu India'. Kakar is more concerned with the spirit of India and what makes the Indianness of Indians rather than with Hindu India. His problem is to understand how one can be an Indian while living with tradition and modernity at the same time. 'I do not look down upon the middle class as betraying the Indian ethos,' observes Kakar, 'because it is creating the ethos for a modern society. The traditional ethos was good for those earlier times. I do not think the Indian identity has emerged yet—this type of contest will go on and on. I think that in society all kinds of changes take place. But there are also parts of it that stay the same.' In other words, what describes the Indian attitude towards life is a certain philosophical relativity and psychological fluidity.

Thus, the Indian *weltanschauung* is one that is beyond the rigid and cynical binary of black and white. Maybe one can say that the Indian ego lives and thinks in that grey zone where there is a permanent exchange between the human soul and the environment. This environment includes the occult and the metaphysical sense of being, and therefore, gurus, shamans, astrologers, and ascetics play an important role in the ongoing reality of the Indian psyche. What makes Indians distinct from the rest of the world is not only the predominance of family, community, and caste in their everyday lives, but also, as Kakar shows in his book *The Indians*, written in collaboration with anthropologist Katharina Kakar, their attitude to sex and marriage, their idea of the 'Other' as we see in the Hindu–Muslim conflict, and their understanding of life and death. However, Kakar is clearly conscious of the complexity and diversity of India when he says, 'How can anyone generalise about a country of a billion people—Hindus, Muslims, Sikhs, Christians, Jains—speaking fourteen major languages and with pronounced differences? How can one postulate anything in common between a people divided not only by social class but also by India's signature system of caste, and with an ethnic diversity characteristic more of past empires than of modern nations?'

And yet, there is an underlying unity in the great diversity of India that needs to be recognized. Interestingly, in India, equality, in the Tocquevillian sense of the term, as a modern social value has not been taken to mean the absence of hierarchy. To quote Sudhir Kakar, 'An Indian has a heightened dependence on external authority figures. An Indian tends to search for authority figures he can idealise, whose "perfection" and omnipotence he can then adopt as his own. Thus, the automatic reverence for superiors is a nearly universal psycho-social fact. And, when it comes to leadership in the larger social institutions of business and government in India, charisma plays an unusually significant role.' As such, old values manifest themselves in the practice of modern values. Indian democracy is strangely adapted to the undemocratic structures of the Indian past. Kakar ascribes the Indian political taste for charisma to 'an unconscious tendency to "submit" to an idealized omnipotent figure, both in the inner world of fantasy and in the outside world of making a living; the lifelong search for someone, a charismatic leader or a guru, who will provide mentorship and a guiding world-view'. The hierarchical nature of the Indian mind applies to all ethnic and caste groups in India. Therefore, democracy in India is not a cultural attitude, but a political value. This is a phenomenon which merits attention.

What makes Kakar's work original is that he presents a composite view of India in which Indians recognize themselves and which helps other people to go beyond their touristic and simplistic view of Indianness. Above all, Kakar remains in dialogue with the key building blocks of Indianness while he interrogates the impact of modernity on Indian society. The works of Sudhir Kakar on the psychosocial tensions underlying Indian identity are a great landmark in understanding the stresses and strains of an unexplored and hidden India which is in the process of aspiring to be authentically traditional and yet is thoroughly modern. Analysing India with Sudhir Kakar, therefore, is not only a way of understanding the Indian way of thinking about the world but also a means to think of the issues in today's world.

Ramin Jahanbegloo
University of Toronto

Introduction

IT IS WITH GREAT PLEASURE that I write an introduction to this well-timed volume. An admirer of Kakar's writings—and I know from personal experience that this is true of many others who find his prose extremely lucid, imaginative, and insightful—I have often resorted to them to understand the tussle between culture and individual, how a discourse of the unconscious can be extended to understand social structures and processes, and the ways in which one can explore the roots of cultural psychoanalysis and find expressions for cross-cultural similarities and angularities around vagaries of human subjectivity.[1] Listening to one of the several talks that Kakar gave in London in 2009, I could relate for the first time with the compelling force of the unsettling experiences of his youth and his determined efforts to work around themes of selfhood and identity. And in a person who looks so serene and self-composed, it reaffirmed for me the transformative role writing must have played in his life.

For me, two questions seem pertinent to Kakar's corpus of writing: the first concerns the place of *culture in psychoanalysis* (especially a non-Western one); the second is centred on the place of *psychoanalysis in culture* (specifically Indian, and broadly non-Western). Both issues of place—culture in psychoanalysis and psychoanalysis in culture—continue to be important concerns for critical engagement and further research. With regard to how the thematic of culture could be addressed in psychoanalysis, Kakar suggests that there is a growing need to integrate cultural and social idioms by developing the psychoanalytic model of symbolizations, such as dream-work and interpretation, further allowing and encouraging social and cultural expressions to be voiced, represented, and worked on within the clinical or social research context. He is concerned with the question of how Indian culture also needs to acknowledge and embrace the psychoanalytic model, which promises richer insights and opens newer terrains of human enquiry, more informed base for social activism and political transformation, along with the promise of a unique model of social research. Amongst the many threats to its existence, psychoanalysis in India is likely to encounter a neo-colonial backlash both from cultural and social science theorists in their rejection of the former to be scientistic and deterministic (it perhaps appears too hedonistic for their intake)[2] and also from the mainstream psychoanalysis that chooses to keep its engine going aculturally.[3]

Kakar has authored more than a dozen books on various aspects of Indian cultural psyche. Informed by psychohistory and influenced by Erikson's theory of identity and its psychosocial development within the lifecycle of an individual in a given society, he has been very vocal in articulating the issues of identity and separation–individuation dynamics operating within Indian psyche and culture. T.G. Vaidyanathan in his introduction to *The Essential Writings of Sudhir Kakar* (2001) manages to raise significant themes that Kakar evolved and developed as an ingenious writer in the last two decades. He begins by elucidating the course of Kakar's journey into the Indian cultural identity discourse as explicated in *The Inner World* (1978), *Culture* and *Psyche* (1997), and also in *The Colours of Violence* (1995) wherein he evolves a clinical methodology and analysis of political action, its actors focusing on the group dynamics in a communally volatile city of Hyderabad. To the luscious details of intimacy, sexual entanglements, power dynamics, and the exhilarating, diabolic, and numbing moments of desire's seething currents as depicted in *Intimate Relations* (1990), Kakar takes this thematic further into the forays of group-identity processes and manifestation of sexuality within the cultural field, in both its inspirational and diabolic strands.

In this Introduction I hope to flag off some of Kakar's key ideas, extend the discussion around his influence of thinking, and provide a critical commentary on how these ideas fit in with the larger psychoanalytic theory and understanding of culture. The book is divided into six sections: Culture and Healing; Psychoanalysis and Culture; Erotic Love;

Psychobiography; Religion and Psyche; Childhood and Identity; and it also includes an interesting conversation between Kakar and Madhu Sarin, wherein Kakar talks about his influences and impressions on varied aspects of Indian culture, psychoanalysis, and the interpenetration of the two in his own life. While the Preface by Ramin Jahanbegloo provides a sociological and philosophical analysis of the influence of Kakar's ideas, I focus on providing an overarching view of the length and breadth of Kakar's thinking and discuss how his work extends the existing connections with psychoanalysis and social theory.

Fascinated by Gandhi's political thinking and philosophy (an influence from the time Kakar spent in Ahmedabad city; perhaps also from Erikson's writings on Gandhi), Kakar offers a psychobiograpical exploration of Gandhi's everyday life and the meaning of his larger political mission. First published in *Intimate Relations*, the chapter entitled 'Gandhi and Women' revolves around Gandhi's relationship with women and the developmental vicissitudes of a qualitatively peculiar encounter with his parents that became a defining moment in Kakar's ideas around Indian male psyche and childhood and led to one of his most important psychoanalytic concept called the maternal–feminine. Kakar's essay is a psychoanalytic deconstruction of the autobiographical writing of Gandhi, *The Story of My Experiments with Truth*, written in 1902. While reading, one cannot help drawing parallels between Gandhi and Freud. I am aware of the hazards of oversimplification and so I shall try to tread cautiously. It appears to me that in several aspects of their lives, particularly in the arena of their childhood, in a sustained search for the 'truth', and in their corresponding ambition to achieve something larger than life, Gandhi and Freud were strikingly similar.

Gandhi's near obsession with food (with elaborate details of what he ate, what should be eaten, what should be prohibited, and practising vegetarianism) gave rise to this popular dictum: 'simple living, high thinking', which remains a favourite with good-old Gandhians even today. His preoccupations with religious and spiritual matters appear symptomatic of the internal turmoil the man in the mahatma was undergoing. The vivacity with which Kakar establishes connections between both these aspects, discussing Gandhi's recurrent struggle with sexuality—primarily a genital one—provides interesting insight into the fault line running between symptom and its subverted formation, sublimation. Bringing his life history back and forth to recount the aspects of his childhood where he grapples with the pervasive Brahaminical morality and his newly acquired Western ideals adds an interesting angle to the 'beginnings of Mahatma' in Gandhi. It is this personal transformation that made Gandhi the leader he was to become later on, electrifying masses with enormous success and following in his famous 'Quit India' movement, bargaining and negotiating for freedom from them in a manner which appeased (or least humiliated!) British pride.

Gandhi's practice of sexual abstinence asked for 'a thoroughgoing desexualization of the male–female relationship', in which he professed 'women should lead'.[4] For Gandhi, women were a symbol of *ahimsa* (non-violence), and Kakar analyses Gandhi's struggle to grapple with the pre-Oedipal mother–infant merger and a concomitant tendency to locate the mother in every woman he encountered in his life. Kakar points out that this could simply be a way of denying overwhelming and puzzling feminine eroticism. He reiterates that Gandhi's relationships with women were 'dominated by the unconscious fantasy of maintaining an idealized relationship with the maternal body'.[5] Even while working rigorously on his doctrine of 'satyagraha' (insistence on truth), right in the thick of the freedom movement, what Gandhi wrote and appeared constantly pre-occupied with was his dietary regimen, testing whether he was a pure celibate, checking if thoughts of sexual pollution entered into his mind during waking hours or sleep and how these hindered his spiritual being and his work in the community. In this sense, he fought a constant battle not so much with the British rulers but with the 'dark god of desire'.[6] By choosing Gandhi as an example, Kakar tries to bring to the fore the place Hindu cultural tradition accords to sexuality and 'spirituality within sexuality'.

These are two themes Gandhi's autobiography opens up for critical as well as sympathetic reader. The dimension most emphasized by the Hindu tradition in relation to the question of sexuality is genital sexuality with its transmutation into a spiritual and sacred order and how in the ultimate analysis all desire and pleasure needs to be channelized towards self-realization in achieving unity with the universe. Kakar elaborates on Hindu conception of 'spirituality within sexuality' further:

> The sexual urges amount to a creative fire—not only for procreation but, equally, in self-creation … further it is a tradition which does not reduce sexual love to copulation but seeks to elevate it into a celebration, even a ritual that touches the partners with a sense of the sacred, and where orgasm is experienced as a symbolic blessing of man by his ancestors and by the nature of things ….[7]

Providing illustrations from the legendary book of *Kamasutra*, Kakar explicates the problematic of Hindu sexuality as it seeks to tap the sacred, grapple with and tame the diabolic through engaging with the most poignant elements of human sexuality.[8] *Kamasutra* opens many vistas towards understanding Hindu versions of sexuality. Some of these versions at once appear representative of the phallocentric and misogynist texts where curious and at the same time inchoate questions around exploration and control into woman's body, desire, and psyche are sermonized. In other instances, the text, at varied moments, illustrates another strand of Hindu theorization on sexuality. It is where the sacred and transcendental, poignant, excessive, and overwhelming aspects of sexuality are shown to be characteristic of a basal need and primal struggle for love and unity in human life. Developing this thematic from *Kamasutra*, Kakar points to the vicissitudes of this struggle effectively: 'The concept is even present in the *Kamasutra*, the text book of eroticism and presumably a subvertor of ascetic ideals, where the successful lover is not someone who is overly passionate but one, who has controlled and stilled his senses through brahmacharya and meditation'.[9]

Through transforming sexual desires into spiritual power (or some power of higher order above the bodily preoccupations), 'Indian "mysticism" is typically intended to be an intensely practical affair, concerned with an alchemy of the libido that would convert it from a giver of death (by wasting the sexual energy through copulation) to a bestower of immortality'.[10] Though the cultural anxiety of 'squandering the sperm' and 'biological self sacrifice' entails ambivalence towards women that verges on misogyny and phobic avoidance.

Much of this philosophy seems to be treated with a reserve by Western rationalist philosophy. Indian spirituality, as Kakar sees it, is pre-eminently a theory of 'sublimation guided by the tight throes of the cultural superego'.[11] In the case of Gandhi, there are two parallels continually in play with each other, while in a loose sense it is the 'fixation' on the mother imago that keeps the genital desire psychically forever unconsummated and one that threatens complete disintegration of a coherent experience of self. On the other hand, Kakar brings out a subtle dimension of Indian cultural tradition and philosophy that Gandhi emulated and had strongly identifications with. For Gandhi, 'lust was not just sinful but poisonous, contaminating the elixir of immortality, one which served to destructuralize, rather than be merely immoral. Gandhi's struggle with sexuality was not one with sin and morality, it was one with psychic death and immortality, on which moral quandary was superimposed'.[12]

One question which Kakar poses repeatedly to us in different (dis)guises is: 'the psychoanalytic question of the vicissitudes of sublimation in Indian culture and, particularly, its role in Gandhi's life but the question also looms around a larger issue of why phallic desire is considered so offensive that he constantly tries to tear it out by its roots'.[13] It is this question that brings in the sensibility of a psychoanalytic clinician who tries to delve into the common pool of triangular relationships—one mediated by actors in familial space—to figure out where this phallic revulsion is created. Oedipal myths in Indian culture have always centred on the duel between the father and son, where father emanates from a long hibernation, and seeks to remove his archrival from the position the latter had acquired in his absence. Most of the myths end with the father killing the son—infanticide appears as the most prominent theme of the Indian grand narrative. On repentance and being in constant threat from the enraged mother whose haven is broken and destroyed, the father in some mystico-magical ways brings the son back to life and the son on being reborn through father vows to be loyal and subservient to him. Thus, father in an Indian culture is a figure full of murderous rage, hatred, and someone who destroys the mother–infant union, asks for his share of the mother, and demands a lifelong submission from the infant.[14] 'The phallic desire (or genital sexuality) thus is considered violent and tumultuous', is primarily the 'way of the fathers'; then, 'genital abstinence, its surrender, provides the tranquil, peaceful path back to the mother',[15] then a return to the womb, becomes compulsive need for the psychic peace. Therefore, the striving for One and there onwards, shall we say, further down to prehistory, to Zero, is a destination yearned for. Returning to Gandhi, Kakar points out that the 'perceived' sexual desire, both of the mother and the child, is the most potent obstacle to the preservation of the union with the maternal principle.

Gandhi and Freud come together in regard to an exhilarating fascination towards the principle of nirvana (aspiring for oneness with the Zero, through the deadening of desires), even when both worked on this idea from opposite ends. I am alluding here to the revolutionary idea of death drive. It must have been Freud's deep dislike for mysticism (which was radically different from his fervour for scientism) that must have prevented him from familiarizing himself with the Hindu philosophy, which to my mind works on similar ideas though treated in rather mythopoeic ways. An interesting definition of mysticism provided by Freud much towards the end of his life helps us to figure out the complex relationship between Id and Ego. For Freud mysticism meant 'the obscure self-perception of the realm outside the ego, of the [I]d'.[16] Hindu spirituality had already a model of primal self-perceptions and consciousness and a rather clear demarcation of the dead end of consciousness, thereby accepting a force of inertia akin to Freudian death-drive.

The Ascetic's Desire?

Kakar's thesis on spirituality is enriched further as he dabbles with lives of two saint-philosophers: the nineteenth-century bhakti saint Ramakrishna Paramhansa and another revolutionary activist, monk-pupil of Ramakrishna, Vivekananda, extending the discussion to the themes of nature and quality of religious experience, mystical experience, and erotic love manifested in their lives. In this, he dabbles with the idea of the 'transitional phenomena' (á'la Winnicott) and the sacred space that is accorded to the cultural experience of mysticism, which is clearly different from the way the religious sacrosanct perceive it.

In the chapter entitled 'Childhood of a Spiritually Incorrect Guru—Osho', Kakar focuses on maverick guru Rajneesh's insistence on importance of sexuality, and, in the process, opens up uninhibited spaces and dialogues:

> Mysticism remains a mainstream idea in Hindu religiosity and the Hindu mystics are generally without the restraints of their counterparts in the monotheistic religions such as Judaism, Islam, and to a lesser extent, Christianity, where mystical experience and insights must generally be interpreted against a given dogmatic ideology. A Hindu mystic is thus normally quite uninhibited in expressing his views and does not have to be on his guard lest his views run counter to the officially interpreted orthodoxy.[17]

Kakar also addresses questions around empathy in 'Empathy in Psychoanalysis and Cultural Healing'.

Mystical states cannot always be understood by placing them in rigid, stereotypical diagnostic categories such as psychotic regression, depersonalization, or severe withdrawal from the world; yet there is an enigma surrounding the mystic's being. Be that as it may, altered states of consciousness have always posed this challenge before psychoanalysis as one is forced into the debate of auto-erotism–objectlessness–objectalization at this point. It was Romain Rolland's work on Ramakrishna's mystical experiences that drew Freud's interest in what he later termed as the 'oceanic feeling'. For instance, Kakar quotes one of Ramakrishna's oft-repeated metaphors of the salt doll that went to measure the depth of the ocean: 'as it entered the ocean it melted, then who is there to come back and say how deep the ocean is'[18]. For Rolland, 'these were the spontaneous religious feelings, or more exactly, religious sensations, which are entirely different from religion proper and much more enduring'.[19] The question that needs to be raised is what enables the mystic to create 'the suspension of many kinds of boundaries and distinctions in both the inner and outer worlds ...' that result in the mystic's increasing '... ability to make ever-finer perceptual differentiations'.[20] How does the mystic become the master of his madness and of his reason alike whereas the schizophrenic remains their slave?[21] Kakar returns to Winnicott, Bion, and Lacan as writers 'who in spite of different theoretical orientations pursued a common antireductionist agenda'.[22] He accords to the mystical experience a status of a manifestation of 'transitional phenomena', where different orders of experience co-exist and are tolerated. Bion's work on the 'O' and his theory of thinking and mental functioning serve as symbols of ultimate reality and seem much influenced by the phenomenology of subjective experience that Indian philosophy often alludes to. The space that Winnicott's work provides to cultural experience, where the incommunicado, true self is experienced more readily, this is the space where this mystical experience can be placed.

Kakar draws the reader's interest as his discussion on 'Ramakrishna and the Mystical Experience' centres on the finer vicissitudes of Ramakrishna's mystical Being and how this experience transformed him with each passing day. Ramakrishna used to often break into song and dance in an uninhibited way, his frequent and repeated ecstasies (visions), his metaphysical discourses full of wisdom and penetrating insight, his parables, jokes, views on sexual abstinence, anxieties (did not touch women at all), pleasure in dressing up and behaving like a woman are aspects Kakar unravels through the psychoanalytic tool of opening the unconscious symbolism behind these acts. He develops this thesis of the all-pervasive maternal–feminine by looking into the origins of the mystical experience. 'The vicissitudes of separation,' he finds, 'lie at the heart of psychoanalytic theorizing on mysticism',[23] and these can be more painful and implicate a life-long-mourned-separation than the one encounter with the mother. It is '... the yearning to be united with a perfect, omnipotent being the longing for the blissful soothing and nursing associated with the mother of the earliest infancy (perhaps as much as the adult myth a co-terminus with infantile reality), has been consensually deemed to be the core of mystical experience'.[24]

The mystical path is thus a way of lessening the agony of separation, mitigating the grief of loss, reducing the sadness of bereavement. In all of this, it is the infant's (may be mother's as well) experience of the basic rupture that constantly creates the spaces in life where one deals (consciously or unconsciously) with the primordial state of mind. It is the separation from the mother's body that leaves an eternal feeling of psychic incompleteness. Lacan calls the fantasies of these (rather universal) insufficiencies, a 'lack' translated as desire and between the becoming of subject and the refinding of the object; it is the play with this desire that seeks to compensate for the eternal loss.

Kakar presents the mystic's search as:

> [T]he mystical quest seeks to rescue from primal repression the constantly lived contrast between an original interlocking and a radical rupture. The mystic, unlike most others, does not mistake hunger for its fulfilment. If we are all fundamentally perverse in the play of our desire, then the mystic is the only one who seeks to go beyond the illusion of The Imaginary and also the Maya of the Symbolic register.[25]

In this sense, the inner world comprises not only of the interjected mother or father images or functions. The primary object of creative experiencing is the unknowable ground of creativeness as such. It is the transitional phenomenon—the primary experience of symbolizing the self (and object) experience. It is the renewed emphasis psychoanalysis has placed on the identification with elements of bisexuality inherent in the self (or the being), that helps to distil these experiences of primary femininity and place the separation–merger dynamic in the mother who triggers this part of an apotheosised experience.

Mother's *Jouissance*: The Object or the Other?

Developing the theme of maternal–feminine further, Kakar looks into the cloistered passion of Radha and Krishna as a medium to understand the experience of Indian male's psychic femininization using the metaphor of the Radha–Krishna love. 'As a tale of romantic love this transformative moment from desire's sensations to love's adoration gives the story of Radha and Krishna its singular impact'.[26] This love is the replay of those very brief moments when the child (primarily boy) begins to understand and discover his and his mother's sexuality[27] (akin to Laplanche's idea of the implanted 'message' of seduction in the process of being metabolized[28]). It is brief because potential rivals have not entered into the scene (thus internal inhibitions not yet culminated into anxieties and moral qualms) to spoil the delight of enjoying mother's eroticism: like a brief interlude of *jouissance*, mother for once is experienced as overarchingly sexual. Relating this to the experience of an analysand who fears sexual intercourse and orgasm, and reconstructing Gandhi and Ramakrishna's experiences on similar lines, Kakar understands this as an unconscious fantasy of eternal sexual excitement.[29] What makes this idea interesting is that, the hate or all the badness is projected onto the act of experiencing orgasm. In effect, in this, while one seeks to get back to the original erotic *play* (her physical, bodily, and mental presence) with the mother where intense sexual arousal and excitement is generated, sexual intercourse with a woman would amount to an unconscious attempt at having one with the mother—it is this which appears incestuous and one that disables pleasurable unity with the mother. In the way Krishna takes over the role of female and Radha that of the male, 'sexual excitement in its unconscious fantasy are decisively formed and coloured by the theme of a forbidden crossing of boundaries'[30]and a violation of primal sexual demarcation.[31] Both unmarried and yet seen as devoted lovers also manifest the unconscious fantasy of illicit love, involving the crossing of boundaries set by social mores and norms. Also, in this fantasy lies the 'magical termination/removal' of the father, and the union of the mother–child unhindered by the father or the family. In a culture where mother–son relationship arouses such passions, one wonders if father's entry actually prevents them from 'consummating' the union. In the depiction of Radha as the woman full of lust and sexual yearnings, there also lies the 'fear of the mother' as the primary seductor. Often, in the images of female deities, the lustful sexual prowess of these goddess(es) is alluded to. While femininization of male takes place at one level, at another level the unconscious fantasy of seeing the woman as the powerful, demoniac 'other' full of breasts, penis, bodily fluids, ever-pregnant, and perversely sexual: hence the creation of a near-masculine split self or the 'bad breast/mother' in Kleinian sense.[32]

Kakar's writing about the nature of relationship between mothers and infants is a vignette taken from *The Inner World*, a momentous work undertaken by Kakar in 1978. In his presentation of the complex, entangled relationship between mothers and infants (essentially sons), what is conspicuous by its absence is the experience of the female child. In another way of looking at it, Indian culture accords nearly marginal (autonomous) existence or identity to the girl child and Kakar's theorization reflects this bias. It is as though she gets her social and individual identity only through becoming a mother. In this work, while Kakar highlights the socio-cultural devaluation of girl child and all-pervasive gender bias predominant in Indian culture, at another level, I feel, he gives into this 'lack' since his theories account for what can basically be thought to reflect primarily a male child's experience.

Though Kakar does look at a wide range of processes and states of mind: from heightened female hostility and envy to strong tones of ambivalence, together with a generally prolonged antagonism between the two sexes as emanating from this gender inequity. The socio-cultural taboos play on the social inferiority of women and on their dependence on men. They also seek to control and regulate the expression of their rage and resentment. Thus, in her relationship with children, especially with the male child, women as mothers direct their unconscious destructive and aggressive impulses. Over-protection, over-indulgence, and a heightened sense of caution, care, and attention towards the male child seeks to indicate the unconscious hate the mother conceals behind the extreme display of affection and oodles of care.

It is in the constant mourning over their lost childhoods that Indian mothers often develop depressive symptoms and increased melancholic disposition (the cultural devaluation of women which, according to Kakar, is translated into a pervasive sense of worthlessness and self depreciation).

> Many psychic tendencies in the young mother ... like the repeated need to be emotionally close to the 'pre-oedipal' mother and the reversal (emulation) of the wish to be loved into the wish to love; hostility towards the her surroundings, are directed towards the protection of the child from the environment; and the longing of her genital sensuality which is temporarily sublimated, is given over to physical ministrations of her child.[33]

The description of the psychic changes and development of a female is more of a narration of the culturally programmed attempts at fragmenting and repressing the individuality of her being and experience into culturally suitable roles.

Kakar shows how Indian culture at many levels survives as a result of creating splits between the good and the bad mother [parental imagos] (this compulsion with splitting in Indian cultural psyche only seeks to indicate the recurrent loud vacillation between paranoid-schizoid and depressive modes of thinking). A 'good mother' then is one who remains most nurturing, deeply attached, and available for her child. In this mould, she tries to draw her basic emotional needs from looking after the child. This experience of protracted contact with the mother lasts three to five years, and it is only after it that the child gradually moves away from the first all-important other. Therefore, the development of the Indian child might lag behind significantly considering the timetable of psychosexual development charted out as normative of the Western cultures. 'The quality of deference and indulgence in Indian motherhood thus has psychological origins in identity development of the Indian women'.[34]

'The "good mother",' according to Kakar, 'is largely a male construction'.[35] Women do not sentimentalize their mothers this way; for them mother is more of an earthy presence, not always benign but always 'present'. 'The preoccupation with themes of loneliness and separation together with the confirming presence of the "M(O)ther" stays with the individual throughout life'.[36] Yet another dimension of the mother is her 'bad self', which is often manifested in the male child's fear of inversion of emotional (sexual) roles—of what can be called the *fear of femininization of male psyche.* In the way the culture deprives and subjugates the woman's identity, a 'bad mother' can be one who induces a lot of forced compliance for she takes her child to be the [unconscious] object of her own unfulfilled desires and wishes. In many ways, the child feels the need to act as her saviour and feels torn apart between moving away from her and remaining rooted within her desires and her unconscious motive of repudiation of his maleness. In many myths and cultural representations of vagina, it is the imagery of entrance into depths of a dead womb, a poisonous dark hole which takes life away or leaves one with wound (fear of castration by the mother or through union with her).

The repetitive 'implantation' of mixed 'enigmatic messages'[37]due to the daily intimacy of contact of the child with her signifies the child's experience of accumulating the mother's inner discontentment and mixed feeling states. Of how these intromissive[38] messages are translated and metabolized by the body–ego vary according to the particular strength and quality of mother–infant relationship. One can also posit the idea of an intergenerational transfer of trauma[tic] symbolisms here. The Indian mother's physical presence is such that the child anxiously struggles to balance the intromissive and the readily interpretable messages, making this relationship forever swelled-up and fuelled with excitation.

It is the predominance of this protracted relationship in the mind of Indian males that keeps two split-images of the mother simultaneously: 'one as the nurturing, fulfilling benefactress and the other as a threatening seductress'.[39] The quick reconciliation between the parents and children over issues of power, sexual mores, and hierarchy represented in the ancient myths, parables, folk tales, and these days in films, depict the contract a child abides by in his/her relationship to parents which is to remain forever subservient to their needs and renunciation of its desires which comes in the way of parental care and duty towards them. Kakar illustrates the main emphasis of the early years of Indian childhood as the avoidance of frustration and the enhancement of the pleasurable mutuality of mother and infant, not encouragement of the child's individuation and autonomy.[40]

In a striking cross-cultural analysis of childhood, Kakar indicates that the process of ego development in Indian children differs sharply in contrast to the Western counterparts:

> The detachment of the mother by degrees that is considered essential to the development of a strong, independent ego, since it allows a child almost imperceptibly to take over his mother's functions in relation to himself is simply not a feature of early childhood in India. The child's differentiation of himself from his mother (and consequently of the ego from the id) is structurally weaker and comes chronologically later than in the West with the outcome: the mental processes characteristic of the symbiosis of infancy play a relatively greater role in the personality of the adult Indian.[41]

Kakar points out how primary process organization and thinking predominates in the Indian than the Western psyche, it is also represented in the way the Indian child is encouraged to continue to live in a mythical, magical world for a long time without much pressure on him to develop logical modes of thinking and communication.[42] This lack of the development of secondary process thinking and organization is mediated through the socio-familial organization around the child. It is then a communal responsibility to look after the ego development of the child and enable the child to adapt to both outer and inner experiences. In this way, 'the ego's responsibility for monitoring and integrating the reality is then transferred onto the mother from her to family-at-large and other institutions'.[43] The individual identity struggle is then an attempt to recapitulate and master the 'psychic unity' and the merger-fusion dynamics that reverberates throughout an Indian child's life (and adult alike).

The role of culture in psychic healing is another issue of concern and one which can provide necessary rejoinders to the primacy given to the alternative healing traditions by traditional societies (over modern psychotherapeutic interventions). Hysteria is one such example of an illness, which is in part generated and in part sustained by the traditional culture itself. The suppression and marginalization of women gives rise to the dislocation and somatic displacement of the 'personal idiom'[44] into conditions and symptoms like spirit-possession, depersonalization, pseudo-cyesis, which when looked into can open up a possibility of relocating suffering and pain in the individual life-histories which simply lack articulation and seek discharge in more primal and convoluted ways. Kakar points out that large numbers of cases of male hysterics often have an interesting side to the origins of their psychological troubles: the first attack beginning a few days after their marriage. The chapter 'Lord of the Spirit World' presents an interesting point of reference in the form of a case-vignette of Sushil. The case illustrates, in great depth, the (Indian) male's fear and repudiation of the maternal–feminine. It points to an *intercourse* with genital sexuality and encountering of a familiar uncanniness in a woman other than one's mother. I am reminded a quote I read in a paper by Robert Young[45]: '[A]ll knowledge is a knowledge of mother's body' and consequently, human struggle to grapple with the maternal–feminine becomes strangely (or perhaps not-so-strangely) extraordinary.

'To *Have* or To *Be*'… and the Psycho-cultural Manifesto

Pre-eminently operating from within the heart of the Western myth, enclosed in the 'mahamaya' (the Great Illusion) of Europe—from myths of the ancient Greece to the 'illusions' of the enlightenment—psychoanalysis has had little opportunity to observe from within and with empathy, the deeper import of the myths of other cultures in the workings of the self.[46]

While the child-rearing practices, social rituals, and institutions vary so much in the Western and non-Western cultures, Kakar aptly poses the question of how can '… the middle class man of north-European and north-American societies become the yardstick for measuring the neurotic deviations of people growing in the non-Western world?'.[47] He is critical of the ways in which Eastern ('Other') cultures are researched and presented in psychoanalytic work. 'The ways in which psychoanalysis has been studying non-Western cultures indicate a similar tendency of neo-colonial mindset where theories and complexes are sought to be superficially confirmed'[48] where Western world often becomes the standard, ideal, and the purveyor of universal truth. Sadly, the hegemonizing shadow lingers on to the relics of the past!

As a result of this schism between what native cultures aspire for and what they undergo, psychoanalysis in India since last two decades has remained moribund. The absence of the 'cultural idiom' in case histories today, such as the patient's use of Indian mythology, Kakar feels, 'are then not only due to a presumed increase in mythological illiteracy as a consequence of modernizing process. It may well also be due to the patient's sensing the analyst's disinterest in such material because of his commitment to "deeper" universalistic models'.[49]

The recent changes in the global economy and with increasing pace of modernization and technological advancement, the West has become the only suitable model for traditional societies, which struggle for existence in this fast pace of change. Offering a psychoanalytic analogy with the Freudian model of mind, Kakar analyses Indian social structure as one where '... this complementary fit between the ego and social organization and mediation remains functional so long as the pace of environmental change is slow ...'[50], with the changes occurring at jet speed the group-mind tends to become autistic and '... the traditional arrangement of social institutions creating consensual modes of decision-making'[51] are no more workable. The already weak and dependent ego is under these conditions very susceptible to mal-adaptation and schizoid breakdown.

What needs to be evolved in the changed global environment is an analysis of psychological changes in cultures that are still in the process of *transformation*—a politically active and socio-culturally vibrant psychoanalysis in the developing world has to be given priority. But this is also a challenging task for it demands creation of an identity, an original body of thought and knowledge, elaboration of an indigenous system and approach to contribute to the pool of psychoanalytic field; not merely replicating the theoretical insights that are emblematic of the Western psychoanalysis.

Kakar's writings in general are full of authentic observations and a real appreciation of the indigenous ways in which a traditional culture evolves collective and individual meaning of personhood and self, how it looks at patienthood and psychological health or well-being, and ways in which psychotherapy can be conceptualized as happening through mediation of the cultural and social practices. After reading *Shamans, Mystics and Doctors* (1982) and *The Analyst and the Mystic* (1992), one soon realizes that the local exorcist or shaman commands equal respect and competence as the clinical psychologist or an experienced psychoanalyst trained in the Western health tradition receives. Kakar's recent ventures into novellas and literary forays as seen in his works such as *The Ascetic of Desire* (2000), *Ecstasy* (2001), *Mira and Mahatma* (2004), and the most recent *The Crimson Throne* (2010) show how uniquely he combines psychoanalytic discourse with a vibrant historical imagination and literary creativity that re-enliven characters such as Dara Shikoh, Aurangzeb, Mira, Mahatma, and Vatsayayana before us. This attempt at a renewed presentation of ideas on our cultural and historical past embodies another vista in which he is developing the part-mythic, part-historical infantile-and-dream-potential of the Indian cultural psyche in a psychologically nuanced way. By all measures, Kakar is a writer, a theoretician whose works should certainly invite critical engagement especially from the Indian psychoanalytic audience, Indian academia, and readers across the world who recognize and are enchanted by the vibrant psychological mettle that Indian cultural imagination is constituted of. Finally, I would like to invite the reader to critically engage with these rich and compelling writings that certainly do enrich the discourses around childhood, religion, culture, politics, and most importantly provide a vibrant framework to develop psychoanalytic theory and praxis in the Indian context. I wish Sudhir Kakar many more years of fruitful thinking and writing and I am certain that as admirers of his prose we will get to savour many-a-exciting and relevant contributions from him in the near future!

Manasi Kumar
University of Nairobi

Notes and References

1 For further examination of some of Kakar's writings, see Kumar, Manasi, 2009, 'Recasting the Primal Scene of Seduction: Envisioning a Potential Encounter of Otherness', in *Psychoanalytic Review*, 96 (3), pp. 485–513..

2 I have elsewhere argued that cultural theory and social sciences literature in India in general has used psychoanalysis merely as a trope only to dismiss psychological interpretations and has not engaged sufficiently with it; see Kumar, Manasi, 2005, 'In a Bid to Restate the Culture-psyche Problematic: Revisiting the Essential Writings of Sudhir Kakar', *Psychoanalytic Quarterly*, LXXIV(2), pp. 561–87. It is to Kakar's credit that attempts have been made to show how psychoanalytic thinking provides a rich and valid methodology of social research (see, in particular, *The Colors of Violence* (1995), *Mira and Mahatma* (2004), and *The Crimson Throne* (2010).

3 Kumar, 2005, 'In a Bid to Restate the Culture-psyche Problematic', pp. 561–87.

4 Kakar, Sudhir, 2001, *The Essential Writings of Sudhir Kakar*, New Delhi: Oxford University Press, p. 238.

5 Ibid.

6 Ibid., p. 234.

7 Ibid., p. 256.

8 Similar ideas have been developed by Andrè Green in Green, 1996, *The Chains of Eros*, translated by Luke Thurston, London: Karnac Books; Ruth Stein has illustrated the poignant and excessive aspects of sexuality through developing links with Laplanche's enigmatic signifiers, his concept of otherness, Green's disobjectal function as seen in negative narcissism and Georges Bataille's anthropological researches on enigmatic and sacred strands of human sexuality, see Stein, R., 1998, 'The Enigmatic Dimension of Sexual Experience: The "Otherness" of Sexuality and Primal Seduction', *Psychoanalytic* Quarterly, 67, pp. 594–625 and 1998, 'The Poignant, the Excessive and the Enigmatic in Sexuality', *International Journal of Psychoanalysis*, 79, pp. 253–68.I have developed these ideas further in Kumar, Manasi, 2009, 'Recasting the Primal Scene of Seduction: Envisioning a Potential Encounter of Otherness', in *Psychoanalytic Review*, 96 (3), pp. 485–513.

9 Kakar, *Essential Writings*, p. 254.

10 Ibid., p. 252.

11 Ibid., p. 25.

12 Ibid., p. 236.

13 Ibid., p. 257.

14 At the same time one can also pick on the theme of homosexuality where an intensely volatile relationship with the father whose absence-presence appears forever tormenting. Lacan's notion of the Law-of-the-father could be another apt metaphor for the Indian situation. See Kakar, *Essential Writings*, chs 11 and 12, where Kakar alludes to the theme of Oedipality, and develops the indigenous version of Oedipus complex, called the Ganesha Complex. It is through discussing the Shiva–Parvati–Ganesha–Skanda mythic nexus that he arrives at the significance of Ganesha–Parvati. He develops themes of Oedipality from various vantage points highlighting parricide, maternal enthrallment, penis-envy, infanticide, etc. as motifs in the familial drama.

15 Ibid., p. 257.

16 Freud, S., 1938[1937], *Findings, Ideas and Problems*, London: Standard Edition, XXIII, p. 300.

17 Kakar, *Essential Writings*, pp. 282–3.

18 Ibid., p. 284.

19 Roland (1927) quoted in Kakar, *Essential Writings*.

20 Kakar, *Essential Writings*, p. 284.

21 Ibid.

22 Ibid., p. 285.

23 Ibid., p. 305.

24 Ibid.

25 Ibid., p. 308.

26 Ibid., p. 201.

27 Ibid., p. 204.

28 Laplanche, J., 1999, *Essays on Otherness*, translated by J. Fletcher, London: Routledge.

29 Kakar, *Essential Writings*, p. 209.

30 Ibid., p. 211.

31 Both Robert Stoller in *Sexual Excitement* (London: Pantheon Books, 1979) and Masud Khan in *In Privacy of the Self* (London: Hogarth Press, 1974) and *Alienation in Perversions* (London: Hogarth Press, 1979) have mapped the trajectory of sexual excitement, risks, thrills, and feelings of *jouissance* felt in transgressing boundaries. Both have consequently worked on the themes of ego-orgasm, ego-identity, and perversions and have developed various strands of sexual identification process.

32 It is interesting to note here that most of the Hindi abuses centre on the imagery of 'mother's penis or a penis inside vagina'.

33 Kakar, *Essential Writings*, pp. 28–9.

34 Ibid., p. 32.

35 Ibid., p. 33.

36 Ibid., p. 35.

37 Laplanche, *Essays on Otherness*.

38 Meaning traumatic and sexualized messages. In *Essays on Otherness*, Laplanche distinguishes intromission from implantation as the former is the result of a perversion of communication between the mother-baby dyad.

39 Laplanche, *Essays on Otherness*, p. 42.

40 Kakar, *Essential Writings*, p. 52.

41 Ibid., p. 53.

42 Ibid., p. 54.

43 Ibid., p. 56.

44 Bollas, C., 1989, *Forces of Destiny: Psychoanalysis and Human Idiom*, London: Free Association Books.

45 Young, R.B., 1998, 'Being a Kleinian is not Straightforward', http://human-nature.com/rmyoung/papers/pap113h.html

46 Kakar, *Essential Writings*, p. 192.

47 Kakar, Sudhir, 1985, 'Psychoanalysis and Non-western Cultures', *International Review of Psychoanalysis*, 12, p. 442.

48 Ibid., p. 441.

49 Kakar, Sudhir, 1995, 'Clinical Work and Cultural Imagination', *Psychoanalytic Quarterly*, 64, p. 433.

50 Kakar, *Essential Writings*, p. 57.

51 Ibid., pp. 56–7.

Culture and Healing

Lord of the Spirit World

TWO HUNDRED AND FIFTY MILES south of Delhi, the Balaji temple is best reached by taking a bus from the nearest town of Bharatpur, a town described in tourist brochures as 'the eastern gateway to Rajasthan.' Founded by the Jat chieftain Suraj Mal, who carved out a kingdom of his own in the eighteenth century, in the twilight of the Moghul Empire, Bharatpur is not unlike other North Indian towns. Except for the presence of Suraj Mal's dilapidated fort and a group of palaces, cannily turned by his descendants into a luxury hotel for tourists, the ecology of Bharatpur's bazaars is universal. In summer, there are the usual flies in dense clusters on the overripe fruit and sweets and dust that steams and not infrequently smells of horse urine once the monsoon comes. There are the irate tonga drivers cursing their scrawny horses, apparently lifeless but for their running sores; the placid oxcarts plodding unhurriedly through crowded bazaars, overloaded with everything from hay to steel girders; the Sikh drivers, strands of hair defying the purpose of their dirty turbans, two feet on the accelerator and two hands on the horns of their ancient trucks. There are the dank eating places with grime-covered clay ovens, radios blaring the latest film songs, and the all-pervasive smell of frying onions and hot curries.

If the impression I have given of Bharatpur is one of sweltering discomfort, an unrelieved drabness, then I should hasten to correct it. For during the four or five months of cold weather at least, Bharatpur is transformed. These months are a feast of brilliant colour and sharp smells, patches of wild bougainvillaea and strings of red chillies drying under the wintry sun. It is the season for fresh spices and the bazaars abound in heaps of gnarled turmeric roots and rich brown tamarind stocked in front of the shops. The air is crisp and the intervening haze of dust no longer dulls the clear sky, which has only a few wisps of gray to mar its blinding blue symmetry. The Ghana bird sanctuary, three miles from the town, lies on the great migratory route to the warm south and is a resting place for the birds from North and Central Asia, the Siberian cranes, the gray-legged geese, and countless others that are the ornithologist's delight. In fact, on our first trip to the Balaji temple in the middle of November, it was the variety of birds in the countryside outside Bharatpur that made the strongest impression on me. Families of peacocks pecking their way through the plowed furrows, sleek blue kingfishers swooping down gracefully to find a sure perch on the telegraph wires that run parallel to the road, and flights of parrots and flamingos were a common sight.

At least for the first few miles outside Bharatpur, the visual impressions one receives as the bus clatters past the villages lining the road are ones that are familiar from the rest of the Indo-Gangetic plain. They are registered as a succession of snapshots: a buffalo, immersed up to its neck in a pond thickly carpeted with green slime, motionless except for the occasional movement of its primeval head; a little girl, wrapped up in a yellow *chudder*, trying to move a recalcitrant ox by pulling at the string that runs through the animal's nose; the deeply pitted mud wall of a hut, plastered with flat cow dung cakes drying in the sun. Gradually, however, as we move deeper into Rajasthan and approach Balaji, the landscape begins to change. Squat hills, with thorny bushes and eroded topsoil that exposes the underlying rock, become more frequent. Some of the hills are crowned by the ruins of equally squat fortresses that loom above the road and once guarded this old invasion route to the medieval Rajput kingdoms to the south. The countryside is sparsely populated. Miles and miles of barren land, dotted with olive-green scrub and scarred by dried-out gullies and narrow ravines, stretch out on either side of the road. It is as if the vast Rajasthan desert, still hundreds of miles to the south, is sending out intimations of its inexorable existence, an impression enhanced by the increasing number of camel carts coming from that direction.

The temple of Balaji lies between two hills in the middle of just such a desolate landscape, three miles off the main road to Jaipur. After a twenty-minute tonga ride through a sun-drugged silence, broken only by the sound of the horse's hooves rhythmically striking against the metalled road, the sudden din on reaching the lane that leads up to the temple comes as something of a shock. In fantasy, I had envisioned the temple having been built in the tradition of the classical Hindu temples—those of Bhubaneshwar or Puri, for instance. I had pictured it being lovingly hewn out of rock by ancient guilds of anonymous craftsmen, strong in their simple faith and devotion. I had thought of it standing in a solitary, if somewhat decayed, splendor in the middle of jungle scrub and rocky hills. Except for the scrub and the hills, the reality does not bear the faintest resemblance to the imaginary product. Flat-roofed, the temple is a simple two-storied structure at the end of a long lane which is lined on both sides by shops and a number of dharmashalas, the free boardinghouses for pilgrims erected by the pious. The temple can be distinguished from its neighbours only by the fact that its facade has been painted a bilious green. In spite of the fluted columns, small arched windows and stone latticed balconies typical of the Rajasthani style of architecture, the building still manages to convey a general impression of shabbiness, enhanced by the patches of green paint peeling off the underlying stucco. There is a total absence of any atmosphere of sanctity both in and around the temple premises. The space in front of the steps that lead into the temple (as also the steps themselves) are littered with banana skins, orange peels, crushed marigolds, and other assorted refuse. The sides of the temple are crowded by eating places, small provision stores and hawkers selling fruit, vegetables, gaudy posters, and painted clay images of the temple deities as well as prayer books and other holy bric-á-brac. The shop on the right side of the temple displays the signboard of an RMP—registered medical practitioner—and the good doctor, a stout unshaven man with a roll of fat bulging out between the end of his vest and the top string of his pajamas, can be seen reclining on a cot, thoughtfully paring his nails as he waits for customers who might have cause to be disappointed with the healing powers of the gods inside the great temple. In Balaji at least, medicine exists as a poor relation to religion, obsequious and faintly disreputable.

Like the ancient Greek temples of Asclepius at Epidaurus, Pergamon and Cos, the temple of Balaji at Mehndipur has acquired more than local prominence as a shrine of healing. To the large number of patients from all over northern India who approach it in 'a spirit of service, faith and devotion,' the temple promises a quick relief from many afflictions, including 'obstacles raised by *bhuta–preta* [malignant spirits], madness, epilepsy, tuberculosis, barrenness and other diseases.' The overwhelming number of patients I interviewed had come to Balaji because of certain bodily symptoms and alterations in behaviour that were diagnosed, by their neighbourhood exorcist (*sayana*) or by knowledgeable elders in the family and community, as manifestations of a mental illness caused by spirit possession. It is its promise of cure from mental illness caused by malignant spirits, illness that has proved intractable to the best efforts of modern doctors and traditional shamanic healers, which gives the temple its distinctive reputation.

The malignant spirits of which I speak here are collectively known as bhuta–preta, though Hindu demonology distinguishes between the various classes of these supernatural beings. The *bhuta*, for instance, originates from the souls of those who meet an untimely and violent death, while a *preta* is the spirit of a child who died in infancy or was born deformed.[1] A third class, that of *pishacha*, derives from the mental characteristics of the dead person: a pishacha being generally the ghost of a man who was either mad, dissolute or violent-tempered. In addition, to complete the malignant pantheon, there are a few female spirits of which the best known is the *churel*—the ghost of an unhappy widow, a childless woman, or, more generally, of any woman who lived and died with her desires grossly unsatisfied. It is emphasized by both laymen and experts alike that a common characteristic of most malignant spirits is the fact that they are souls of persons who could not live out their full life and potential. In other words, they are all *atripta* spirits—*ghosts with unsatisfied desires*—and this of course makes them of professional interest not only to the exorcist but also to the psychoanalyst.

The bhuta–preta are said to exist in a halfway house between the human world and the world of ancestral spirits (*pitri–lok*). Until they have been judged, have paid their Karmic debts and are allowed into the world of ancestral spirits, the bhuta–preta continue to yearn for a human body which they can enter and contrive to make sick through their nefarious activity. I was, however, struck by the fact that both the individual's guarded apprehensiveness in relation to the malignant spirits and his longing for guidance from the benign ancestral spirits had an underlying tone of easy familiarity. In his relationship with these spirits, the person did not seem to feel the terror and the awe often evoked by the village and local deities; nor did he have the feelings of reverence that are due to the major gods such as Ganesha and Hanuman, and he certainly had none of the distant devotion with which the great gods and goddesses (and their incarnations) are apt to be regarded. Perhaps this psychological proximity is due to the fact that these spirits, occupying the lowest rungs in the Hindu hierarchy of supernatural beings, are closest to the human state. Whatever the reason, both the bhuta–preta and the pitri are a tangible, living presence for most people. They seem to populate a mental region that is contiguous and has open borders with the land of ordinary consciousness in which normal everyday life takes place. Persons may occasionally have encounters with the spirit world without these encounters being necessarily regarded as auditory or visual hallucinations of the pathological kind.

The Legend of the Divine Healer

Balaji, the chief deity of the temple, is better known throughout India as Hanuman, the monkey god who was Rama's main assistant in his epic battle against Ravana. The myth goes that Balaji was born of Anjana, a heavenly nymph who married a noble monkey and was cursed by the gods with a simian form. One day, while standing on top of a mountain, lost in a pleasant reverie, Anjana was ravished by Vayu, the god of the winds. Balaji was the offspring of this forced union. Like Bhima, the mighty warrior of the Mahabharata and another son of Vayu, Balaji was distinguished right from the start by great strength and gargantuan appetites. As an infant, he was perpetually hungry. Once he ran after the sun with all intentions of swallowing the orb to appease his hunger pangs. This caused great consternation among the gods and elicited vociferous protests from Rahu, whose right to periodically swallow the sun and cause the solar eclipse was being so insolently violated. In anger, Indra, the king of gods hurled his thunderbolt at the greedy infant, who fell down on a mountain top, breaking his jaw or *hanu*; hence also his name of Hanuman. The father, Vayu, picked up his unconscious son, retired into a cave, and in sorrow and protest over the treatment meted to his offspring, refused to carry out his assigned tasks. With Vayu on strike, there was a sudden absence of the ten forms of wind (*prana*, *apana*, *samana*, *udana*, etc.) and thus a stoppage of such functions as breathing, elimination, digestion, sleep, and so on, with the result that creation ground to an abrupt halt. Thrown into a panic, the gods came rushing to the grieving Vayu's cave, begging for forgiveness and offering to make the necessary amends. As a first step, each god blessed Balaji with a special power. At the end of this process, Balaji had not only become immortal and invulnerable but also the very personification of all the powers—mental and physical—of the gods. Perhaps the most important blessing given to him, at least from our viewpoint of tracing his status as a divine healer for those afflicted with possession by malignant spirits, was Brahma the Creator's blessing of total *fearlessness.* Indeed, these are the two qualities—power and freedom from fear—that Balaji displayed in abundance in his later exploits on behalf of Rama.

From this point onward, the all-India myth of Balaji gets diverted into a local channel to become the legend of the temple at Mehndipur.[2] In the local legend, the Vedic gods and the masculine preoccupations with power and fearlessness are given short shrift as the legend chooses to focus on Balaji's mother. For while the father gods are fighting the infant, grudgingly relinquishing their powers to him and otherwise acting out the unconscious script of an immemorial paternal fantasy towards sons, the mother is longing to reclaim her darling boy. As the local legend has it, the mother waited at a spot between two hills (yes, the spot where the present temple is located) and was beside herself with joy when she could finally take Balaji in her lap. She 'kissed his face repeatedly, gave him both her breasts to drink from and then after seating him in her lap, both mother and son were soon absorbed in their spiritual practices.'[3] Here, it seems to us, the local additions and elaborations of the original myth intuitively recognize the fact that the worship of Balaji as a god of power and fearlessness alone makes him much too masculine and distant to fulfil ideally the role of the divine healer. Like the female members of Asclepius's family to whom prayers for cure could be addressed,[4] the local legend recognizes the need to surround Balaji with the feminine–maternal principle and the 'feminine' powers of nurturance, warmth, concern, intuitive understanding, and relatedness which, many psychotherapists claim, are essential in every healing encounter and for the success of the healing process.[5]

For millions of years and many world ages, the legend goes on, Balaji sat here in the lap of his mother, accessible only to the gods who approached him for removal of their troubles. Then one day, a thousand years ago, a young prince was murdered at the spot where the temple now stands. His soul, taking the form of a preta, cried out for justice and clamored for liberation into the world of ancestral spirits. Moved by the preta-prince's plight and seeing that the bhuta–preta were a source of such misery to mankind, Balaji decided to make his 'court' (*darbar*) accessible to troubled human beings. He sent a vision to a young priest of Mehndipur village, intimating this decision and requiring that a temple be built. The descendants of this priest are even today the priests of the Balaji temple.

To help him in his task of bringing order in the chaos of the spirit world and in regulating the relations between humans and the bhuta–preta, Balaji invited two other deities to take up their abode in the temple. The first god who accepted the invitation and moved to the Balaji temple with his own court was Preta-raja ('lord of the preta'), which is another name of Dharma-raja, the god of death and the guardian of dharma. As lord of the pretas, Preta-raja is expected to consider the problems and difficulties of a preta before deciding upon his fate, determine the preta's proper quantum of punishment and decide the time when its soul is to be liberated from the preta order into the next order of the spirit world. The second deity to take up his residence within the temple was Mahakal Bhairav, an incarnation of Shiva, who was entrusted with the task of administering the punishments.

Following the inexorable laws of bureaucracy which seem to apply impartially to both the human and the divine worlds, the original trio of gods has since then mushroomed into a whole department of spirits. The three chief gods have added on assistants who specialize in different functions relating to the bhuta–preta and some of whom have further acquired assistants of their own. The origins of these minor gods and how they became a part of the temple are unknown, even to the temple priest, who expressed his frank bafflement at the proliferation of deities. It is, however, indisputable that people have allotted these minor gods temple space and rituals of their own and that these deities take a vigorous part in the healing process and in the life of the temple: in fact, there are many patients whose cures would not be complete without the full collaboration of these suprahuman functionaries. Here, I am specifically thinking of *Bhangiwara*, a minor god in the court of Preta-raja who specializes in dealing with the Muslim bhuta and those belonging to the untouchable castes. When a patient comes out of the bhangiwara enclosure after having exorcised one of these bhutas, it is imperative that he take a ritual bath to rid himself of the pollution. Otherwise it is held that if the patient touches someone else after his bhangiwara sojourn, it is almost certain that his bhuta will be transferred to the other person.

The Temple and the Healing Rituals

The shabbiness of the temple's surroundings and its unimpressive architecture become of minor importance once we enter the temple premises. The moment one steps inside the halls and courtyards of Balaji there is little time and even less inclination for contemplating aesthetic issues.

The senses are taken hold of violently and wrenched out of their normal grooves by strange sights and unfamiliar sounds and smells, embedded in a whirling crowd of pilgrims, patients, and their families in various stages of self-absorption. If I look back to my own first impressions before the bizarre became the familiar, I am struck by the wide gulf in the range of behaviour permitted and encouraged in a healing space—in this case, the court of the Lord of the Spirit World—as compared to rooms and spaces where everyday life is carried on.

Passages from the journal of a colleague describing his first visit to the temple vividly illustrate the drama of the healing process and the colourfulness of the surroundings in which it takes place.

> Climbing up the temple steps to enter the outer courtyard, I am greeted by an unfamiliar aroma. It takes me a few seconds to identify the sweet, smoky smell coming from the direction of the main hall as being produced by burning rice, grain, sugar crystals, coconut and other offerings that the patients are required to make to Balaji. The courtyard is crowded, mostly by young women, many of them sitting or lying on the floor in odd, contorted postures. A young girl, perhaps eighteen years old, quite attractive despite the unnatural pallor of her face, is lying on her back. Her loose hair is spread around her head which is violently jerking from one side to another as expressions of pain flit across her face. Her lips move in an inaudible murmur, interspersed by full-throated shouts of 'Baba, Baba, I won't go, I won't go!'—the *bhuta* (a male to judge by the timbre of his voice and the gender he uses in the verbs) expressing his refusal to vacate her body. My attention is caught by another young girl. She is crouching on her knees, her hips thrust back, the pelvis moving provocatively to both invite and repel an unseen violator. 'Get away! Get away from me, leave me!' she is crying out in a strong voice. She then bursts into deep moans of 'Oh, Baba! Oh, Baba!' her tightly closed eyes shutting out the world from her private struggles with the possessing spirit. I look around but no one else seems to be noticing the girl and my gaze slides off incurious eyes. Another girl, barely into her teens, is standing on her head against the wall. I hear a swishing movement and a shoulder brushes against the back of my legs. I turn around to see a girl bounding away in high, leaping somersaults; the acrobatic somersaults taking her from one end of the courtyard to another and then back again.

From the outer courtyard, I step into the main hall. This room is much larger, squarer in shape, and the grilled roof at the top makes it bright and airy. On the left side, beyond the columns of the temple, there is a narrow, dark corridor from where I get a good view of what is happening in the main hall. As my eyes get accustomed to the darkness I notice that I am not alone. An old woman is squatting next to me, surrounded by the paraphernalia needed for the ritual worship.

There are two copper pots in front of her, both of them filled with water. She is counting beads from a rosary in her lap and with every count she dips a spoon into one of the pots, takes out a spoonful of water and pours it into the second pot. I suddenly notice the presence of yet another person. This is another old woman, with a dark-complexioned face that almost merges into the surrounding darkness. As I move nearer, I am startled to see an unusually long and purple tongue protruding out of her mouth. She is being Kali, I tell myself, and reflexively bow to her. The woman raises a withered hand in benediction and I could almost swear that she has pushed her tongue out a little more for my benefit. Feeling somewhat uneasy I quickly move back into the main hall and step into the path of a dog who swerves to avoid me. The dog is hurrying towards the front of the hall to the dense crowd pressing against an iron grill behind which lie the food offerings heaped into a mound. A part of the offerings is being burned by a priest in a large brass lamp, producing sacred ash and the thick acrid smoke which I had smelled at the temple entrance. Through the smoke, the squares of the iron grill and over the heads of people clamoring to get nearer, I can see the idol of Balaji, which is in fact a triangular piece of stone, vaguely reminiscent of the shape of a human head, painted in ochre and silver colours and with two large black eyes painted on it to give it the appearance of a face.

On the right side of the main hall, there is another corridor in which the temple of Mahakal Bhairav is located. The god of punishment is again represented by a large round stone, enclosed in a protective grill, painted the same ochre and silver colours and with eyes drawn on the surface of the stone. Next to the grill there is a circular cavity in the floor, barely six inches deep and little bigger than a man's head in circumference. An old man, noticing my show of interest, enlightens me as to the cavity's purpose. 'This is where the hangings take place. If you are here for some days you must see a hanging.' Later in the evening I would indeed get a chance to witness a 'hanging.' In fact it was the old Kali woman of my earlier encounter. She had put her head in the cavity and with the help of a female companion who held up her legs, she stood on her head for a full thirty minutes. Her muffled groans of pain indicated both the bhuta's distress and her own physical discomfort, which must have been considerable indeed: 'It's enough, Baba,' she kept on repeating during her ordeal. 'Forgive me now!' 'Don't let him go, Baba,' her companion would shout back. 'Leave him only after you have choked him to death.'

In the open courtyard I join a group of five women and a boy sitting around an elderly man. The man's eyes are closed, a faint smile plays around the corners of his mouth, and the whole atmosphere is charged with a suppressed merriment that is very different from the solemnity of a modern psychotherapist's office. The elderly man, whom they call 'Panditji', is supposedly in a trance and the women seem to be enjoying themselves as they engage his bhuta in an animated conversation. 'O *re Mussulman*!' one of them says. 'Tell us quickly from where you have come.' Panditji murmurs something in reply and the woman repeats it aloud for our benefit. 'He says he is a Sayyad [a particularly strong Muslim bhuta],' and then turning to Panditji she says, 'Just now you were telling us that you want to eat kababs. Don't you know that you won't get any kababs as long as you are on this pandit? Do you understand? Run along now!'

Panditji is now distinctly agitated. His head moves up and down vigorously and his voice is stronger, though it has the quality of a stubborn child, 'I'll eat kababs; I'll eat kababs! I'll certainly eat kababs! I have been hungry for three years. This idiot pandit has neither eaten kababs himself nor has he given me some to eat.' Panditji's wife, who is sitting next to him, takes umbrage at the bhuta's rude tone and starts scolding him, but I am more interested in the women's conversation. 'These Mussulmans! They have ruined our dharma,' says one of the women, referring to the bhuta. 'I don't know where they all come from!' 'First check up whether he is a Mussulman at all,' the second woman retorts, and she is supported by another one: 'Perhaps he is trying to fool us. Sometimes he says he is a Rajput, sometimes he says he is a Mussulman.' As I muse over the fact that Muslim bhutas are considered to be the strongest and the most malignant of evil spirits, indicating perhaps the psychological depths of the antipathy between Hindus and Muslims, I hear Panditji speak: 'I *am* a Mussulman. My home is the shrine of Islaudin. Burn an oil lamp for me there every day or I won't leave.' I ask one of the women about Panditji's problems. 'Panditji stays at our boardinghouse,' she confides in me without hesitation. 'His whole family has the *sankat* [literally stress, predicament]. Sometimes Panditji also gets possessed by a Mussulman who asks to be fed kababs and then we bring him here.' Sankat or distress, I have gathered by now, is the word used in Balaji to describe possession by a malignant spirit.

It is almost three in the afternoon when I leave the group and climb up the staircase to the second floor where the 'court' of Preta-raja is being held. Since the 'King of the Spirits' is most intimately involved in the affairs of bhuta–preta, the second-floor hall is crowded and humming with a suppressed energy. Most people are sitting in an orderly fashion, their prayer books open in front of them, singing hymns in praise of Preta-raja's miracles. The singing is led by a boy of fifteen, under the approving eyes of the priest sitting in front of Preta-raja's stone representation and enclosed by the inevitable iron fence that prevents the patients from touching the stone. The singing is full of devotional excitement, punctuated by the sound of dull thuds produced by patients who are hitting their backs rhythmically against the walls. I go up to the back of the hall, which has three iron gates, similar in appearance to those that bar prison cells. I lean back against one of the gates and notice that the space in front of the other two is already occupied by two girls whose legs are chained to the iron bars. A couple of yards to my right, a woman is lying on her face with heavy stones piled on her back. She lifts up her head and calls me in a pleading voice, asking me to shift one of the stones, which is hurting her. With some effort I lift the heavy stone and put it down on the floor. 'Who told you to remove that stone?' she asks angrily. 'Put it back at once!' A couple of men and a woman—her family, I presume—loudly reproach me at my effrontery and the older of the two men seems very annoyed. I try to explain my action but he is shaking his head angrily muttering abuses against 'good-for-nothing interferers.' Noticing my consternation, a kindly man explains the situation. 'Actually when the girl called you, her bhuta was in considerable pain. If you had not lifted the stone he might have perhaps confessed his origin and his wishes. The family has been waiting here for three months for the bhuta's confession.' I sulkily retire to my place, warning myself never to interfere again and to be on my guard against expressing any human impulse of sympathy and fellow feeling.

The chained girl beside me, whom I have studiously ignored so far, is getting noisier. She is rattling her chains loudly and occasionally she starts shouting in a hoarse voice, 'Stop it! Shut up and stop this nonsense or I'll reduce you all to ashes.' Some people in the crowd who hear her turn their heads but hurriedly look away as she grimaces at them and makes obscene gestures. She then calls her husband, a young man who is desperately trying to ignore her and concentrate on his hymn singing. She loudly asks him to have intercourse with her right away and then attempts to lift up her sari. This produces the desired result since the husband rushes to her side to stop her. As if she had been waiting for this, the girl catches hold of her husband's arm and sinks her teeth into his forearm. The husband gives her a hard slap which sends her sprawling against the gate. 'I am fed up,' the young man is saying, addressing no one in particular. 'I don't know what happens to her. Rot here for all I care! Show everyone your dramas, I am going home!' The girl, recovered from the blow, is sitting up and laughing delightedly.

Looking out of the gate, I see the high cliffs against which the temple nestles. In fact it has been carved out of the hillside. There are big stone steps leading to the top of the cliffs. Names of pretas who have been exorcised and have joined Preta-raja's court as his servants and helpers are chiseled in these stone slabs. Next to the first step there is a raised platform, on which boiled rice, dhal and other edibles from the offerings made by the devout are heaped. Stray dogs and street urchins are gathered around the heap, rushing in to snatch the delicacies—*burfis* or laddoos—when a fresh offering is added to the growing mound. Dogs, I learn, are Mahakal Bhairav's mount and are thus sacrosanct within the temple precincts. Slightly higher than the platform and towards its left, there is a small water cistern which is supposed to be the home of another god known as Kundi Wale Baba. The dirty water of the cistern (it is a favourite bathing place of the dogs) is drunk by those whose spirit proves to be particularly stubborn.

The direct attack on the possessing spirit takes place through a series of temple rituals that seem to be patterned after judicial procedures. The first step is called the 'application' (*darkhwast*), in which a patient makes an offering of rice and dhal worth one and a quarter rupees and gives two laddoos to an attendant every morning and evening before the start of the temple service. During these services, a priest touches the laddoos to a part of Balaji's idol and then gives them back to the patient to eat. It is believed that with the eating of the laddoos the power of Balaji goes into the patient and forces the bhuta to make his 'appearance' in the court (peshi)—the dramatic high point of the healing rituals. If the application is unsuccessful and the spirit does not appear, then the patient can make a 'petition' (*arzi*) in which the 'court costs' are seventeen and a quarter rupees' worth of laddoos for Balaji, boiled rice for Preta-raja and boiled *urad* for Mahakal Bhairav. If the bhuta proves to be stubborn and does not appear even once during the morning and evening services for Balaji or in the afternoon service for Preta-raja, then the petition money is raised to twenty-one and a quarter rupees (*badi arzi*).* In addition, the patient may be asked to make offerings of sweets

*In Hindu ritual, the number of quantities ending in quarters, that is, broken numbers, denotes the magnitudes of misfortunes transferred to the gods.

to various minor deities such as Bhangiwara. Meanwhile, the family members too have been active. Many of them are asked by the priest to chant specific mantras or to read aloud certain passages from the Ramayana and the Hanuman Chalisa. Others are found in the temple halls, chanting mantras over spoonfuls of water that they keep transferring from one pot to another. The mantras supposedly impart divine energy to the water, which is later drunk by the patient, presumably to the further dismay of the possessing spirit. It is quite understandable that the bhuta is rarely able to withstand the concerted onslaught of so many 'divine energies.' In secular language we would say that the application and petition rituals incorporate the awesome authority of the gods in their demand that the patient go into the trancelike state of peshi. The demand is reinforced by the expectations of the priests and family members and is encouraged by the contagious effect of observing other patients having their peshi in the midst of approving groups.

The start of a peshi is marked by well-defined signs of which the rhythmic swaying of the upper half of the body and the violent sideways shaking of the head are the surest evidence of the bhuta's 'appearance.' Beating of the floor with hands, hitting the back against the wall, lying down on the floor with heavy stones piled on the back, and other acts of self-punishment are further signs of peshi. In essence, peshi is a trance-like, altered state of consciousness (not of unconsciousness) where the focus of the patient's awareness of the environment is radically narrowed but not completely erased. In this state, technically known as dissociation, the patient can generally carry out a conversation with members of the audience, though the conversation is often subject to later amnesia. He is careful not to cause himself serious injury in his acts of self-punishment and the peshi stops automatically with the end of the temple service. If the peshi is interrupted for any reason, patients report a fullness in their chests and a choking sensation in their throats 'as if something wanted to come out.'

In many patients, the next phase of peshi is marked by a struggle between the patient's bhuta and one of the temple's presiding deities. 'You have called me here,' the spirit may challenge the god, 'but if you had any courage you should have come to me and then I'd have shown you my strength!' The people around the patient try to provoke the spirit by shouting slogans in praise of the god. Excited, the spirit often becomes angry and abusive, hurling obscenities at the god and mocking the piety of the onlookers. The torrent of aggressive abuse, especially when it is issuing out of the otherwise demure mouths of frail young girls and women, leaves little doubt that we are witnessing a convulsive release of pent-up aggression and a rare rebellion against the inhibiting norms and mores of a conservative Hindu society of which its gods are the most obvious representatives. Temporarily, some of the patients even opt out of the Hindu fold by their bhuta claiming that it is a Muslim, a Sayyad in fact, who is as powerful as Balaji and would never admit defeat. The excitement crescendos as the community now brings its full weight to bear upon the rebellious and wayward spirit, 'You'd fight Baba, will you?' the audience shouts. 'Baba, give it a good thrashing, otherwise this villain will not listen!' Indeed the patient begins to hit himself, which simultaneously increases the volume of his spirit's protesting screams, 'I shall not submit! I'll see you and all of them [the audience] in hell first!' After some time, the patient, patently tired, stops beating himself and the spirit admits defeat: 'Fine, you have won. You starved me and you thrashed me, but after all you are my father. I'll obey you.' There is obvious relief among the onlookers at the reestablishment of the normal cosmic order and the patient's acceptance of old values and old authorities. Many begin to laugh, 'Baba, this is a clever one! Just because you thrashed him, he recognizes you as his father.' The ritual now goes into its next phase of 'statement' (*bayan*), where the spirit begs for forgiveness and, at the urging of the crowd, identifies itself. The spirit then promises to leave the patient alone and to throw itself at the mercy of the god. Sometimes the god might send a reformed, benign spirit—the *duta*—to protect the patient against the onslaught of other malignant spirits; the coming of the duta is signaled by a short trancelike state in which the patient repeatedly prostrates himself before the idol.

The Patients and their Illnesses

As I attempted to enter the inner world of the patients, reflecting on their life histories and observing the possessing spirits at close quarters, many of the bhutas turned out to be familiar acquaintances from clinical psychoanalytic work; the happenings that seemed so mysterious on the first visit gradually lost their sense of the strange and the uncanny. Perhaps a few case histories will not only add to our understanding of possession illness from a dynamic psychoanalytic viewpoint—as distinguished from the more psychiatric, sociological, and cultural contributions of other writers[6]—but also highlight certain kinds of culturally unacceptable behaviour and make vivid the psychic stresses to which the individual is subjected in Indian society.

Shakun's Aunt

Shakun was a nineteen-year-old girl from a small town in Bihar who came to Balaji with her mother and her three brothers. A shy and pretty girl, Shakun was sixteen when she was first possessed by a bhuta. One afternoon she had gone out to the courtyard to urinate and had called to her mother to help her with her underwear since she had freshly dyed her hands with henna, a cosmetic primarily used by girls on the eve of their wedding. On the same night, after everyone had gone to bed, the family heard Shakun's frightened screams. It seems that in the hypnagogic state before falling asleep, Shakun 'saw' a laughing woman come up to her. The girl was frightened and claimed that the woman then danced on her head, giving her a violent headache. The dancing woman's visitations and Shakun's consequent headaches and severe anxiety states occurred at regular intervals for the next three years. The diagnosis of the family and the exorcists brought in for consultation was unanimous in attributing Shakun's state to possession by a female bhuta. Since the local exorcist's efforts at exorcism proved fruitless (though in one of the rituals the bhuta had identified herself as the spirit of Shakun's father's brother's wife), it was decided that the girl be taken to Balaji.

In contrast to Shakun, who was painfully self-conscious and reticent, her mother willingly provided details of her daughter's illness. The dead aunt—Shakun's possessing spirit—the mother said with an air of conspiratorial secrecy, had committed suicide when Shakun was only three years old. 'Surely Shakun was too young to remember her,' the mother said. The suicide of the aunt, who was married to the elder brother of Shakun's father and who lived in the same household, had taken place in scandalous circumstances and the mother's salacious delight was unmistakable as she went on to describe the exciting details. The aunt, it seemed, was quite promiscuous and took her lovers indiscriminately from among all comers, including the low-caste labourers who worked in the family's small cigar-making enterprise. Though everyone else in the family knew and strongly disapproved of the aunt's affairs—Shakun's father had forbidden his wife even to talk to the woman—the husband had proverbially remained unaware of his wife's amorous adventures to the very end. One day, however, he caught his wife in *flagrante delicto* with one of his labourers and there was a violent quarrel between the couple. The aunt committed suicide on the same night. 'But, of course, Shakun doesn't know anything about her aunt. We haven't even mentioned her name in Shakun's presence,' the mother repeated.

Here, I am afraid, I must disagree with Shakun's mother. I cannot imagine that the three-year-old child, at a stage of life when curiosity is at its highest, remained unaware and unaffected by an exciting yet also violently disapproved-of aunt who died in such mysterious circumstances. At that time (and even later), there must have been whispered conversations between her parents and other family elders—conversations that simultaneously reflected their condemnation and vicarious sexual excitement—and which would suddenly cease when the child came within hearing distance of the adults. There must have been many references to the family tragedy, which Shakun overheard, and explicit taunts by other children which left Shakun in little doubt about the aunt's promiscuity and its disastrous fate. For Shakun, the memory of her aunt must have remained vividly alive in the unconscious, becoming involved with all that is both strongly forbidden and overwhelmingly exciting, harbouring that 'secret of life' which every child yearns to unravel.

The aunt, I am suggesting, gradually became the personification of the growing girl's *negative identity*[7]—all that Shakun 'knew' she should never be but feared she might become, especially when her sexual impulses started asserting themselves during the tumult of adolescence. Changing from the Eriksonian to the Jungian idiom, one would say the aunt is the *shadow*, the inferior, dark part of the personality which is repressed to the unconscious and consists of all those forbidden desires that are incompatible with the values and strivings of the conscious persona. Shakun's bhuta is, then, a figure of her unconscious, an iconic representation (in the form of the aunt) of the girl's own sexual (even homosexual?) wishes. Because of the social standards of her community but especially because of the horrible fate of the aunt who gave in to *her* sexual wishes, Shakun, I believe, has struggled desperately to keep these desires from becoming conscious. At sixteen, a time of heightened sexual impulses, the repression failed for the first time, resulting in a psychological possession that led to great anxiety as this inhibited girl's ego fought desperately against being overwhelmed by the feared unconscious content.

Asha and her Spirits

Asha was a twenty-six-year-old woman from a lower-middle-class family in Delhi who had come to Balaji accompanied by her mother and her uncle. A thin, attractive woman with sharply chiselled features and a dusky complexion, Asha had a slight, girlish figure that made her look younger than her age. She had suffered from periodic headaches ever since she could remember, though her acute distress began two and a half years ago when a number of baffling symptoms made their first appearance. Among these were violent stomachaches that would convulse her with pain and leave her weak and drained of energy. Periodically, she had the sensation of ants crawling over her body, a sensation that would gradually concentrate on her head and produce such discomfort that she could not bear even to touch her head. There were bouts of gluttony and fits of rage in which she would break objects and physically lash out at anyone who happened to be near her. 'Once I even slapped my father during such a rage,' Asha told us. 'Can you imagine a daughter hitting her father, especially a father who I have loved more than anyone else in this world?'

Treatment with drugs (her uncle was a medical doctor) and consultations with an exorcist did not make any appreciable difference to her condition, but what really moved Asha to come to Balaji was her discovery, six months after her father's death, that her skin had suddenly turned dark. This caused her intense mental anguish, since she had always prided herself on her fair complexion. Asha now felt that she had become very unattractive and toyed with the idea of suicide.

After coming to Balaji, Asha's peshi was immediate. She had barely finished eating the two laddoos in Balaji's 'court' when she fell down on the floor and revealed that she was possessed by two spirits. The first spirit, who caused the stomachaches, stated that it was sent by Asha's brother's wife. Its name was Masan, it said, a ghost that inhabits cemeteries and cremation grounds and whose 'specialty' is the eating of unborn babies in the womb. The second spirit admitted its responsibility for the sensation of crawling ants and for Asha's rages, and further revealed that it had been sent by the elder brother of Asha's fiancé. After their first confession, both the spirits were silent and did not make any further statements. On subsequent occasions Asha's peshi was a gentler affair consisting of a dreamy swaying of the body from which Asha emerged with a feeling of heightened well-being and the conviction that her skin had become lighter. Asha, it seems, had become addicted to peshi. She was not overly concerned with the punishment of her bhuta and indeed seemed indifferent to the prospects of her cure. If for any reason the peshi did not take place for more than two to three days, Asha's eyes screwed up into narrow slits, her headaches became worse and she inevitably had one of her fits of rage. In a more theoretical formulation, Asha was attempting to exchange her possession symptoms, a pathological reaction to individual conflict, for the ritual trance of peshi, a socially sanctioned psychological defense.[8]

Though Asha was anything but secretive and talked animatedly about her life and her problems, the talk was mostly diffused and scattered. She flitted from one experience to another, from the present to the past and back to the present again so that a chronological piecing together of her life history became a difficult task. Dramatic impressions and nostalgic memories, described with elaborate gestures and in a theatrical voice, succeeded each other with bewildering rapidity, making it difficult to sift facts from impressions, reality from fantasy.

As the youngest child in the family and the only daughter after a succession of five boys, Asha had always been her father's favourite. The memories of her childhood were pervaded by images of a father–daughter closeness and of their delight in each other that had excluded other members of the family from their charmed circle. The first thing the father did on coming home from the office every evening was to ask for his beloved daughter and play with her till it was time for dinner. Even when she was twenty, Asha remembers that her father inevitably brought her sweets in the evening, and then, lifting the now not-so-little girl upon his shoulders, he would romp around the house, often exclaiming, 'O my darling daughter, what would I do when you get married and leave this house! My life would be ever so empty!'

The only discordant note in the 'idyllic' father–daughter relationship occurred when Asha was fifteen. She fell in love with a young college student who had been engaged as her tutor. When her father came to know of their budding romance, he was furious and packed Asha off to her aunt in Saharanpur. Here she was so closely watched that she could neither write nor receive letters. For one year the girl pined away in virtual imprisonment and came back to Delhi only when her father fell sick and refused to be nursed by anyone except his favourite daughter. Asha devotedly nursed him back to health and the subject of the young tutor was never mentioned by either one of them; in fact, the episode seemed to have brought the father and daughter even closer.

The sequence of events that led to Asha's possession by the two spirits seems to have been as follows. Three years before, Asha's favourite brother had got married, and according to Asha, under the influence of his wife he became quite indifferent to his sister. Asha felt very unhappy at her brother's 'betrayal' but continued to perform all her sisterly duties. Once, when she had gone to her brother's house for a short stay—her sister-in-law was pregnant—Asha found some of her own clothes in her sister-in-law's cupboard, which made her very upset at her 'thieving' sister-in-law. Her stomachaches started shortly afterward.

It was during this time that a young man from the neighbourhood began to take a pronounced romantic interest in Asha. Every day the man dropped in at the clinic where Asha helped her uncle in his work and would talk to her for hours. Asha was uninterested in her ardent suitor, she claims, but this did not faze the young man in the least. In their long and frequent conversations the man openly declared his love for the girl. When Asha's father came to know of the young man's pursuit of his daughter, he was, once again, furious. Accompanied by two of his sons, the father went to the man's house to remonstrate with his family. The man's mother persuaded Asha's father and her brothers that Asha should be married into their family and it was decided (it was not clear how and by whom) that Asha would marry not her suitor but his younger brother instead. Asha felt very unhappy at this arrangement but her father fell sick and she could not give vent to her feelings as that might have worsened his cardiac condition. Once again she devotedly nursed her father through his illness, even 'holding and cleaning the organ which a girl never holds in her hand.'

The elder brother of her fiancé had now become bolder and even more insistent in his sexual advances towards the girl. He seemed unmoved by Asha's repeated plea that since she would soon become the wife of his younger brother he should, like a good Hindu, begin to look upon her as his daughter. It was during this period that Asha was attacked by her second spirit for the first time. She had gone to her mother-in-law's house for a visit but found that everyone was out except her lovelorn admirer. He had asked her to come up to his room and Asha had fainted. Her rages, the sensation of crawling ants, and the headaches began soon afterward.

As a psychoanalyst, trying for the moment to understand the basic underlying psychic processes rather than the cultural significance of Asha's behaviour and symptoms, I would say that apart from its Indian stage and Punjabi middle-class setting, Asha's case seems to be a part of the same genre that is often encountered in the early psychoanalytic literature on young women who fell ill while caring for an older, sick relative. Torn between her duty and her love for her father and her own unacknowledged sexual wishes towards another man, Asha's conflict is similar to that of many girls in the European bourgeoisie society of the late nineteenth century—that of Freud's patient Elisabeth von R., for instance.[9] With her need for intense closeness to her father, Asha seems to have had little choice but to deny the hostile component of her feelings towards him—as she must have denied her rage during her first, abortive love affair with the tutor. Given the present stressful circumstances—her father's illness, her engagement, and the man's importunate demands—Asha's defense of denying her aggressive and sexual wishes was no longer sufficient but needed to be supplemented by having these wishes split off from consciousness and attributed to the machinations of a bhuta. Naturally, the spirit was 'sent' by the lovelorn swain who is unconsciously held to be responsible for the conflicting emotions that constantly threaten to overwhelm her. Asha's other distressful symptom of a darkening of her skin, I would say, springs from her identification with her father, since we learn that just before the father died, *his* skin had turned blue-black in colour. Such identification is not only intended as a compensation for the loss of the beloved father but can also be the expression of Asha's vain attempt to free herself from him. Asha's other bhuta—the embryo-eater Masan—too represents a similar symbiosis of destructive and sexual wishes. Her stomachaches, I would suggest, are an expression of her unconscious pregnancy fantasy, created by means of identification with the 'fortunate rival', the sister-in-law. The ghost killer of unborn babies then symbolizes the idea, 'It is not I who would like to destroy my sister-in-law's unborn baby but she who wants to kill my [fantasized] baby.' Asha's bouts of gluttony would seem to reinforce this interpretation. As many creative writers have also known, neurotic greed is the reflection not of the need for food but of unconscious wishes that cannot be satisfied, and thus can never be assuaged by eating. In his novel *Two Women*, for instance, Balzac, in describing a pregnant woman's passion for rotten oranges, intuitively recognizes the cannibalistic nature of her wishes directed against the child in her body.

I have suggested above that Asha (but also Shakun) has much in common with Freud's women patients from the Viennese bourgeoisie. The similarity does not lie in their symptoms but in the underlying *hysteric personality* which they share. The elements of this 'ideal type' hysteric personality are well known: an intense, erotic attachment to the father and an unresolved Oedipal conflict, a fear of sexuality accompanied often by a strong but hidden interest in it, overly great concern with conventional values and social proprieties, an impressionistic way of experiencing the world, dramatized and exaggerated behaviour, a capacity for multiple identifications, and so on. Indeed, a majority of the patients interviewed at Balaji—fifteen out of twenty-eight, eleven of whom were women—evidenced such a core hysteric personality. Significantly, though many of the other patients did not have a peshi in the temple, nor did their bhuta appear to make a 'statement,' in the case of all the fifteen hysterical patients the possessing bhutas appeared without exception to give their 'statements'. Although possession is more than hysteria, the hysterical personality seems to make the best use of possession states.

Where Asha and other Indian hysterical personalities differ from their European counterparts is in the display of a rich, dramatic and concrete imagery of the bhutas, this kind of visual imagery being diffuse, if not completely absent, in the recorded cases of *la grande hystérie* in the West. Here, the culture comes in. The rich mythological world, peopled by many gods, goddesses, and other supernatural beings, in which the Indian child grows up, his early experiences of multiple caretakers, all contribute to the imagery of possessing spirits. Hysteria, as Alan Krohn has pointed out, is uniquely a neurosis that takes on the colouring of a specific historical and cultural setting.[10] 'Vapours', fainting fits, inexplicable paralyses and convulsions in the Victorian era, the devil or a witch wresting control of the body to use it for its own purposes in the Middle Ages, are some of the many costumes that the hysterical personality has worn in its time in the West. In fact, the hysterical personality is probably unique in aligning itself with what Krohn calls the prevailing 'myth of passivity' of its culture. I am the 'passive' vehicle of gods, or of the devil, of my twitching, or my bhutas, which make me do these things, not my own desires.

It may well be that the hysterical personality has not largely disappeared in the West but has merely adapted itself to the culture's present myth of passivity. 'To be the helpless victim of one's society, the stars, one's unconscious, or mental disease,' Krohn writes, 'are now our culturally sponsored myths of passivity and this forms the basis of current hysterical alternatives.'[11] In any event, for an Indian psychoanalyst, Freud's libido theory, derived from his studies of hysteria, which often tends to be relegated these days to the realm of an aesthetic metaphor, is still central to much of his clinical work. In spite of the newer theoretical developments, such as Heinz Kohut's 'psychology of the self', which may preoccupy his colleagues in the West, for the Indian analyst, psychoanalysis remains preeminently the child of a hysterical woman.

We saw above that the single largest category of patients, comprised mostly of young women who come to Balaji in search of healing, are suffering from a hysterical disorder; or, if one prefers to use the traditional idiom, they are possessed by the ghosts of forbidden sexual and aggressive wishes. Though the individual variations in all these cases are of great interest from the clinical angle, the wide prevalence of hysterical personality among Indian women and their use of this particular cultural myth of passivity are also reflections of certain social conditions prevailing in the society. In other words, there is no individual anxiety that does not also reflect a latent concern common to the group, a fact that Erik Erikson pointed out long ago but which we clinicians often tend to underplay in our pursuit of the uniquely individual in case history.[12] For, in going through my Balaji case histories, especially of rural women, I am struck by their accumulated and repressed rage, the helpless anger of young women at the lack of their social emancipation being the canvas on which the individual picture of hysterical illness is painted.[13] Let us look at another case which illustrates this clearly.

Urmilla's Rage

Urmilla is an attractive eighteen-year-old from a village in Rajasthan who had come to Balaji with her husband. A couple of years ago, immediately after her marriage, she started complaining of body aches accompanied by difficulties in breathing. Shortly thereafter she began to get into uncontrollable fits of rage. During these fits of rage she would heap abuse on everyone who came near her, though reserving her choicest epithets for her husband, towards whom she often became physically violent. 'She gets such strength at these times that it takes two or three strong men to restrain her,' the husband reported with grudging admiration. 'She also gets so hungry that she'd eat up the food cooked for the whole family and so thirsty that she'd drink up a full bucket of water.' 'Yes, Doctor Sahib,' Urmilla confirmed her young husband's account. 'Before marriage I did not get angry even once. But when the bhuta comes I don't remember what happens to me. Later, they tell me the filthy abuses I have used against my husband but I have no memory of such a shameful act.'

Urmilla was possessed not only by a malignant bhuta but also by a benign spirit—that of her dead father—who would come to protect her when her bhuta-inspired rages threatened to cause grievous injury. The father had died when Urmilla was five years old and had the reputation of being a short-tempered man. The father's spirit, though also hot-tempered, was perceived by Urmilla as a guiding and benevolent pitri and it was at *his* advice that the couple had made the pilgrimage to Balaji. The couple had been in Balaji for some time now and though the bhuta came often he had yet to confess his origins and his wishes. The husband was getting impatient to go home but Urmilla insisted that she would not go back till her father's spirit instructed her to do so. When the husband insisted, Urmilla became possessed by her father's spirit and roundly abused her husband, threatening to break his legs for even daring to think of leaving his daughter behind. The spirit also told everyone in the boardinghouse where the couple was staying that the man was perhaps planning to take a second wife and that he (Urmilla's father) would see to it that he was severely punished. Occasionally, Urmilla also got possessed by another benevolent spirit—that of her dead mother-in-law—who complained of the family's neglect in carrying out the proper rituals for the welfare of her soul and ordered them to make up the deficiencies.

For the past few days, Urmilla had increasingly got the feeling that her bhuta was leaving her. One day she announced that they would all go to a nearby temple of the Mother Goddess Vaishno Devi—two miles from Balaji—where the Mother (the goddess) would come to possess her and tell them whether the bhuta had really left or whether he was playing one of his tricks for which the bhutas are so notorious. Next morning, a small group consisting of Urmilla, her husband and another couple from a neighbouring village went up to the temple and waited for the Mother in the small room where the idol was kept. Urmilla went on staring at the Mother's face while the others kept up a rhythmical shouting of 'Victory to the Mother!' Urmilla's breathing was becoming faster and expressions of pain and anger flitted across her face in quick succession. Suddenly we noticed a transformation on her face, which became quite still and devoid of all expression; the Mother had come. In a loud and confident voice, Urmilla began to speak rapidly. Urmilla: 'What do you want? Speak. What do you want? Why have you called me?'

The husband (in a low, respectful tone): 'Please tell us if we should leave on Saturday.'

Urmilla: 'Yes, go away. Leave.'

The husband: 'Please also tell us whether her distress is over. Sometimes she is fine but sometimes she starts getting angry again.'

Urmilla (in an excited tone): 'Haven't I told you to leave? We'll look after the girl there. Have faith. We are with her.'

The husband: 'One more favour ... the bhuta's name—' This sentence was left incomplete since Urmilla thundered back angrily: 'Why do you want to know the name, you villain? We'll tell the names when we go back. The whole family is torturing this poor girl! How many names do you want?'

The husband was intimidated and mumbled his assent. Urmilla sought to confirm her domination by ordering him to rub his nose on the floor, the sign of abject surrender. The husband caught the lobes of his ears with his hands and bowing down before the idol rubbed his nose three times on the ground. The other woman who was sitting with folded hands now addressed Urmilla, 'Mother, tell me something about myself too.'

Urmilla (speaking very rapidly): 'The villain eats babies in the womb. Has ruined this poor woman. But everything will be fine. Say "Victory to the Mother." I'll take care of the Mussulman.'

The woman bowed to her and after a couple of minutes Urmilla came to herself. She looked exhausted but at the same time her face glowed with satisfaction at her recent experience. As they walked back to the boardinghouse, Urmilla told us that they would leave Balaji this Saturday. There was no fear of the bhuta returning, she said, since the Mother had decided to be with her and she could protect Urmilla even better than the spirit of her father.

The evidence is strong that Urmilla harboured within her a violent rage, which she suppressed till her marriage, until finally her inability to control the rage provoked the mysterious aches and the motor discharge in possession states. In these states, assured of the protection afforded by the clouding of consciousness and the subsequent amnesia, Urmilla was able to give an otherwise forbidden satisfaction to her pent-up fury. Under the pretext that she herself was not the subject of the rages, she could refuse to acknowledge them as her own and split herself off from her other 'selves'—the bhuta, the father spirit, the mother-in-law spirit and the Mother Goddess. The question then arises: what was the cause of Urmilla's rage and against whom was it aimed, since such rages can be directed not only against actual persons but also against parental images and other inner figures from childhood? As I do not have enough information on Urmilla's past, I can only look at her present circumstances and suggest that Urmilla's expression of rage against her husband and his family is also a rage against her feelings of powerlessness. It is indeed a striking fact that her identifications are with the powerful figures of the father, the mother-in-law and the Mother Goddess. In a Rajput village community where the young daughter-in-law is expected to be completely subservient and not even think angry thoughts about her husband's family and especially about her 'lord and master,' possession by spirits who behave otherwise seems to be one way for a young girl to express and yet not acknowledge the resentment against the powerlessness of her condition. Anger against 'superior' family members seems to be particularly difficult to express. Even 'she hates me', as in the case of Asha and her sister-in-law, is not easy to acknowledge, while one has to be terribly ill and possessed by all manners of spirits to be able to express 'I hate him [or her].' The coin that depicts the *Bharatiya nari*—the 'Indian woman'—in all her sentimentalized chasteness and calm fortitude on one side, shows the same woman engaged in a desperate struggle with her inner demons on the other.

Sushil's Possession

Whereas powerlessness is the social denominator of female hysteria—the cumulative trauma of Indian women, so to speak—the demands of autonomous functioning and anxiety at the prospect of individuation seem to be the social correlates of male hysteria. Instead of reproducing detailed individual case histories in support of this contention, perhaps a vignette will serve the purposes of illustration.

Sushil was a twenty-seven-year-old man who was possessed by a spirit when he was twenty-two. A year earlier, after Sushil graduated from his college in Agra, his father had set him up in a small pharmaceutical business which he expected his son to manage on his own. Things had gone well for a couple of months till Sushil was married. A few days after the marriage, Sushil found that he had lost all interest in business. Instead of going to the shop in the mornings, Sushil would wander around in the bazaar in a daze. Then one day, in this dazed state, Sushil 'saw' his younger brother—who had died in an accident when Sushil was ten—walk towards him, his school bag swinging from a thin, jaunty shoulder. From that day onward Sushil frequently became possessed by his younger brother's spirit. In these possession states, which he did not find unpleasant, Sushil's voice changed into a childish treble, his vocabulary dwindled to that of an eight-year-old and his whole demeanor took on a pronounced childish cast in which his renunciation of independent adulthood was complete.

In the *timing* of his illness, Sushil's case was identical with that of other male hysterics who also had invariably suffered their first attack of possession a few days after their marriage. It was as if they had experienced the sexual activity and the demand of establishing a close emotional bond with a strange woman as the first truly individual act of their lives in which the family could not participate and which had threatened to isolate them from the web of their familial and group emotional ties.

Healing at Balaji—Psychotherapeutic Perspectives

In the West, a big step in the treatment of mental disorders was taken at the end of the last century with the realization—primarily attributed to Charcot and Freud—that hysterical 'illnesses' were the symbolic expression of a definite emotional content; that the person's bodily symptoms could be seen as bits of behaviour intended to convey a message. In other words, the essential and distinctive feature of a hysterical disorder was the substitution of a bodily state for a personal problem which enabled the individual to ignore and escape the anxiety caused by the personal problem. Moreover, Freud demonstrated that the roots of the personal, emotional problem lay in the individual's past of which he or she was normally unconscious. The psychoanalyst's task was to foster a self-reflective attitude in the patient towards his bodily signs or symptoms so as to facilitate their translation into ordinary language. As Thomas Szasz has aptly put it, those who want to deal with so-called hysterical patients must therefore learn not how to diagnose or treat them but how to understand their special idiom and how to translate it into ordinary language.[14] The assumption of psychoanalysis is that by helping a person to decode his symptoms and become explicitly aware of past events that have influenced their genesis, the persistent effects of these events in his future can be mitigated and indeed radically modified.

This approach to the cure of hysteria later became the dominant psychoanalytic paradigm for dealing with other types of mental illness. In short, psychoanalysis and western psychotherapies influenced by psychoanalysis concentrate on what I would call the *text* of the mental illness—on its understanding, translation, and genesis. In contrast, as we shall see below, the healing rituals of the Balaji temple follow radically different principles of therapy. They seem to be more concerned with the *context* of the illness. In traditional therapy, the special idiom underlying the visitations of Shakun's aunt, Asha's spirits, and Urmilla's rages is left at the symbolic level without any attempt at translation. Instead, the healing efforts seem to be directed more towards changing the context of the problem by changing the person's feelings about himself or herself. Basically, the healing rituals seek to connect (or reconnect) the individual with sources of psychological strength available in his or her life situation and thus counteract the more or less conscious feelings of despair, shame, guilt, inferiority, confusion and isolation in which the 'illness' is embedded. Let me illustrate the essentials of the contextual approach to healing through an analysis of the healing process at Balaji.

Typically, a patient whose illness started with disturbing bodily and mental symptoms has exhausted all the local resources before he makes the decision to come to Balaji. He has tried out home remedies, consulted doctors—both of traditional and of modern medicine—and has perhaps undergone the exorcism rituals of one or more exorcists. The decision to go to Balaji is then an admission, both by the patient and by his family, that things are seriously wrong and that the temple represents perhaps the last chance of a cure. The journey to Balaji then acquires an added emotional significance and given the considerable distance a patient and his family must travel, with all the attendant inconvenience and hardship, the long trip to Balaji becomes a sacred journey, a pilgrimage in search of healing. From the medical metaphor of illness, the patient has shifted to a religious–spiritual, metaphor of the pilgrim's progress towards wholeness. All of this represents a strong emotional investment by both the patient and the family in the success of the pilgrimage. We find this increased investment in dreams that some patients had before they came to Balaji. The dreams typically involved a personal summons from the divine healer, either through the god speaking directly in the dream or through the dream image of one or more monkeys—the symbol of Hanuman. Thus even before they embarked on the healing journey, some patients had begun to send themselves messages of reassurance from the unconscious depths, increasing their hope and confidence in the success of the healing mission. Many other patients reported that once the decision was made, their bhuta, knowing of his imminent demise, began to raise obstacles which the patient had to overcome before he could come to Balaji. Obviously such a patient no longer feels himself as a passive recipient of healing ministrations—whether the doctor's medicines or the exorcist's incantations—but has become a more active participant in the process of his own cure.

Expectations and hope are greatly strengthened by the culture prevailing in the Balaji community. Patients and their relatives constantly extol the powers of the divine healer and describe to each other (and especially to the newcomers) the details of miraculous cures that have taken place over the years. The fact that these cures are neither ephemeral nor hearsay is underlined by the presence of a large class of ex-patients. Many of these ex-patients come to Balaji at periodic intervals or on special festive occasions in order to sustain their link with the healing temple and to remain free from distress. Others come to fulfil their commitment of *sava–mani* in which a patient promises to feed the poor with food weighing fifty kilograms after he has been cured. All these former sufferers are living witnesses and reinforcers of the patient's growing faith that the temple healing really 'works'.

A second important characteristic of the temple's healing culture is the involvement and integration of the patient's relatives in the healing process. According to the temple rules a patient can stay in a boardinghouse only if he is escorted by at least one caretaker. In practice there are often three or four family members who accompany the 'sick' person on his pilgrimage. Many rituals that need to be carried out in the temple require the active participation of these family members. Accompanying the patient from morning till late in the evening through the various healing rituals and living in an environment where sankat (and its vicissitudes) is the central theme of community life, the distinction between a 'sick' and a 'normal' member of the family is gradually eroded. There were many cases where a person who had come to Balaji with a possessed relative soon discovered that he too was in distress from a bhuta and in need of healing. Another bridge between the 'normal' and the 'sick' is through the concept of sankat transfer. According to this belief, if a close relative of the patient prays to Balaji that he is ready to take on the distress then the bhuta often leaves the patient and possesses the supplicant. However, in the three cases of sankat transfer that I observed, the family member began to show signs of bhuta possession without any corresponding relief for the original sufferer.

The importance of the wall between 'sickness' and 'health' becoming porous and the blurring of the distinctions between 'normal' and 'possessed' lies in the fact that it helps the patient considerably to overcome his feelings of isolation and moral worthlessness. Even though possession by a bhuta is not culturally alien to the patient, who has seen and heard of many others who have been similarly afflicted, possession by a malignant spirit nevertheless isolates and bars the individual from sources of collective strength residing in his or her group and community. The feeling of isolation is attributable to the fact that possession is also seen as a stigma, a kind of leprosy of the character that cuts off the individual from members of his immediate and extended community. This becomes evident when we read of the kinds of people that Hindu culture considers especially susceptible to possession by bhuta–preta. These are 'the impotent, the lustful, the lately widowed, bankrupts, sons and brothers of whores, convicts, the idle, the brooders on the unknowable, gluttons and starvers. ... Intelligent and educated men and healthy intelligent women are free from spirit attacks.'[15]

The temple regulations, verbally communicated to the patient by the priest and available in a printed brochure, lay considerable stress on the patient's achieving a state of purity before any appeal to the deities can be made. These rules enjoin a strict observation of celibacy during the whole of his or her stay at Balaji, prohibit the use of spices, onion, garlic and other impure foods and require daily morning baths and a fresh change of clothes every time the patient enters the temple precincts. Elsewhere, I have suggested that the feeling of being dirty and polluted is the Indian form of experiencing guilt. The purification rituals, then, with their washing and cleansing the inner 'filth,' seem to be directed towards a symbolic expiation of the patient's feeling of guilt, while at the conscious level they prepare the patient to receive the superior power of the god.

Yet another quality of Balaji's communal culture is the openness with which sankats are discussed. Patients (and their families) exchange detailed case histories within and outside the temple premises and when two patients encounter each other in the street, 'How is your sankat doing?' is both an acceptable greeting and a mode of inquiry about the other's well-being. The possible responses to such an inquiry—'There is no change', 'It is turning out well'—are very much like the matter-of-fact exchanges between two graduate students in physics on the progress of their experiment. The point is that possession illness and the presence of bhuta–preta are accepted in a plain, uncomplicated way. In the boardinghouses, after their gates are closed for the night, patients and their families spontaneously form into small groups to discuss each other's distress. In such therapeutic group sessions, the most intimate details of the individual's distress are revealed, speculations on the probable origins of the spirit are advanced and the possible outcome of a particular healing ritual debated. Besides lessening any residual feelings of shame, the public sharing of the illness certainly makes the malignant spirits lose their private terrors. Anxious and fearful emotions that we would normally expect to be associated with the bhuta–preta are quite conspicuous by their absence as the patients begin to address their possessing spirits derisively with the diminutive '*bhutra*'. What one's bhutra did on a particular day during the healing ritual in the temple is related to others in an indulgent manner, as if the bhuta were a naughty child whose antics had to be suffered patiently. This marks a distinct change in the individual's attitude towards the illness, for it is no longer the bhuta who is possessing the patient but the patient who has to bear with the bhuta. From our own clinical experience, we can appreciate the difference it makes (and the big step it constitutes towards cure) when a person begins to feel he has the neurosis instead of the earlier feeling that the neurosis has him. We can now understand better how a 'standard ritual'—as Obeyesekere in his excellent study of exorcism in Sri Lanka has called such healing practices[16]—can help patients who are suffering from various kinds of mental illnesses. Ignoring the different texts of the illness, the standard ritual works chiefly through the context in which the feelings aroused by the illness are embedded. This approach 'works' since the context is also the nexus for those universal human strengths whose restoration in the individual makes for his wholeness.

Of the multiple perspectives on mental illness—illness as an expression of alienation from the bodily order, illness as an alienation from the self, and illness as alienation from the social order—we see from the above description that healing at Balaji lays an emphasis on ending the patient's alienation from his social (and cosmic) order. The judicial court of the god recognizes two parties who are clamouring for the possession of the individual: his or her cut-off 'selves' (the bhutas) and the representatives of the family and community. The judicial (and therapeutic) task, in the judgement of the court, is not only, or even primarily, the reintegration of the cut-off parts of the self, as in western psychotherapy, which therefore demands that an isolated neurotic be put into an isolated setting under a treatment dominated by a scientific theory. Instead, the 'court' also sees as its task the reintegration of the individual with his community. This requires a polyphonic social drama that attempts a ritual restoration of the dialogue, not only within the patient but with the family. By participating in rituals together with the patient, and especially by having the patient's sankat transferred onto themselves, the family members too seem to be accepting their share of the blame for the patient's problems.

As far as the cut-off parts of the self are concerned, the therapy proceeds along two separate lines. One, the individual's tolerance of the bhuta is sought to be increased by lessening the spirit's fearsomeness. The spirit's potentially benign nature—the bhuta being replaced by a duta, the god's 'messenger'—is pointed out and it is reemphasized that malignant spirits are only unfortunate pitris or ancestral spirits deserving compassion rather than anxious reactions. In other, psychoanalytic words, the unconscious content of the psyche is considered neither fixed and immutable nor malignant and threatening, as in the notion of the psychoanalytic id, but as fundamentally capable of a benign transformation. And we must remember that the bhuta–preta are only defendants in Balaji's court and not outside the pale of society. Preta-raja, after all, is as much a defense lawyer who must look after the bhuta–preta's interests, as a judge who must punish them.

Second, peshi ritual attempts to transform the patient's belief into a conviction that his bad traits and impulses are not within but without; that they are not his own but belong to the bhuta. The fact that fifteen out of twenty-eight patients were possessed by a Muslim spirit indicates the extent of this projection in the sense that the Muslim seems to be *the* symbolic representation of the alien in the Hindu unconscious. Possession by a Muslim bhuta reflects the patient's desperate efforts to convince himself and others that his hungers for forbidden foods, tumultuous sexuality and uncontrollable rage belong to the Muslim destroyer of taboos and are farthest away from his 'good' Hindu self.

Like every other system of therapy—western or eastern—which can help some but not all of its clients, the temple healing finds reasons for not being as universally effective as it would like or as its adherents might claim.[17] In cases where a patient has successfully gone through the complete course of 'application', 'appearance', and 'statement' and yet retains many of his original symptoms, he is declared to have multiple sankats, with more than one possessing spirit being involved. In such cases, the patient is expected to go through the complete ritual all over again and to repeat it as many times as the number of bhutas that possess him. The record is held by a man who had twenty-one possessing spirits! In other cases, where the patient is obviously relieved of his symptoms but falls ill soon after he gets back home, the relapse is attributed to the inherently deceitful nature of the bhuta, who has sneakily reneged on its solemn promise to Balaji. For more severe disorders where in spite of all efforts the peshi is at best limited to a swaying of the body, without the dramatic struggles between Good and Evil and *without* the bhuta making the 'statement,' the solution offered is 'imprisonment' of the spirit for a year at the temple. The patient may then go about his normal affairs, but must return to Balaji before the end of the year to once again go through the healing rituals. As a direct suggestion to the patient to remain well for at least a year, the sankat imprisonment seems like a last desperate measure and has correspondingly little success.

In conclusion, without going into a comparison of the effectiveness of the temple healing vis-à-vis modern psychotherapy in the treatment of the various classes of mental disorder, I would only like to underline their radically different assumptions. The assumptions underlying western psychotherapy are also the highest values of modern individualism. They are epitomized in psychoanalysis (in Kenneth Keniston's words) as 'its almost limitless respect for the individual, faith that understanding is better than illusion, insistence that our psyches harbour darker secrets than we care to confess, refusal to promise too much, and a sense of the complexity, tragedy and wonder of human life'.[18] The underlying values of the traditional temple healing, on the other hand, stress that faith and surrender to a power beyond the individual are better than individual effort and struggle, that the source of human strengths lies in a harmonious integration with one's group, in the individual's affirmation of the community's values and its given order, in his obedience to the community's gods, and in his cherishing of its traditions.

Notes and References

1 For a detailed description of various kinds of Indian spirits, see Hastings, J. (ed.), 1908–16, *Encyclopaedia of Religion and Ethics*, 13 vols, Edinburgh, vol. 4, pp. 602 ff.

2 For the local legend of the temple and its deities, see Anon., n.d., *Shri-Balaji-dham-mahatmya*, Vrindavan: Matrapith.

3 Ibid., p. 48.

4 The classic work on the Asclepius cult is Meier, C.A., 1967, *Ancient Incubation and Modern Psychotherapy*, Evanston, Ill.: Northwestern University Press.

5 See, for instance, Sanford, John A., 1977, *Healing and Wholeness*, New York: Paulist Press, pp. 49–51.

6 For psychiatric and sociological views on spirit possession in India, see Freed, Stanley S. and Ruth S. Freed, 1964, 'Spirit Possession as Illness in a North Indian Village', *Ethnology*, 3, pp. 152–71; Harper, Edward B., 1963, 'Spirit Possession and Social Structure', in B. Ratnam (ed.), *Anthropology on the March*, Madras: The Book Centre, pp. 165–97; Teja, J.S., B.S. Khanna, and T.B. Subhramanyam, 1970, 'Possession States in Indian Patients', *Indian Journal of Psychiatry*, 12, pp. 71–87. For a cultural view of spirit possession, see Claus, Peter, 1979, 'Spirit Possession and Spirit Mediumship from the Perspective of Tulu Oral Traditions', *Culture, Medicine and Psychiatry*, 3 (1), pp. 29–52.

Of the twenty-eight patients interviewed at Balaji, ten were male and eighteen female. They ranged in age from sixteen to sixty-five years, with a median age of twenty-seven years. They hailed from large metropolises, small towns, and villages in almost equal number. All of them belonged to the upper castes and were predominantly of middle and lower-middle class status. Almost all had a few years of schooling and seven had even some college education.

7 On the concept of negative identity, see Erikson, Erik H., 1968, *Identity: Youth and Crisis*, New York: W.W. Norton, pp. 172–6.

8 See Ward, Colleen, 'Spirit Possession and Mental Health: A Psychoanthropological Perspective', *Human Relations*, 33 (1), pp. 149–63.

9 Freud Sigmund, 1895, 'Studies on Hysteria', in J. Strachey (ed.), 1958, *The Standard Edition of the Complete Psychological Works of Sigmund Freud*, vol. 2, London: Hogarth Press, ch. 2.

10 Krohn, Alan, 1978, *Hysteria: The Elusive Neurosis*, New York: International University Press.

11 Ibid., p. 188.

12 Erikson, Erik H., 1954, *Childhood and Society*, New York: W.W. Norton, p. 36.

13 The link between spirit possession among women and their social powerlessness has been also emphasized by Harper, 'Spirit Possession and Social Structure', and Teja *et al.*, 'Possession States in Indian Patients'.

14 Szasz, Thomas S., 1974, *The Myth of Mental Illness*, New York: Harper and Row, p. 230.

15 Hastings, *Encyclopaedia of Religion and Ethics*, p. 604.

16 Obeyesekere, Gananath, 1976, 'Psychocultural Exegesis of a Case of Spirit Possession in Sri Lanka', in V. Crapanzano (ed.), *Case Studies in Spirit Possession*, New York: John Wiley, p. 289.

17 For whatever it is worth, eleven of the twenty-eight patients (and their relatives) reported 'considerable improvement' in their condition at the end of their stay at Balaji. The breakdown of those reporting improvement was hysteria, eight; manic depressive, one; obsessive-compulsive, one; and undiagnosed (complaining symptom, white patches on skin), one.

18 Quoted in Adams, Virginia, 1979, 'Freud's Work Thrives as Theory, Not Therapy', in *The New York Times*, 14 August.

Empathy in Psychoanalysis and Spiritual Healing*

AT FIRST GLANCE, the spiritual practices of the main Eastern religions—Hinduism, Buddhism, Taoism—directed towards an 'absolute' rather than the phenomenal self of modern psychotherapy seem far removed from the concerns of psychoanalysis. If we except the Jungians, there is a venerable psychoanalytic tradition going back to Freud that tends to view religious or spiritual domains of experience as antithetical to psychoanalytic thought.[1] In spite of some respectful and non-reductionist treatment of religious–spiritual phenomena in the last quarter of the century, Freudian analysts have been often loath to acknowledge any similarities between the two.[2] Yet, these spiritual practices—mainly forms of meditation—also have an implicit psychotherapeutic function in that the absolute self is said to be manifested through the phenomenal self which obscures and entangles the former in a web of distortions and illusions that need to be removed. Both psychoanalysis and the spiritual traditions acknowledge the primacy of the human mind in the production of suffering. They also accept that the mind can help in processing and containing disturbed thoughts and feelings that lead to emotional distress. Thus, in Hinduism, it is the workings of the five passions, sexual desire, rage, greed, infatuation, and egotism which are held responsible for mental illness.

Similarly, Buddhists describe human suffering as due to causes internal to the individual mind: cognitive factors such as a perceptual cloudiness

*From *Mad and Divine: Spirit and Psyche in the Modern World,* Delhi: Viking-Penguin, 2008; University of Chicago Press, 2009.

causing misperception of objects of awareness as well as affective causes such as agitation and worry and the elements of anxiety, greed, avarice, and envy which form the cluster of what the Buddhists call 'grasping attachment'. Eastern spiritual traditions, thus, converge with psychoanalysis and psychodynamic therapies in the shared conviction that life does not happen to us but through us, and that it is false to believe that someone outside us is responsible for our distress.

Here, it should be made clear that the terms 'spiritual' and 'religious' are not identical. Religion and spirituality are not synonyms, even if they are often regarded as such by many who have been brought up in the Judeo–Christian worldview. The theological belief in God may be of great help in the striving for spiritual progress but it is not a necessity. In many Hindu, Buddhist and Taoist schools, an experiential understanding of the 'true' nature of the self is sought through an intensive practice of certain meditative-contemplative disciplines which do not require the presence of religious belief. In some early forms of Upanishadic and Yogic mysticism, for example, there is no trace of love or yearning for communion with God which is considered the highest manifestation of spiritual mood in the Christian and Islamic mystical traditions (as also in the Hindu *bhakti* devotionalism), without which no spiritual illumination is conceivable. Zen Buddhist practice, too, is silent on the question of a Divine Being. In many Eastern traditions, then, spiritual progress is achieved entirely through the seeker's own efforts and without the intervention of divine grace.

Spiritual disciplines regard themselves as scientific in the sense that they describe the stages and processes of transformation of consciousness through specific practices. And, indeed, as we shall see later, their descriptions of mental states reached through spiritual, meditative practices are no longer solely dependent on the subjective but credible reports through the ages of advanced practitioners but have begun to gather tentative support from recent brain research in the emerging discipline of 'neurotheology' which seems to have identified the state of consciousness in advanced meditation through its traces in the brain: the quieting of parietal lobes and the lighting up of the frontal lobe during the intense concentration of meditation when all sensory inputs are blocked.[3]

At the outset, let me state that my focus here is not on a psychoanalytic understanding of meditative practices and psychic states reached by adepts of Eastern spiritual disciplines. The literature on this aspect is considerable, ranging from an emphasis on the (mostly earlier) characterization of these states as regressive in the pathological sense,[4] to a more (mostly later) positive view of these states as integrative and adaptive.[5] My own thrust is more on the healing aspect of the interaction between the teacher–healer and the seeker–patient in the Eastern traditions and the contribution this understanding, including the self-understanding of the traditions, can make to psychoanalysis and the analyst–analysand interaction.

In theory, Eastern spiritual traditions generally view their healing function, both of mind and body, as incidental to and as a byproduct of their main task: the purification of the mind, the removal of its distortions, and illusions—its ignorance—in Buddhist terms. A purified mind is calm (or mindful) and thus a fit receptacle for the flow of a higher, transcendent consciousness. In most forms of yoga, for instance, the body, though important, is considered as subordinated to the mind. The gross body, our material sheath, is viewed as a shadow or creation of the subtle body we call the mind. The body is a mould into which the mind pours itself, a mould that has been prepared and can be changed by the mind.[6] Impurities of the mind not only lead to mental distress and illness but also, physically translated, manifest themselves in the body as disease. The removal of the cause—the impurities—also means the cessation of the effect: distress and disease. A purified mind makes for a pure body, a perfected mind for the perfection of the body. The perfection of the body, however, is not simultaneous with that of the mind but delayed till the impure precipitates of the mind, including karmic traces from past lives, have worked themselves out. This is a process which should not disturb the spiritual seeker, although some may attempt to accelerate the purification of the body by certain forms of yoga, such as Hathayoga. Moreover, the spiritual disciplines are believed to be accompanied by profound alterations in brain physiology and chemistry, in the nervous system, in the digestive and secretive processes. These cannot be effected without some physical disturbances which, however, are temporary and never more than is necessary for the process.

In practice, of course, for most people, the attraction of a spiritual discipline, especially if a famous spiritual guide imparts it—the guru, rinpoche, *roshi* or any other kind of teacher—lies more in an expectation of immediate healing by the spiritual teacher than in an indeterminate promise of a purified mind and eventual spiritual perfection through meditation. Although there is a large variety of Eastern meditative practices, the differences between them perhaps insufficiently appreciated in psychoanalytic literature,[7] there is a much greater uniformity in the way the spiritual teacher is regarded across the Eastern traditions. The complete devotion and unquestioning faith expected of the seeker by the Hindu guru, for instance, is identical with the expectations entertained by the Tibetan Buddhist master, in spite of the differences in their respective yogic and tantric meditation practices. In other words, the teacher, more than the meditative discipline itself, incorporates a therapeutic potential which draws to him the many seeking relief from emotional distress or physical suffering.

This is certainly true of the devotees of well-known Indian gurus I have studied over the years.[8] The prominence of the healing offer is especially marked in the case of some contemporary gurus like Sathya Sai Baba, with a worldwide following numbering in tens of millions, who may fairly be described as the healer guru *par excellence*. An unusually large number of stories told about him by devotees are narratives of 'miraculous' healing. To a lesser extent, this is also true about spiritual guides whose healing offer is less conspicuous. In a study of Ma Anandamayi ('Mother of Bliss'), a famous female saint of North India with a large following, including the former Indian Prime Minister Indira Gandhi, 11 of 43 interviews with her disciples contained incidents of her healing exploits.[9] Even in the case of an 'intellectual', modern guru like Jiddu Krishnamurti, with a following among the most modern and highly educated sections of society, it is not his teaching that excited the greatest interest[10] but the news about his miraculous cures.

Reading or listening to a number of healing stories, it becomes evident that the psychoanalytic theory which provides the most useful concepts in understanding therapy in the spiritual traditions, is not the Freudian equation of cure with the patient's attainment of a mature genitality through his or her engagement with and a resolution of early Oedipal conflicts. Nor does the Kleinian goal of re-experiencing and ultimately overcoming the archaic layers of depression and paranoia do justice to cure in the Eastern traditions. This does not mean that the aspects of human experience highlighted by Freud or Klein are absent from the spiritual setting. In a long interaction with the guru, stretching over many years, a re-experiencing of early Oedipal conflicts and of archaic depression, suspicion and rage may indeed take place without being subjected to conscious insight, except perhaps in a most fragmentary manner. What I wish to emphasize is that the theory of cure that makes the best *psychoanalytic* sense of spiritual healing, is the self psychology of Heinz Kohut.[11] According to this theory, analysis cures by restoring to the self the empathic responsiveness of the 'selfobject', of which the most important is the mother of infancy.[12] Of course, this does not mean that self psychology shares the self-transcendental concerns of Eastern spiritual traditions. In its pronounced relational orientation, self psychology is closer to Confucianism among the Eastern traditions rather than the more 'mystical' traditions of Hinduism, Buddhism, and Taoism. Confucianism, too, conceives of the self in fundamentally relational terms. The self may begin with a physical individuality but expands along a web of related existences[13]—selfobjects—until theoretically it could identify with the whole universe. The Confucian tradition, though, does not seek the mystical perfection of the self's identification with the whole world but is content to recommend an ideal of mental health and psychological maturity where the self is appropriately responsive to and in tune with the situations and persons of daily life: family, friends, colleagues at work, without an artificial boundary that shrinks the existence of the self to that of an individual unit.

The disciples' accounts of healing interaction with the spiritual guide also make it evident that the seeker–patient's interactions with the teacher have the aim of establishing him as a highly reliable, always available selfobject for merging experiences. The teacher furthers this process by his willingness to let the seeker merge with what the latter perceives to be the teacher's greatness, strength, calmness, just as the mother once did when she lifted the anxious infant and held him against her body. Sai Baba constantly reminds his devotees that they are not separate from him: 'I am in you, outside you, in front of you, above you, below you. I am all the time around you, in your proximity,'[14] and 'Anything coming out of the depth of your heart reaches me. So never have any doubt on this account'.[15]

Teachers in many Eastern spiritual traditions have always known that a prolonged phase of meditation on the guru's face or form—practised, for instance, in the Guru Yoga of Vajrayana Buddhism or in the Siddha Yoga of Kashmir Shaivism (a Hindu tradition), as also the contemplative uses of the guru's photograph in such modern sects as the Radhasoami Satsang and Sahaja Yoga—will contribute to and hasten the merging experience.[16] As a Siddha Yoga guru, Swami Muktananda, observes: 'The mind that always contemplates the guru eventually becomes the guru. Meditation on the guru's form, immerses the meditator in the state of the guru'.[17] As I have described elsewhere in a discussion of the Hindu guru as healer, other aspects of the guru–disciple interaction, such as the taking in of *prasada* (food offerings touched or tasted by the guru) or drinking water used to wash his feet, perform a similar function in the loosening of the seeker–patient's self boundaries and accelerate his experience of merging with the guru.[18] Gradually, the seeker–patient seems to acquire the capacity of summoning the guru's image with a hallucinatory intensity when in distress. Thus, one patient, when lying sick with jaundice, feverish and in a state of drowsiness, reports: 'I do not know if I used to dream or it was reality. I always felt Baba constantly with me. He was caressing me, touching my hands. I never felt lonely. He was there all the time.'[19] This access to archaic modes of contact in which a hallucinatory image of the guru is created to sustain a self in danger of losing its cohesion is reported by many seeker–patients and seems to be an integral part of the spiritual healing discourse.

With the spiritual healer's focus on a merger selfobject experience—in contrast to the analyst's effort to consolidate a sense of personal agency—the guru is initially much more active than the analyst in fostering the seeker–patient's idealization of his person. This is because of the signal importance most spiritual traditions attach to *surrender* as indispensable for mutative changes in the self, a surrender which can only be driven forward by intense forces of idealization.

Surrender of the self is, of course, also to be found in other religious traditions of the world. William James called it regeneration by relaxing and letting go. He characterized it as giving one's private convulsive self a rest and finding that a greater self is there.[20] The regenerative phenomenon which ensues on the abandonment of effort remains a fact of human nature.

He added: '... you see why self-surrender has been and always must be regarded as the vital turning point of religious life. ... One may say the whole development of Christianity in inwardness has consisted in little more than greater and greater emphasis attached to this crisis of self-surrender.'[21]

In Sufism, too, surrender to the master is a necessary prerequisite for the state of *fana fil-shaykh* or annihilation of oneself in the master. Of the *iradah*, the relationship between the Sufi master and his disciple, the Sufi poet says: 'O heart, if thou wanted the Beloved to be happy with thee, then thou must do and say what he commands. If he says, "Weep blood!" do not ask "Why?"; if He says, "Die!" do not say "How is that fitting?"'[22]

Psychologically, surrender is the full flowering of the idealizing transference, with its strong need for the experience of merging into a good and powerful, wise and perfect selfobject—the guru. The seeker, in wanting to experience his self as part of the guru's self, hearing with the guru's ears, seeing with the guru's eyes, tasting with the guru's tongue, feeling with the guru's skin, may be said to be striving for some of the most archaic selfobject experiences.

In interviews with seeker–patients, and in reading their accounts, what I found most striking about the healing encounter in the spiritual traditions is the seeker–patient's conviction of being profoundly understood by the guru. In case after case, sometimes even in the first encounter, we hear reports of how the guru saw deep into the patient's heart, looked into the innermost recesses of her being, and the effect this understanding had on her. Mahamaya is a middle-aged Bengali woman who first met Sai Baba in 1992 and has remained a devoted follower ever since. She grew up in a middle-class household in Calcutta and remembers that both her parents had strong devotional and spiritual leanings. The outer shell of her biography—the events of her life including her education, arranged marriage, children, part-time work as a teacher while her husband climbs the bureaucratic ladder in a state-owned insurance company—follows the conventions of an Indian middle class success story. There are, however, tantalizing hints of unhappiness in the marriage during its early years, some episodes of depression, especially one following the surgical removal of a malignant tumour in the kidney just before she met Sai Baba.

Mahamaya may be sparing in the narration of painful events of her life but not in the description of her emotional state prior to the first meeting with Swami (master): 'I was steeped deep in crisis, and altogether shattered in body and mind. At that stage of my life, I was weak and had physically broken down, mentally in utter darkness. I was groping for true and abiding support.'[23]

Visiting Baba's ashram together with her husband, she is sitting among a number of other visitors when Baba motions the couple to move to a smaller room adjoining the main hall for a private interview. Let me take the story forward in her own words:

As soon as my eyes met Swami's, He said, 'So you have come, with how much love I have called you'. What a moment! A storm raged within me. I was stunned, dazed, and then broke down into a storm of tears. Since 1988, life had been a struggle for me beset with moments of trouble, mental agony, anguish, and depression overcoming me now and then. But never had I opened my heart to any one, not even my husband. God was the sole companion of my broken heart. An introvert from childhood, I had not even opened my heart to my parents. Something happened to me the moment I looked into the divine eyes, all restraint, and all constraints just vanished, tears welled up in my eyes and poured down my cheeks. I was sobbing like a child. I felt my heart was purified through and through.[24]

Baba then tells her that

I [Mahamaya] should not worry about my son who, being busy with studies, was not writing letters. Secondly, I need not bother about my arthritis. In due course the pain would be reduced even though it would not go altogether. Thirdly, my younger daughter would have a safe delivery. These thoughts were in my mind no doubt but I had not uttered a word to him on these matters. He is the indweller. He knows all that goes on in our mind.[25]

Over the years, Mahamaya's healing is evident in a marked increase in her zest for life and a creative outpouring in which she writes many poems and songs in Bengali and Hindi.

The patient's feeling of being deeply understood by the guru, of the Swami being the 'indweller'—of the guru's empathy, the analyst will say—is a primary feature of the healing discourse in Eastern, especially Hindu and Tantric Buddhist spiritual traditions. I shall argue in the rest of this chapter that an exploration of the basic features of the spiritual guide's empathy can make a significant contribution to the psychoanalytic discussion of empathy.

It seems to me that empathy, Freud's *Einfuehlung*, the 'feeling into' another person, has been the object of a good deal of ambivalence in psychoanalytic literature, an ambivalence that has perhaps to do with what Freud, in a letter to Ferenzci, called its 'mystical character'.[26] The Oxford English Dictionary's definition of empathy seems unabashedly 'mystical' when it defines it as 'the power of projecting one's personality into (and so fully comprehending) the object of contemplation'. Although empathy constitutes the foundation of psychoanalytic work, of essence for gathering data for analytic interpretation, its connection to poorly understood unconscious processes in the analyst has surrounded the concept with a degree of unease in psychoanalytic discussion. Its general usage in psychoanalysis as one person's capacity to partake of the inner experience of another through unconscious attunement skims over the underlying mystery of the process. In other words, how does our normal non-empathic state, a state of self-experience with thoughts which are usually self-related,[27] change into a state where we can transcend the boundaries of the self to share the conscious and unconscious feelings and experiences of another self? Even the analyst's psychic state that is conducive to the operation of empathy, namely his evenly suspended, free-floating attention, when examined closely, seems to belong as much (if not more) to the meditative practices of spiritual traditions as to a 'scientific' psychoanalysis.

Consider, for instance, Freud's description of this psychic state:

Experience soon showed that the attitude which the analytic physician could most advantageously adopt was to surrender himself to his own unconscious mental activity, in a state of evenly suspended attention, to avoid as far as possible reflection and the construction of conscious expectations, not to try to fix anything that he heard particularly in his memory, and by these means catch the drift of the patient's unconscious with his own unconscious.[28]

Ehrenzweig has called free-floating attention 'unconscious scanning' which depends on a conscious blankness and is liable to be disturbed by introspection.[29] Unconscious scanning clearly has a meditative character, very different from the process of introspection. Ehrenzweig compares unconscious scanning to Paul Klee's 'multidimensional attention' or to 'horizontal listening' in music where one hears polyphonic voices as opposed to normal 'vertical' listening where one follows a single melody underscored by a harmonic background of accompanying voices. Horizontal hearing, in which several voices contending for exclusive attention cancel each other out, is totally blank in so far as conscious memory is concerned. This conscious blankness, however, does not preclude precision and fullness of information. In such comparisons and descriptions of (an ideal) free-floating attention, expert meditators will not fail to recognize advanced stages of meditative contemplation in certain Hindu and Buddhist spiritual disciplines. In other words, the analyst's potential for unconscious scanning or what Ogden calls the use of reverie experience, namely his unobtrusive thoughts, feelings, fantasies, ruminations, daydreams, bodily sensations, and so on, seemingly unconnected to what the patient is saying at the moment,[30] may well be related to his capacity for metaphysical openness. It is this openness which bears on the analyst's capacity 'to feel the alive moments of an analytic session in a visceral way, to be able to hear that a word or a phrase has been used, has been made anew in an interesting, unexpected way.'[31]

The increasing psychoanalytic ambivalence towards the phenomenon of empathy seems to have its origins in Freud's changing views towards it as he aged. Paul Roazen, in his Introduction to a paper by Hélène Deutsch, suggests that Freud took a far more distant and detached view of his patients in his later years than in an earlier, healthier period.[32] In his draft of 'Psychoanalysis and Telepathy' (1921), the 'secret essay' that was published posthumously in 1941, Freud had been sympathetic to the operation of such occult phenomenon as telepathy and thus, presumably, to the non-rational, intuitive, aspects of empathy. By 1927, though, he was taking a much more unambivalent stance on behalf of positivist science:

'The riddles of the universe reveal themselves only slowly to our investigation; there are many questions to which science today can give no answer. Nevertheless, scientific work is the only road which can lead us to knowledge of reality outside ourselves. It is once again merely an illusion to expect anything from intuition and introspection; they can give us nothing but particulars about our own mental life, which are hard to interpret, but never any information about the questions which religious doctrine finds it easy to answer.'[33] Not all his close followers shared Freud's criticism of intuition and introspection; Hélène Deutsch, for instance, viewed the analyst's intuition as a powerful therapeutic tool.[34] Yet, with hardening attitudes towards the 'occult' in the wake of Freud's distancing from it, empathy, too, became an object of suspicion since there were no satisfactory criteria that distinguished it from telepathy in the analytic situation.[35]

In contemporary psychoanalysis, the unease with empathy is expressed variously. Many psychoanalytic contributions on the nature of empathy seek to temper its self-transcendental character by emphasizing that the analyst's identification with the patient is transient, non-regressive, and under the analyst's ego control.[36] Beginning with Freud,[37] other analysts have emphasized the intellectual and rational aspects of empathy.[38] They have sought to domesticate its highly subjective, experiential character by enlarging the scope of the concept to include more neutral and cognitive aspects. Empathy, they assert, is not only an unconscious process in which the analyst shares the patient's experience for a short time but also includes the placing of this experience in a larger, more objective and complex understanding of the patient and then responding with an appropriate interpretation.[39] The analyst's unconscious resonance with the patient oscillates with a more intellectual attitude,[40] to produce what has been called 'generative empathy',[41] 'vicarious introspection',[42] or 'emotional knowing'.[43]

Others, again going back to Freud who pointed out the difficulty of knowing whether or not our empathy is merely the projection of our own feelings on to the patient,[44] have surrounded empathy with danger signals.[45] What we often take for empathy may only be an 'empathic fantasy',[46] a 'projective distortion'.[47] Empathy is also imprecise in that the range of empathic immersion into another person can extend from a state of minimal feeling with him to the extreme of nearly becoming the other person and thus psychotic.[48] A prolonged identification with the patient is quite likely to be a pathological gratification of the analyst's own unconscious needs.[49]

The overwhelming majority of psychoanalytic contributions on the nature of empathy, then, have tried to distance it (perhaps also defensively) from its moorings in unconscious, still poorly understood but no longer completely mysterious mental states. These mental states, as we shall see later, seem to be quite similar to those traversed during the meditative process.

In psychoanalysis, the analyst's understanding of the patient's inner state is primarily conveyed through a verbalizable and verbalized interpretation. In other words, the analyst's communication of empathy for the patient's inner state is primarily conveyed through words. Other means of communication, employing the aural, visual, tactile, and olfactory senses, have received a limited attention in analytic literature[50] although analysts have long known that it is these other nonverbal means which constitute the fundamental layer of human communication in infancy.[51] To take the aural sense first, the *music* of healing, the prosodic aspects of the analyst's discourse—tone, accent, pauses, silences, intonation—may amplify or belie the empathy of his words. The importance of prosody differs with individuals but may also vary across cultures. In the major Eastern civilizations, for instance, the formal mode of communication required within the family and especially in hierarchical relationships and specifically the reliance placed on prosody to divine the real meaning of a speaker's words, may be greater than in cultures which hold 'saying what one means' and 'meaning what one says' as highly desirable virtues.

The psychoanalytic setting, with the patient lying on the couch and an absence of eye contact between the patient and the analyst during the analytic hour, is actively inimical to the visual aspects—expression in eyes, gestures, facial mimicry, positions of body—of communicating empathy. The psychoanalytic emphasis on free association, fostered through a restriction of the visual channel, then has the disadvantage that it outlaws the *dance* of healing. And, of course, because of the rule of abstinence and the dread of 'crossing boundaries', amplified by psychoanalytic lore around the transgressions of once heroic and now tragic figures in the history of the discipline,[52] the tactile aspects of empathic communication between the analyst and the patient must perforce be completely excluded. Not for the analyst the clasping of a shoulder, the taking of a hand between one's own, the consoling stroke on the head—which convey empathic connection to a person as nothing else can in her periods of acute distress—for the analyst is acutely aware that a touch of understanding can soon become a caress of desire or a stab of anxiety, a risk that spiritual teachers routinely take, sometimes with disastrous consequences for the seeker.

I must also add that, like the experience of many people deprived of sight who develop acute aural or tactile perceptions, the emphasis on words in the analytic situation increases the patient's (and the analyst's) sensitivity to the nuances and particularities of language. At least this has been my own experience when, in the full throes of transference during my training in analysis in Germany, I not only began to dream in German but also to write fiction in that language, a gift that was snatched away when the analysis ended. This enhanced linguistic sensitivity receded when the transferential context which had made it possible disappeared.

Compared to the analyst, then, the spiritual teacher is relatively uninhibited (but also more endangered) in employing the full register of communication to convey his empathic understanding of the patient–seeker's internal state. In describing their experiences of the guru's empathy, patient–seekers in the Eastern traditions often emphasize factors other than the content of his words. 'I did not understand but I came away with the words alive within me', is a typical reaction.[53] The Indian spiritual traditions even have a technical term for the teacher's look, *darshanat*, 'through the guru's look', in which the seeker–patient is believed to be seen 'in every detail as in a clear mirror.'[54]

Like analysts, spiritual teachers, too, differ among themselves in their innate empathic capacities. Yet, with their meditative practices designed to weaken what Brickman calls the encapsulation of the self,[55] not in an uncontrolled regression but in controlled de-centring experiences, a spiritual discipline seems to open the doors to an empathic responsiveness, that can extend to a high degree of identification with another person. Analysts, too, may have these 'transcendental' moments during an analytic hour. However, these do not follow from being a part of a rigorous training explicitly designed to foster the mental state of what Bion called 'ignorance' and whose first stage is what Keats called 'negative capability', a passive, receptive state where there is no irritable reaching after fact and reason and no search for meaning.[56] For the nineteenth century poet John Keats, it is the presence of the 'negative capability' that makes an empathic participation in the existence of other persons possible. The poet, perhaps a person of particularly strong empathic development, grasps the 'truth' about the animate and inanimate 'Other' through this empathy and then reproduces it in literary images.[57] A radical increase in empathy for another person, claimed by spiritual adepts, is a part of their heightened responsiveness—empathy in its widest sense—towards the animate and inanimate worlds. In the *homini religiosi*, this empathy is also translated into a heightened metaphysical openness towards the Divine.

In their empathic identifications, analysts can perhaps never go as far as a few spiritual teachers are reputed to have done. In describing Anandamayi as a 'spiritually realized' person, for instance, a devotee explains: 'It means you have no personal centre. The centre of the realized person is everywhere. She can identify with whoever comes in contact with her. She becomes yourself and has your problems at the very moment and can help you from inside.'[58] Another disciple describes her as: 'She had no sense of "I" or "mine" and often simply mirrored the emotions of those around her; she seemed to have no desires of her own, so the incentives to her behaviour took shape out of the wishes of her companions'.[59] Here, Anandamayi approaches the ideal of the spiritual master met with in almost all the Eastern traditions. In the Sufi tradition, for instance, the Shaykh's 'own bodily form has been annihilated and he has become a mirror; within it are reflected the faces of others ... If you see an ugly face, that is you; and if you see Jesus and Mary, that is you. He is neither this nor that, he is plain; he has set your own reflection before you.'[60]

Compare these portraits of the 'enlightened' spiritual teacher with Keats's description of the identity—he called it 'character'—of the poet:

> As to the poetic Character itself—it is not itself—it has no self—it is everything and nothing. It has no character—it enjoys light and hate; it loves in gusto, be it foul or fair, high or low—it has as much delight in conceiving an Iago as an Imogen. What shocks the virtuous philosopher, delights the chameleon Poet—A Poet is the most unpoetical of anything in existence; because he has no identity—Not one word I ever utter can be taken for granted as an opinion growing out of my identical nature—the identity of everyone begins to press upon me.[61]

The reflecting mirror ideal of the spiritual guru, then, is quite different from the earlier psychoanalytic ideal of the analyst as a blank screen; the analyst's self is hidden, unlike that of the spiritual master which often appears to be absent. Anandamayi, like some spiritual teachers, but unlike many analysts, can accompany the patient to the land of pre-psychological chaos met with in psychosis and borderline states. It is perhaps only Bion's ideal analyst who has eschewed memory and desire (in a later amendment, has also abandoned understanding)[62] and is a twin of the (also ideal) spiritual teacher.

Hindu spiritual traditions give detailed descriptions of the process that augments empathy to a point where there is no affective obstacle to an identification with another's experience. A complete empathic knowledge of another person, they claim, involves the activation of a normally dormant 'higher' faculty or consciousness. In yogic practice, for instance, reason, imagination, memory, thought, and sensations have first to become sufficiently quiet for the higher faculty of *buddhi* to become active and to know itself as separate and different from the lower qualities.[63] Buddhi is the yogic analogue of Bion's 'sense organ' of psychical qualities which responds to the broadcast of a 'sender', which dwells in the domain of the inner world, and to which psychoanalysts need to develop a keener reception. Analysts, Bion maintained, needed to screen out the noise of sensible life so as to become more receptive to other messages from the psychical world.[64] This receptivity leads to expansion of preconscious communication channels and a greater capacity for retrieval from the depths of the psyche.[65]

In conclusion, one can say that, from a spiritual viewpoint, the chief obstacle to an analyst's empathy is his phenomenal, sensual self. Fuelled by the senses, the sensual self prevents the emergence of buddhi. The meditative practices of the Eastern spiritual traditions are directed precisely towards the reduction of noise and glare produced by the sensual self. Thus, although empathy is common to both spiritual healing and psychoanalytic cure, the concept itself veers towards its 'mystical' (in a non-pejorative sense) pole in the former case and towards its rational, intellectual pole in the latter. If we concede the spiritual teacher's claim, supported by personal testimony of spiritual adepts over the centuries, that the activation of buddhi is accompanied by an extraordinary increase in his empathic capacity, then it follows that some kind of spiritual training may significantly enhance an analyst's potential for empathic identification. Such a training not only contributes to a greater ease with the setting aside of ego functions, making one less defensive against the anxiety of 'drowning', but can also expand the analyst's potential for 'reverie' or implicit listening, and thus, for deep empathy.

Yet another way of increasing our empathic capacity may well be a constant and conscious practice of compassion till it becomes an ingrained way of approaching all living beings. In this endeavour, one does not have to aim for the heights of empathy reached by Alain Passard, an icon of French cuisine. Passard, who famously converted to vegetarian cooking a few years ago describes his conversion thus: '… every day I was struggling to have a creative relationship with a corpse, a dead animal! And I could feel inside me the weight and sadness of the *cuisine animale*. And since then (the change) … gone.'[66] To be consequence in one's practice of compassion is not an easy task. The Dalai Lama, who has been meditating for at least three hours every day for over fifty years, tells this story about himself. In Dharamshala, where he lives, there are many mosquitoes. When the first mosquito alights on his bare arm, his thought is, 'Fine, my friend, you must also live. Have your meal of my blood.' With the second one, he is a bit irritated. When the third one comes buzzing to the dining table, he squashes it flat. The Buddhists believe that your thoughts when you are dying have a huge effect on how you are reincarnated in your next birth—pure, spiritual thoughts ensuring a higher form of consciousness in the next life. 'When I am dying,' Dalai Lama says with his trademark smile, 'I will make sure that my bed is covered with a mosquito net.'[67]

For psychotherapists, then, the augmentation of their empathic capacity is of signal importance. This is true even if one does not regard empathy as a primary curative agent as Kohut does, but is prepared to concede that it is indeed a very significant tool for gathering data in the treatment situation. After all, even the most sophisticated interpretation in psychoanalysis can only be as good as the data on which it is based. Empathy, and the meditative state that underlies it, may well be the sluice through which the spiritual enters the consulting room and where it flows together with the art and science of psychoanalysis in the practice of psychotherapy. This is not to suggest that psychoanalysis should lose its distinctive character by an indiscriminate borrowing from Eastern spiritual traditions. Psychoanalysis itself can be viewed as a singularly modern meditative praxis, unique in its emphasis on being a meditation that is joint rather than individual. Yet, in the spirit of Freud's legacy of openness to other disciplines (Freud recommended the study of anthropology, folklore, and mythology to the budding analyst), analysts need to remain open to the possibility that an Eastern meditative discipline could become a part of their training if, as claimed by its practitioners, it demonstrably contributed to an enhancement in empathic capability. The traditional Freudian suspicion of the spiritual domain and the cultural pride in psychoanalysis as a uniquely valuable product of Western civilization and imagination, should not come in the way of such borrowings.

Notes and References

1. See also Brickman, H.R., 1998, 'The Psychoanalytic Cure and its Discontents: A Zen Buddhist Perspective on "Common Unhappiness" and the Polarized Self', *Psychoanalysis and Contemporary Thought*, 21, pp. 3–32.

2. Some of these are Jones, J.W., 1991, *Contemporary Psychoanalysis and Religion*, New Haven: Yale University Press; Kakar, S., 1991, *The Analyst and the Mystic*, Chicago: University of Chicago Press; Meissner, W.W., 1984, *Psychoanalysis and Religious Experience,* New Haven: Yale University Press; Rizzuto, A.M., 1979, *The Birth of the Living God*, Chicago: University of Chicago Press; Vergote, A., 1988, *Guilt and Desire*, New Haven: Yale University Press.

3. Newberg, A., *et al.*, 2001, *Why God Won't Go Away: Brain Science and the Biology of Belief*, New York: Random House.

4. See Alexander, F., 1931, 'Buddhist Training as an Artificial Catatonia', *Psychoanalytic Review*, 18, pp. 129–45; Freud, S., 1927, 'The Future of an Illusion' and 1930, 'Civilization and its Discontents', *SE*, 21; Fingarette, H., 1958, 'Ego and Mythic Selflessness', *Psychoanalytic Review*, 45, pp. 5–40; Jones, E., 1923, 'The Nature of Auto-suggestion', in *Papers on Psychoanalysis*, Boston: Beacon Press, 1961, pp. 273–93; Masson, J.M., 1980, *The Oceanic Feeling: The Origins of Religious Sentiment in Ancient India*, Dordrecht: Reidel; Ross, N., 1975, 'Affect as Cognition: With Observations on the Meaning of Mystical States', *International Review of Psycho-Analysis*, 2, pp. 79–93.

5. See, for instance, Fromm, E., 1960, 'Psychoanalysis and Zen Buddhism', in D.T. Suzuki, E. Fromm, and R. De Martino (eds), *Zen Buddhism and Psychoanalysis*, New York: Harper, pp. 77–141; Horton, P.C., 1974, 'The Mystical Experience: Substance of an Illusion', *Journal of the American Psychoanalytic Association*, 22, pp. 364–80; Shafii, M., 1973, 'Silence in Service of the Ego: Psychoanalytic Study of Meditation', *International Journal of Psychoanalysis*, 45, pp. 431–43; Brickman, 'Psychoanalytic Cure'; Meissner, *Psychoanalysis and Religious Experience.*

6. Sri Aurobindo, 1911, 'Yogic Sadhan', *Sri Aurobindo Archives and Research*, 10:1, pp. 55–83.

7. See Epstein, M., 1990, 'Beyond the Oceanic Feeling', *International Review of Psychoanalysis*, 17, pp. 159–64.

8. Kakar, S., 1982, *Shamans, Mystics and Doctors*, New York: Knopf; Kakar, *Analyst and Mystic.*

9. Hallstrom, L.L., 1999, *Mother of Bliss: Anandamayi Ma*, Delhi: Oxford University Press, p. 10.

10. Jayakar, P., 1987, *J. Krishnamurti: A Biography*, Delhi: Penguin, p. 211.

11. Kohut, H., 1971, *The Analysis of the Self*, New York: International Universities Press; 1977, *The Restoration of the Self*, New York: International Universities Press; 1984, *How Analysis Cures*, Chicago: University of Chicago Press.

12. Selfobjects are those 'others' (and their symbolic equivalents) who are deeply internalized and experienced as part of one's own self.

13. Kalton, M., 1995, 'Self Transformation in the Confucian Tradition', in *Psychotherapy East and West*, Seoul: Korean Academy of Psychotherapist.

14. Agarwal, M., 2000, *Sai Ek, Roop Anek* ('Sai is one but forms are many'), Calcutta: Sri Satya Sai Book and Publications Trust, p. 54.

15. Ibid., p. 116.

16. Kakar, *Analyst and Mystic*, Ch. 3.

17. Swami Muktananda, 1983, *The Perfect Relationship*, Ganeshpuri: Gurudev Siddha Vidyapeeth, p. 3.

18. Kakar, *Analyst and Mystic*, p. 52.

19. Agarwal, *Sai Ek, Roop Anek*, p. 72.

20. James, *The Varieties of Religious Experience*, p. 102.

21. Ibid., p. 176.

22. Nurbakhsh, D., 1978, 'Sufism and Psychoanalysis', *International Journal of the Society of Psychiatrists*, 24, p. 208.

23. Agarwal, *Sai Ek, Roop Anek*, p. 7.

24. Ibid., p. 28.

25. Ibid., pp. 29–30.

26. Grubrich-Simitis, I., 1986, 'Six Letters of Sigmund Freud and Sandor Ferenczi on the Interrelationship of Psychoanalytic Theory and Technique', *International Review of Psychoanalysis*, 13, p. 271.

27. Satran, G., 1991, 'Some Limits and Hazards of Empathy', *Contemporary Psycho-analysis*, 27, p. 739.

28. Freud, S., 1923, 'Two Encyclopaedia Articles', *SE*, 18, p. 239.

29. Ehrenzweig, A., 1964, 'The Undifferentiated Matrix of Artistic Identification', in W. Muensterberger and S. Axelrad (eds), *The Psychoanalytic Study of Society*, vol. 3, New York: International Universities Press.

30. Ogden, T., 1997, 'Reverie and Metaphor', *International Journal of Psychoanalysis*, 78, pp. 719–32.

31. Ibid., p. 719.

32. Roazen in Deutsch, H., 1989, 'On Satisfaction, Happiness and Ecstasy', *International Journal of Psychoanalysis*, 70, p. 715.

33. Freud, 'Future of an Illusion', pp. 31–2.

34. Deutsch, H., 1926, 'Okkulte Vorgaenge waehrend der Psychoanalyse', *Imago*, 12, pp. 418–33.

35. Rycroft, C., 1954, 'Review of G. Devereux ed., "Psychoanalysis and the Occult"', *International Journal of Psychoanalysis*, 35, pp. 70–1.

36. Levy, S., 1985, 'Empathy and Psychoanalytic Technique', *Journal of the American Psychoanalytic Association*, 33, pp. 353–78.

37. Grubrich-Simitis, 'Six Letters', p. 272.

38. Pigman, G., 1995, 'Freud and the History of Empathy', *International Journal of Psychoanalysis*, 76, pp. 237–56.

39. Levy, 'Empathy and Psychoanalytic Technique', p. 356.

40. Reich, A., 1973, 'Empathy and Countertransference', in *Psychoanalytic Contributions*, New York: International Universities Press, pp. 344–60.

41. Schaefer, R., 1959, 'Generative Empathy in the Treatment Situation', *Psychoanalytic Quarterly*, 28, p. 342.

42. Kohut, H., 1959, 'Introspection, Empathy and Psychoanalysis', *Journal of the American Psychoanalytic Association*, 7, p. 459.

43. Greenson, R., 1960, 'Empathy and its Vicissitudes', *International Journal of Psychoanalysis*, 41, p. 418.

44. Freud, S., 1912–13, *Totem and Taboo*, *SE*, 13, p. 103.

45. See Buie, D., 1981, 'Empathy: Its Nature and Limitations', *Journal of the American Psychoanalytic Association*, 30, pp. 959–78; Moses, I., 1988, 'The Misuse of Empathy in Psychoanalysis', *Contemporary Psychoanalysis*, 24, pp. 577–94; Shapiro, T., 1974, 'The Development and Distortions of Empathy', *Psychoanalytic Quarterly*, 43, pp. 4–25; Spence, D, 1988, 'Discussion of I. Moses: The Misuse of Empathy in Psychoanalysis',*Contemporary Psychoanalysis*, 24, pp. 594–98; Tuch, R., 1997, 'Beyond Empathy: Concerning Certain Complexities in the Self Psychology Theory', *Psychoanalytic Quarterly*, 66, pp. 259–82.

46. Satran, 'Some Limits and Hazards of Empathy', p. 739.

47. Spence, 'Discussion of I. Moses', p. 596.

48. Satran, 'Some Limits and Hazards of Empathy', p. 739.

49. Greenson, 'Empathy and its Vicissitudes', p. 420.

50. However, see Jacobs, T.J., 1973, 'Posture, Gesture and Movement in the Analyst: Cues to Interpretation and Countertransference', *Journal of the American Psychoanalytic Association*, 21, pp. 72–92; 1994, 'Non-verbal Communications: Some Reflections on their Role in the Psychoanalytic Process and Psychoanalytic Education', *Journal of the American Psychoanalytic Association*, 42, pp. 741–62; 1995, 'When the Body Speaks: Psychoanalytic Meaning in Kinetic Clues', *Psychoanalytic Quarterly*, 64, pp. 784–8.

51. Spitz, R., 1957, *No and Yes*, New York: International Universities Press.

52. Ross, J.M., 1995, 'The Fate of Relatives and Colleagues in the Aftermath of Boundary Violations', *Journal of the American Psychoanalytic Association*, 43, pp. 959–61.

53. Jayakar, *J. Krishnamurti*, p. 8.

54. Muktananda, *The Perfect Relationship*, p. 37.

55. Brickman, 'Psychoanalytic Cure'.

56. Keats, J., 1958, *Letters of John Keats*, edited by H.E. Rollins, Cambridge, Mass.: Harvard University Press, p. 193.

57. Levy, S., 1970, 'John Keats' Psychology of Creative Imagination', *Psychoanalytic Quarterly*, 39, pp. 173–97.

58. Hallstrom, *Mother of Bliss*, p. 98.

59. Ibid., p. 26.

60. Chittick, W.C., 1983, *The Sufi Path of Love: The Spiritual Teachings of Rumi*, Albany: SUNY Press, p. 145.

61. Keats, *Letters of John Keats*, pp. 386–7.

62. Bion, W.R., 1967, 'Notes on Memory and Desire', *Psychoanalytic Forum*, 2, pp. 271–80.

63. Aurobindo, 'Yogic Sadhan'.

64. Grotstein, J.S., 1981, 'Wilfred R. Bion: The Man, the Psychoanalyst, the Mystic: A Perspective on his Life and Work', *Contemporary Psychoanalysis*, 17, pp. 501–36.

65. Bolognini, S., 2001, 'Empathy and the Unconscious', *Psychoanalytic Quarterly*, 70, pp. 447–71.

66. Gopnik, A., 2005, 'Two Cooks', *The New Yorker*, 5 September, p. 97.

67. Dalai Lama in a Workshop on Buddhism, held in New Delhi, 21–3 December 2006.

Psychoanalysis and Culture

Clinical Work and Cultural Imagination*

THE PERENNIAL QUESTION of the cross-cultural validity of psychoanalysis actually has two parts: Is psychoanalysis at all possible in a traditional non-Western society with its different family system, religious beliefs, and cultural values? Is the mental life of non-Western patients radically different from that of their Western counterparts?

Over the years, in my own talks to diverse audiences in Europe and the United States, the question of trans-cultural validity of psychoanalysis has invariably constituted the core of animated discussions. The sharp increase in scepticism about this particular question has, in recent years, been correlated with the rise of relativism in the human sciences. Intellectually, the relativistic position owes much of its impetus to Foucault's powerful argument on the rootedness of all thought in history and culture and in the framework of power relations. Adherents of this perspective are not a priori willing to accept why psychoanalysis, a product of nineteenth century European bourgeois family and social structure, should be an exception to the general rule of the incapacity of thought to transcend its roots. In this essay, I propose to discuss the issue of the cultural rootedness of psychoanalysis with illustrations from my own clinical practice in India.

Ramnath was a 51-year-old man who owned a grocery shop in the oldest part of the city of Delhi. When he came to see me some eighteen

* From *Culture and Psyche*, Delhi: Oxford University Press, 1997.

years ago, he was suffering from a number of complaints, though he desired my help for only one of them—an unspecified 'fearfulness'. This anxiety, less than three years old, was a relatively new development. His migraine headaches, on the other hand, went back to his adolescence. Ramnath attributed them to an excess of 'wind' in the stomach, which periodically rose up and pressed against the veins in his head. Ramnath had always had a nervous stomach. It was now never quite as bad as it was in the months following his marriage some thirty years ago, when it was accompanied by severe stomach cramps and an alarming weight loss. He was first taken to the hospital by his father, where he was X-rayed and tested. Finding nothing wrong with him, the doctors prescribed a variety of vitamins and tonics which were not of much help. Older family members and friends then recommended a nearby *ojha*—'sorcerer' is too fierce a translation for this mild-mannered professional of ritual exorcism—who diagnosed his condition as the result of magic practised by an enemy, namely, his newly acquired father-in-law. The rituals to counteract the enemy magic were expensive, as was the yellowish liquid emetic prescribed by the ojha, which periodically forced Ramnath to empty his stomach with gasping heaves. In any event, he was fully cured within two months of the ojha's treatment, and the cramps and weight loss have not recurred.

Before coming to see me about his 'fearfulness', Ramnath had been treated with drugs by various doctors: by allopaths (as Western-style doctors are called in India) as well as homeopaths, by the *vaids* of Hindu medicine, as well as the *hakims* of the Islamic medical tradition. He had consulted psychiatrists, ingested psychotropic drugs, and submitted to therapy. He had gone through the rituals of two ojhas and was thinking of consulting a third who was highly recommended.

His only relief came through the weekly gathering of the local chapter of the Brahmakumari (literally 'Virgins of Brahma') sect which he had recently joined. The communal meditations and singing gave him a feeling of temporary peace and his nights were no longer so restless. Ramnath was puzzled by the persistence of his anxious state and its various symptoms. He had tried to be a good man, he said, according to his dharma, which is both the 'right conduct' of his caste and the limits imposed by his own character and predispositions. He had worshipped the gods and attended services in the temple with regularity, even contributing generously towards the consecration of a Krishna idol in his native village in Rajasthan. He did not have any bad habits, he asserted. Tea and cigarettes, yes, but for a couple of years he had abjured even these minor, though pleasurable, addictions. Yet, the anxiety persisted, unremitting and unrelenting.

Since it is culture rather than psyche which is the focus of this presentation, let me essay a cultural—rather than a psycho—analysis of Ramnath's condition. At first glance, Ramnath's cognitive space in matters of illness and well-being seems incredibly cluttered. Gods and spirits, community and family, food and drink, personal habits and character, all seem to be somehow intimately involved in the maintenance of health. Yet, these and other factors such as biological infection, social pollution, and cosmic displeasure—all of which most Hindus would also acknowledge as causes of ill health—only point to the recognition of a person's simultaneous existence in different orders of being ... of the person being a body, a psyche, and a social being at the same time. Ramnath's experience of his illness may appear alien to Europeans only because, as I have elaborated elsewhere,[1] the body, the psyche, and the community do not possess fixed, immutable meanings across cultures. The concept of the body and the understanding of its processes are not quite the same in India as they are in the West. The Hindu body, portrayed in relevant cultural texts, predominantly in imagery from the vegetable kingdom, is much more intimately connected with the cosmos than the clearly etched Western body which is sharply differentiated from the rest of the objects in the universe. The Hindu body image stresses an unremitting interchange taking place with the environment, simultaneously accompanied by ceaseless change within the body. The psyche—the Hindu 'subtle body'—is not primarily a psychological category in India. It is closer to the ancient Greek meaning of the 'psyche', the source of all vital activities and psychic processes, and considered capable of persisting in its disembodied state after death. Similarly, for many Indians, the community consists not only of living members of the family and the social group but also of ancestral and other spirits as well as the gods and goddesses who populate the Hindu cosmos. An Indian is inclined to believe that his or her illness can reflect a disturbance in any one of these orders of being, while the symptoms may also be manifested in the other orders. If a treatment, say, in the bodily order fails, one is quite prepared to reassign the cause of the illness to a different order and undergo its particular curing regimen—prayers or exorcisms, for instance—without losing regard for other methods of treatment.

The involvement of all orders of being in health and illness means that an Indian is generally inclined to seek more than one cause for illness in especially intractable cases. An Indian tends to view these causes as complementary rather than exclusive and arranges them in a hierarchical order by identifying an immediate cause as well as others that are more remote. The causes are arranged in concentric circles, with the outer circle including all the inner ones.

To continue with our example. Ramnath had suffered migraine headaches since his adolescence. Doctors of traditional Hindu medicine, Ayurveda, had diagnosed the cause as a humoral disequilibrium—an excess of 'wind' in the stomach which periodically rose up and pressed against the veins in his head—and prescribed Ayurvedic drugs, dietary restrictions, as well as liberal doses of aspirin. Such disequilibrium is usually felt to be compounded by bad habits which, in turn, demand changes in personal conduct. When an illness like Ramnath's persists, its stubborn intensity will be linked with his unfavourable astrological conditions, requiring palliative measures such as a round of prayers (puja). The astrological 'fault' probably will be further traced back to the bad karma of a previous birth about which, finally, nothing can be done except, perhaps, the cultivation of a stoic endurance with the help of the weekly meetings of the Virgins of Brahma sect.

I saw Ramnath thrice a week in psychoanalytic therapy for twenty-one sessions before he decided to terminate the treatment. At the time, although acutely aware of my deficiencies as a novice, I had placed the blame for the failure of the therapy on the patient or, to be more exact, on the cultural factors involved in his decision. Some of these were obvious. Ramnath had slotted me into a place normally reserved for a personal guru. From the beginning, he envisioned not a contractual doctor–patient relationship but a much more intimate guru–disciple bond that would allow him to abdicate responsibility for his life. He was increasingly dismayed that a psychoanalyst did not dispense wise counsel but expected the client to talk, that I wanted to follow his lead rather than impose my own views or directions on the course of our sessions. My behaviour also went against the guru model which demands that the therapist demonstrate his compassion, interest, warmth, and responsiveness much more openly than I believed is possible or desirable in a psychoanalytic relationship. I did not know then that Ramnath's 'guru fantasy', namely the existence of someone, somewhere—now discovered in my person—who will heal the wounds suffered in all past relationships, remove the blights on the soul so that it shines anew in its pristine state, was not inherent in his Indian-ness but common across many cultures. Irrespective of their conscious subscription to the ideology of egalitarianism and a more contractual doctor–patient relationship, my European and American patients, too, approached analysis and the analyst with a full-blown guru fantasy which, though, was more hidden and less accessible to consciousness than in the case of Ramnath.

More than Ramnath's expectations, it was the disappointment of mine, I now realize, on which the analysis floundered. I had expected Ramnath to be an individual in the sense of someone whose consciousness has been moulded in a crucible which is commonly regarded as having come into existence as part of the psychological revolution in the wake of the Enlightenment in Europe. This revolution, of course, is supposed to have narrowed the older, metaphysical scope of the mind, to a mind as an isolated island of individual consciousness, profoundly aware of its almost limitless subjectivity and its infantile tendency to heedless projection and illusion. Psychoanalysis, I believed, with some justification, is possible only with a person who is individual in this special sense, who shares, at some level of awareness and to some minimum degree, the modern vision of human experience wherein each of us lives in our own subjective world, pursuing personal pleasures and private fantasies, constructing a fate which will vanish when our time is over. The reason why in most psychoanalytic case histories, whether in Western or non-Western worlds, analysands, except for their different neurotic or character disturbances, sound pretty much like each other (and like their analysts), is because they all share the post-Enlightenment world-view of what constitutes an individual. In a fundamental sense, psychoanalysis does not have a cross-cultural context but takes place in the same culture across different societies; it works in the established (and expanding) enclaves of psychological modernity around the world. We can, therefore, better understand why psychoanalysis in India began in Calcutta [now Kolkata]—the first capital of the British empire in India where Indians began their engagement and confrontation with post-Enlightenment Western thought—before extending itself and virtually limiting itself to Bombay [now Mumbai] which prides itself on its cosmopolitan character and cultural 'modernity'. It is also comprehensible that the clientele for psychoanalysis in India consists overwhelmingly—though not completely—of individuals (and their family members) who are involved in modern professions like journalism, advertising, academia, law, medicine, and so on. In its sociological profile, at least, this clientele does not significantly differ from the one that seeks psychoanalytic therapy in Europe and America.

Ramnath, I believed, was not an individual in the sense that he lacked 'psychological modernity'. He had manfully tried to understand the psychoanalytic model of inner conflict rooted in life history that was implied in my occasional interventions. It was clear that this went against his cultural model of psychic distress and healing wherein the causes for his suffering lay outside himself and had little to do with his biography—black magic by the father-in-law, disturbed planetary constellations, bad karma from previous life, disturbed humoral equilibrium. He was thus not suitable for psychoanalytic therapy and perhaps I had given up on him before he gave up on me. However, Ramnath, I realized later, like many of my other traditional Hindu patients, had an individuality which is embedded in and expressed in terms from the Hindu cultural universe. This individuality is accessible to psychoanalysis if the therapist is willing and able to build the required bridges from a modern to a traditional individuality. The Indian analyst has to be prepared, for instance, to interpret the current problems of such a patient in terms of his or her bad karma—feelings, thoughts, and actions—not from a previous existence but from a forgotten life, the period of infancy and childhood, his or her 'pre-history'. Let me elaborate on this distinction between traditional and modern individuals who both share what I believe is the essence of psychological modernity.

Psychological modernity, although strongly associated with post-Enlightenment, is nevertheless not identical to it. The core of psychological modernity is internalization rather than externalization. I use internalization here as a sensing by the person of a psyche in the Greek sense, an animation from within rather than without. Experientially, this internalization is a recognition that one is possessed of a mind in all its complexity. It is the acknowledgement, however vague, unwilling or conflicted, of a subjectivity that fates one to episodic suffering through some of its ideas and feelings—in psychoanalysis, murderous rage, envy, and possessive desire seeking to destroy those one loves and would keep alive—simultaneously with the knowledge, at some level of awareness, that the mind can help in containing and processing disturbed thoughts—as indeed can the family and the group as well.[2] In Hindu terms, it is a person's sense and acknowledgement of the primacy of the subtle body—the *sukshmasharira*—in human action and of human suffering as caused by the workings of the five passions: sexual desire, rage, greed, infatuation, and egotism. Similarly, Buddhists, too, describe human suffering as being due to causes internal to the individual: not only cognitive factors such as a perceptual cloudiness causing mis-perception of objects of awareness but also affective causes such as agitation and worry—the elements of anxiety, and greed, avarice, and envy which form the cluster of grasping attachment. This *internalization* is the essence of 'individuation', and of psychological modernity, which has always been a part of what Hindus call the 'more evolved' beings in traditional civilizations. The fact that this core of individuation is expressed in a religious rather than a psychological idiom should not prevent us from recognizing its importance as an ideal of maturity in traditional civilizations such as Hindu India; it should also give us pause in characterizing, indeed with the danger of pathologizing India or any other civilization as one where some kind of familial self[3] or group mind[4] reigns in individual mental life. The 'evolved' Hindu in the past or even in the present who has little to do with the post-Enlightenment West, thus interprets the Mahabharata as an account of inner conflict in man's soul rather than of outer hostilities. The 'evolved beings' in India, including the most respected gurus, have always held that the guru, too, is only seemingly a person but actually a function, a transitional object in modern parlance, as are all the various gods who, too, are only aspects of the self. 'The Guru is the disciple, but perfected, complete,' says Muktananda.[5] 'When he forms a relationship with the guru, the disciple is in fact forming a relationship with his own best self' (p. ix). At the end of your *sadhana*, burn the guru, say the Tantriks; kill the Buddha if you meet him on the way, is a familiar piece of Zen Buddhist wisdom. All of them, gurus or gods (as also the analyst), have served the purpose of internalization—of a specific mode of relating to and experiencing the self, and are dispensable.

Psychological modernity is thus not coterminous with historical modernity, nor are its origins in a specific geographical location even if it has received a sharp impetus from the European Enlightenment. My biggest error in Ramnath's case was in making a sharp dichotomy between a 'Hindu' cultural view of the interpersonal and transpersonal nature of man and a modern 'Western' view of man's individual and instinctual nature and assuming that since Ramnath was not an individual in the latter sense, he was not an individual at all. Although suggestive and fruitful for cultural understanding, the individual/relational differences should not be overemphasized. Even my distinction between traditional and modern individuality is not a sharp one. In reference to his satori or enlightenment, occasioned by the cry of a crow, Ikkyu, a fifteenth century Zen master, known for his colourful eccentricity, suggests the presence of a 'modern' biographical individuality when he writes:

> *ten dumb years I wanted things to be different furious proud I*
> *still feel it*
> *one summer night in my little boat on lake Biwa*
> *caaaawwweeeee*
> *father when I was a boy you left us now I forgive you.*[6]

In spite of the cultural highlighting of the inter- and transpersonal I found my traditional Indian patients more individual in their unconscious than they initially realized. Similarly, in spite of a Western cultural emphasis on autonomous individuality, my European and American patients are more relational than *they* realize. Individual and communal, self and other, are complementary ways of looking at the organization of mental life and exist in a dialectical relationship to each other although a culture may, over a period of time, stress the importance of one or the other in its ideology of the fulfilled human life and thus shape a person's *conscious* experience of the self in predominantly individual or communal modes. It is undeniable that Indians are very relational, with the family and community (including the family of divinities) playing a dominant role in the experience of the self. It is also undeniable, though less evident, that Indians are very individualistic and, at least in fantasy, are capable of conceiving and desiring a self free of *all* attachments and relationships.

In positing some shared fundamentals for the practice of the psychoanalytic enterprise, I do not mean to imply that there is no difference between analysands from Bombay, Beirut, or Birmingham. The middle-class, educated, urban Indian, although more individualized in his experience of the self and closer to his Western counterpart on this dimension, is nevertheless not identical with the latter. Contrary to the stance popular among many anthropologists of Indian society, the traditional Hindu villager is not the only Indian there is with the rest being some kind of imposters or cultural deviants. The urban Indian analysand shares with others many of the broader social and cultural patterns which are reflected in the cultural particularities of the self. One of these particularities, frequently met with in case histories and a dominant motif in Hindu myths and other products of cultural imagination, is the centrality of the male Hindu Indian's experience of the powerful mother.[7] Let me first illustrate this more concretely through a vignette.

Pran, a thirty-five year old journalist, came to analysis suffering from a general, unspecified anxiety and what he called a persistent feeling of being always on the 'edge'. Until March of that year, Pran's 320 sessions have been pervaded by his mother to a degree unsurpassed in my clinical work. For almost two years, four times a week, hour after hour, Pran would recollect what his mother told him on this or that particular occasion, what she thought, believed, or said, as he struggled to dislodge her from the throne on which he has ensconced her in the deepest recesses of his psyche. She was a deeply religious woman, a frequenter of discourses given by various holy men, to which Pran accompanied her and which contributed significantly to the formation of his traditional Hindu worldview. In contrast to the mother, Pran's memories of his father, who died when he was eleven, are scant. They are also tinged with a regret that Pran did not get a chance to be closer to a figure who remains dim and was banished to the outskirts of family life when alive. He is clearly and irrevocably dead while the mother, who died ten years ago, is very much alive. The father was a man about town, rarely at home, and thoroughly disapproved of by the mother who not only considered herself more virtuous and intelligent, but also implied to the son that the stroke which finally killed his father was a consequence of his dissolute, 'manly' ways.

Pran's memories of his closeness to his mother, the hours they spent just sitting together, communing in silence, a feeling of deep repose flowing through him, are many. He remembers being breastfed till he was eight or nine, although, when he thinks about it a little more, he doubts whether there was any milk in the breasts for many of those years. In any event, he distinctly recollects peremptorily lifting up her blouse whenever he felt like a suck, even when she was busy talking to other women. Her visiting friends were at times indulgent and at others indignant, 'Why don't you stop him?' they would ask his mother. 'He does not listen,' she would reply in mock helplessness.

Pran slept in his mother's bed till he was eighteen. He vividly recalls the peculiar mixture of dread and excitement, especially during the adolescence years, when he would manoeuvre his erect penis near her vagina for that most elusive and forbidden of touches which he was never sure was a touch at all, where he never knew whether his penis had actually been in contact with her body. Later, his few physical encounters with women were limited to hugging, while he awkwardly contorted the lower part of his body to keep his erection beyond their ken. For a long time, his sexual fantasies were limited to looking at and touching a woman's breasts. As his analysis progressed, his most pleasurable sexual fantasy became one of the penis hovering on the brink of the labial lips, even briefly touching them, but never of entering the woman's body.

After his studies, at which he was very good, Pran joined a newspaper and became quite successful. The time for his marriage had now arrived and there began the first open though still subdued conflicts with his mother on the choice of a marriage partner. His mother invariably rejected every attractive woman he fancied, stating bluntly that sons forget their mothers if they get into the clutches of a beautiful woman. Pran finally agreed to his mother's choice of a docile and plain-looking woman. For the first six months, he felt no desire for his wife. (The fact that his mother slept in the room next to the bridal couple and insisted that the connecting door remain open at all times except for the hours of the night, did not exactly work as an aphrodisiac.) When the family used the car, the wife would sit at the back, the mother not holding with new-fangled modern notions which would relegate her to the back seat once the son had brought a wife home. Even now, his sexual desire for his wife is perfunctory and occasional. He feels excited by women with short hair who wear make-up and skirts rather than a long-tressed Indian beauty in the traditional attire of *salwar kameez* or sari. Such a woman is too near the mother. For many years, Pran has been trying to change his wife's conservative appearance, so reminiscent of the mother's, towards one which is closer to the object of his desire.

It was only after his mother's death that Pran experienced sexual intercourse with his wife as pleasurable. Yet, after intercourse there is invariably a feeling of tiredness for a couple of days and Pran feels, as he puts it, that his body is 'breaking'. His need for food, especially the spicy-sour savouries (*chat*) which were a special favourite of the mother and are popularly considered 'woman's food', goes up markedly. In spite of his tiredness, Pran can drive miles in search of the spicy fare.

The need for sleep and spicy food, together with the feeling of physical unease, also occurs at certain other times. A regular feature of his work day is that after a few hours of work, he feels the need for something to eat and a short nap. The physical unease, the craving for food, and sleep increase dramatically when he has to travel on business or to take people out for dinner. It is particularly marked if he ever has a drink at a bar with friends.

Relatively early in his analysis, Pran became aware of the underlying pattern in his behaviour. Going to work, travelling, drinking and, of course, sexual intercourse, are 'manly' activities to which he is greatly drawn. They are, however, also experienced as a separation from the mother which give rise to anxiety till he must come back to her, for food and sleep. He must recurrently merge with her in order, as he put it, to strengthen his nervous system. The re-establishment of an oral connection with the mother is striking in its details. Pran not only hankers after the mother's favourite foods but feels a great increase in the sensitivity of the lips and the palate. The texture and taste of food in the mouth is vastly more important for the process of his recuperation than is the food's function in filling his belly. His sensual memories of his mother's breasts and the taste of her nipples in the mouth are utterly precise. He can recover the body of the early mother as a series of spaced flashes, as islands of memory. The short naps he takes after one of his 'manly' activities are framed in a special ritual. He lies down on his stomach with his face burrowed between two soft pillows, fantasizes about hugging a woman before he falls asleep, and wakes up fresh and vigorous.

It took a longer time for Pran to become aware of the terror his mother's overwhelming invasiveness inspired in the little boy and his helpless rage in dealing with it. He railed, and continues to do so, at her selfishness which kept him bound to her and wept at memories of countless occasions when she would ridicule his efforts to break away from her in play with other boys, or in the choice of his workplace, clothes, or friends. She has destroyed his masculinity, he feels. As a boy, she made him wash her underclothes, squeeze out the discharge from her nipples, oil her hair and pluck out the grey ones on an almost daily basis. The birth of his four daughters, he felt, was due to this feminization which had made his semen 'weak'. He realized that all his 'manly' activities were not only in pursuit of individuation as a man, or even in a quest for pleasure, but also because they would lacerate the mother. 'I always wanted to hurt her and at the same time I could not do without her. She has been raping me ever since I was born,' he once said.

Often, as he lies there, abusing the mother, with a blissful expression on his face reflecting her close presence, I cannot help but feel that this is *nindastuti*, worship of a divinity through insult, denigration, and contempt, which is one of the recognized relationships of a Hindu devotee with a divinity.

I have selected this particular vignette from my case histories because in its palette of stark, primary colours and in its lack of complex forms and subtle shades, it highlights, even caricatures, a dominant theme in the analysis of many male Hindu Indians. Judged by its frequency of occurrence in clinical work and in its pre-eminence in the Hindu cultural imagination, the theme of what I call maternal enthrallment and the issue of the boy's separation from the overwhelming maternal–feminine—rather than the dilemmas of Oedipus—appears to be the hegemonic (to use the fashionable Gramscian term) narrative of the Hindu family drama.[8] It is the cornerstone in the architecture of the male self. The reason why I mention cultural imagination in conjunction with clinical work when advancing a generalized psychoanalytic proposition about the Indian cultural context, is simple. Clinical psychoanalysis is generally limited to a small sample from three or four large Indian metropolises. It cannot adequately take into account the heterogeneity of a country of eight hundred million people with its regional, linguistic, religious, and caste divisions. Clinical cases can, at best, generate hypotheses about cultural particularities. The further testing of these hypotheses is done (and remains true to psychoanalytic intention and enterprise) by testing them in the crucible of the culture's imagination.

The kind of maternal enthrallment and the prolonged mother–son symbiosis I have described in this particular vignette, including the peek-a-boo, was-it-or-was-it-not incest, would ordinarily be associated with much greater pathology in analytic case conferences in Europe and North America. Pran's level of functioning, however, is quite impressive in spite of his many inhibitions and anxieties, especially sexual. I wonder how much of this kind of psychoanalytical expectation that Pran is sicker than what I believe to be actually the case, is due to a cultural contamination creeping into the clinical judgement of his sexual differentiation and separation–individuation processes. For instance, is the psychoanalytic evaluation of Pran's undoubted feminization and a certain lack of differentiation also being influenced by a Western cultural imagination on what it means to be, look, think, and behave like a man or a woman? This becomes clearer if one thinks of Greek or Roman sculpture with their hard, muscled men's bodies and chests without any fat at all and compares it with the sculpted representations of Hindu gods or the Buddha where the bodies are softer, suppler and, in their hint of breasts, nearer to the female form.

I have no intention of relativizing Pran's pain and suffering out of existence. I only wish to point out that there is a whole range of positions, each occupied by a culture which insists on calling it the only one that is mature and healthy.

Compared to a model Western analysand, then (and one needs to postulate such a being if civilizational comparisons are to be made) his Hindu counterpart highlights different intra-psychic issues and places different accents on universal developmental experiences. Yet, perhaps because of an underlying similarity in the psychoanalytic clientele across cultures, as discussed earlier, cultural 'other-ness' does not spring the psychoanalytic framework, made increasingly flexible by a profusion of models. Clinical work in India is thus not radically different from that in Europe and America. An analyst from outside the culture, encountering the strangeness of the cultural mask rather than the similarity of the individual face, may get carried away into exaggerating differences. However, if he could listen long enough and with a well-tuned ear for the analysand's symbolic and linguistic universes, he would discover that individual voices speaking of the whirling of imperious passion, the stabs of searing, burdensome guilt, the voracious hungers of the urge to merge, and the black despair at the absence of the Other, are as much evident here as in the psychoanalysis of Western patients.

Clinical work in another culture, however, does make us aware that because of the American and European domination of psychoanalytic discourse, Western cultural (and moral) imagination sometimes tends to slip into psychoanalytic theorizing as hidden 'health and maturity moralities', as Kohut[9] called them. Cultural judgements about psychological maturity, the nature of reality, 'positive' and 'negative' resolutions of conflicts and complexes often appear in the garb of psychoanalytic universals. Awareness of the cultural contexts of psychoanalysis would therefore contribute to increasing the ken and tolerance of our common discipline for the range of human variations and a much greater circumspection in dealing with notions of pathology and deviance.

Notes and References

1 Kakar, S., 1982, *Shamans, Mystics and Doctors*, New York: Alfred Knopf.

2 Bollas, C., 1992, *Being a Character: Psychoanalysis and Self-experience*, New York: Hill and Wang.

3 Roland, A., 1990, *In Search of Self in India and Japan*, Princeton: Princeton University Press.

4 Kurtz, S., 1992, *All the Mothers are One: Hindu India and the Cultural Reshaping of Psychoanalysis*, New York: Columbia University Press.

5 Muktananda, S., 1983, *The Perfect Relationship*, Ganeshpuri: Guru Siddha Vidyapeeth.

6 Berg, S., 1989, *Crow with No Mouth: Ikkyu — 15th Century Zen Master*, Port Town-send: Copper Canyon Press, p. 42.

7 Kakar, S., 1978, *The Inner World: A Psychoanalytic Study of Childhood and Society in India*, Delhi: Oxford University Press.

8 Kakar, S., 1989, 'The Maternal-feminine in Indian Psychoanalysis', *International Review of Psychoanalysis*, 16 (3); 1990, *Intimate Relations: Exploring Indian Sexuality*, Chicago: University of Chicago Press.

9 Kohut, H., 1979, 'The Two Analyses of Mr Z', *International Journal of Psychoanalysis*, 60.

The Maternal–Feminine in Indian Psychoanalysis*

ON 11 APRIL 1929, Girindrasekhar Bose, the founder and first president of the Indian Psychoanalytical Society, wrote to Freud on the difference he had observed in the psychoanalytic treatment of Indian and Western patients:

> Of course I do not expect that you would accept offhand my reading of the Oedipus situation. I do not deny the importance of the castration threat in European cases; my argument is that the threat owes its efficiency to its connection with the wish to be female [Freud in a previous letter had gently chided Bose with understating the efficiency of the castration threat]. The real struggle lies between the desire to be a male and its opposite, the desire to be a female. I have already referred to the fact that castration threat is very common in Indian society but my Indian patients do not exhibit castration symptoms to such a marked degree as my European cases. The desire to be female is more easily unearthed in Indian male patients than in European ... The Oedipus mother is very often a combined parental image and this is a fact of great importance. I have reason to believe that much of the motivation of the 'maternal deity' is traceable to this source.

Freud's reply is courteous and diplomatic: 'I am fully impressed by the difference in the castration reaction between Indian and European patients and promise to keep my attention fixed on the opposite wish you accentuate. The latter is too important for a hasty decision'.[1]

* From *Culture and Psyche*, Delhi: Oxford University Press, 1997.

In another paper, Bose elaborates on his observations and explains them through his theory of opposite wishes:

During my analysis of Indian patients I have never come across a case of castration complex in the form in which it has been described by European observers. This fact would seem to indicate that the castration idea develops as a result of environmental conditions acting on some more primitive trend in the subject. The difference in social environment of Indians and European is responsible for the difference in modes of expression in two cases. It has been usually proposed that threat of castration in early childhood days, owing to some misdemeanour, is directly responsible for the complex, but histories of Indian patients seem to disprove this.[2]

Bose then goes on to say that though the castration threat is extremely common—in girls it takes the form of chastisement by snakes—the difference in Indian reactions to it is due to children growing up naked till the ages of 9 to 10 years (girls till 7) so that the difference between the sexes never comes as a surprise. The castration idea, which comes up symbolically in dreams as decapitation, a cut on a finger, or a sore in some parts of the body, has behind it the 'primitive' idea of being a woman.

Indeed, reading early Indian case histories, one is struck by the fluidity of the patients' cross-sexual and generational identifications. In the Indian patient, the fantasy of taking on the sexual attributes of both the parents seems to have relatively easier access to awareness. Bose, for instance, in one of his vignettes tells us of a middle-aged lawyer who, with reference to his parents, sometimes

took up an active male sexual role, treating both of them as females in his unconscious and sometimes a female attitude, especially towards the father, craving for a child from him. In the male role, sometimes he identified himself with his father and felt a sexual craving for the mother; on the other occasions his unconscious mind built up a composite of both the parents towards which male sexual needs were directed; it is in this attitude that he made his father give birth to a child like a woman in his dream.[3]

Another young Bengali,[4] whenever he thought of a particular man, felt with a hallucinatory intensity that his penis and testes vanished altogether and were replaced by female genitalia. While defecating, he felt he heard the peremptory voice of his guru asking, 'Have you given me a child yet?' In many of his dreams, he was a man whereas his father and brothers had become women. During intercourse with his wife, he tied a handkerchief over his eyes as it gave him the feeling of being a veiled bride while he fantasized his own penis as that of his father and his wife's vagina as that of his mother.

In my own work, fifty years after Bose's contributions of which, till recently, I was only vaguely aware, I am struck by the comparable patterns in Indian mental life we observed independently of each other, and this in spite of our different emotional predilections, analytic styles, theoretical preoccupations, geographical locations, and historical situations. Such a convergence further strengthens my belief, shared by every practising analyst, that there is no absolute arbitrariness in our representation of the inner world. There is unquestionably something that resists, a something which can only be characterized by the attribute 'psychical reality' which both the analyst and the analysand help discover and give meaning to.

It is the ubiquity and multiformity of the 'primitive idea of being a woman', and the embeddedness of this fantasy in the maternal configurations of the family and the culture in India, which I would like to discuss from my observations. My main argument is that the 'hegemonic narrative' of Hindu culture, as far as male development is concerned, is neither that of Freud's Oedipus nor that of Christianity's Adam. One of the more dominant narratives of this culture is that of Devi, the great goddess, especially in her manifold expressions as mother in the inner world of the Hindu son. In India at least, a primary task of psychoanalysis, the science of imagination or even (in Wallace Stevens' words) 'the science of illusion'—*Mayalogy*—is to grapple with *Mahamaya*, 'The Great Illusion', as the goddess is also called. Of course, it is not my intention to deny or underestimate the importance of the powerful mother in Western psychoanalysis. All I seek to suggest is that certain forms of the maternal–feminine may be more central in Indian myths and psyche than in their Western counterparts. I would then like to begin my exposition with the first ten minutes of an analytic session.

The patient is a 26-year-old social worker who has been in analysis for three years. He comes four times a week with each session lasting fifty minutes and conducted in the classical manner with the patient lying on the couch and the analyst sitting in a chair behind him. He entered analysis not because of any pressing personal problems but because he thought it would help him professionally. In this particular session, he begins with a fantasy he had while he was in a bus. The fantasy was of a tribe living in the jungle which unclothes its dead and hangs them on the trees. Mohan, the patient, visualized a beautiful woman hanging on one of the trees. He imagined himself coming at night and having intercourse with the woman. Other members of the tribe are eating parts of the hanging corpses. The fantasy is immediately followed by the recollection of an incident from the previous evening. Mohan was visiting his parents' home where he had lived till recently, when he married and set up his own household. This step was not only personally painful but also unusual for his social milieu where sons normally brought their wives to live in their parental home. His younger sister, with her three-year-old son, was also visiting at the same time. Mohan felt irritated by the anxious attention his mother and grandmother gave the boy. The grandmother kept telling the child not to go and play outside the house, to be careful of venturing too far, and so on. On my remarking that perhaps he recognized himself in the nephew, Mohan exclaimed with rare resentment, 'Yes, all the women [his mother, grandmother, his father's brother's wife, and his father's unmarried sister who lived with them] were always doing the same with me'.

Beginning with these ten minutes of a session, I would like to unroll Mohan's conflicts around maternal representations and weave them together with the central maternal configurations of Indian culture. Because of his particular objective, my presentation of further material from Mohan's analysis is bound to be subject to what Donald Spence[5] has called 'narrative smoothing'. A case history, though it purports to be a story that is true, is actually always at the intersection of fact and fable. Its tale quality, though, arises less from the commissions in imagination than from omissions in reality.

Born in a lower-middle-class family in a large village near Delhi, Mohan is the eldest of three brothers and two sisters. His memories of growing up, till well into youth, are pervaded by the maternal phalanx of the four women. Like his mother, who in his earliest memories stands out as a distinct figure from a maternal–feminine continuum to be then reabsorbed into it, Mohan, too, often emerges from and retreats into femininity. In the transference, the fantasies of being a woman are not especially disturbing; neither are the fantasies of being an infant suckling at a breast which he has grown on to my exaggeratedly hairy chest. One of his earliest recollections is of a woman who used to pull at the penises of the little boys playing out in the street. Mohan never felt afraid when the woman grabbed at his own penis. In fact, he rather liked it, reassured that he had a penis at all or, at least, enough of one for the woman to acknowledge its existence.

Bathed, dressed, combed, and caressed by one or the other of the women, Mohan's wishes and needs were met before they were even articulated. Food, especially the milk-based Indian sweets, was constantly pressed on him. Even now, on his visits to the family, the first question by one of the women pertains to what he would like to eat. For a long time during the analysis, whenever a particular session was stressful because of what he considered a lack of maternal empathy in my interventions, Mohan felt compelled to go to a restaurant in town where he would first gorge himself on sweets before he returned home.

Besides the omnipresence of women, my most striking impressions of Mohan's early memories is their diurnal location in night and their primarily tactile quality. Partly, this has to do with the crowded, public living arrangements of the Indian family. Here, even the notions of privacy are absent, not to speak of such luxuries as separate bedrooms for parents and children. Sleeping in the heat with little or no clothes next to one of his caretakers, an arm or a leg thrown across the maternal body, there is one disturbing memory which stands out clearly. This is of Mohan's penis erect against the buttocks of his sleeping mother and his reluctance to move away, struggling against the feelings of shame and embarrassment that she may wake up and notice the forbidden touch. Later, in adolescence, the mothers are replaced by visiting cousins sharing mattresses spread out in the room or on the roof, furtive rubbings of bodies and occasional genital contact while other members of the extended family were in various stages of sleep.

Embedded in this blissful abundance of maternal flesh and promiscuity of touch, however, is a nightmare. Ever since childhood and persisting well into the initial phases of the analysis, Mohan would often scream in his sleep while a vague, dark shape threatened to envelop him. At these times, only his father's awakening him with the reassurance that everything was all right helped Mohan compose himself for renewed slumber. The father, a gentle retiring man, who left early in the morning for work and returned home late at night, was, otherwise, a dim figure hovering at the outskirts of an animated family life.

In the very first sessions of the analysis, Mohan talked of a sexual compulsion which he found embarrassing to acknowledge. The compulsion consisted of travelling in a crowded bus and seeking to press close to the hips of any plump, middle-aged woman standing in the aisle. It was vital for his ensuing excitement that the woman have her back to him. If she ever turned to face Mohan, with the knowledge of his desire in her eyes, his erection immediately subsided and he would hurriedly move away with intense feelings of shame. After marriage, too, the edge of his desire was often at its sharpest when his wife slept on her side with her back to him. In mounting excitement, Mohan would rub against her and want to make love when she was still not quite awake. If, however, the wife gave intimation of becoming an enthusiastic partner in the exercise, Mohan sometimes ejaculated prematurely or found his erection precipitately shriveled.

It is evident from these brief fragments of Mohan's case history that his desire is closely connected with some of the most inert parts of a woman's body, hips and buttocks. In other words, the desire needs the woman to be sexually dead for its fulfillment. The genesis of the fantasy of the hanging corpse with whom Mohan has intercourse at night has at its root the fear of the mothers' sexuality as well as the anger at their restraint on his explorations of the world. My choice of Mohan's case, though, is not dictated by the interest it may hold from a psychoanalytical perspective. The choice, instead, has to do with its central theme, namely the various paths in imagination which Mohan traverses in the face of many obstacles to maintain an idealized relationship with the maternal body. This theme and the fantasized solutions to the disorders in the mother–son relationship are repeated again and again in Indian case and life histories. Bose's observation on the Indian male patient's 'primitive idea of being a woman' is then only a special proposition of a more general theorem. The wish to be a woman is one particular solution to the discord that threatens the breaking up of the son's fantasized connection to the mother, a solution whose access to awareness is facilitated by the culture's views on sexual differentiation and the permeability of gender boundaries. Thus, for instance, when Gandhi (1943) publicly proclaims that he has mentally become a woman or, quite unaware of Karen Horney and other deviants from the orthodox analytic position of the time, talks of man's envy of the woman's procreative capacities, saying 'There is as much reason for a man to wish that he was born a woman as for woman to do otherwise', he is sure of a sympathetic and receptive audience.

In the Indian context, this particular theme can be explored in individual stories as well as in the cultural narratives as we call myths, both of which are more closely interwoven in Indian culture than is the case in the modern West. In an apparent reversal of a Western pattern, traditional myths in India are less a source of intellectual and aesthetic satisfaction for the mythologist than of emotional recognition for others, more moving for the patient than for the analyst. Myths in India are not part of a bygone era. They are not '*retained* fragments from the infantile psychic life of the race' as Karl Abraham[6] called them or '*vestiges* of the infantile fantasies of whole nations, secular dreams of youthful humanity' in Freud's words.[7] Vibrantly alive, their symbolic power intact, Indian myths constitute a cultural idiom which aids the individual in the construction and integration of his inner world. Parallel to patterns of infant care and to the structure and values of family relationships, popular and well-known myths are isomorphic with the central psychological constellations of the culture and are constantly renewed and validated by the nature of subjective experience.[8] Given the availability of the mythological idiom, it is almost as easy to mythologize a psychoanalysis, such as that of Mohan, as to analyse a myth; almost as convenient to elaborate on intrapsychic conflict in a mythological mode as it is in a case historical narrative mode.

Earlier, I advanced the thesis that the myths of Devi, the great goddess, constitute a 'hegemonic narrative' of Hindu culture. Of the hundreds of myths on her various manifestations, my special interest here is in the goddess as mother, and especially the mother of the sons, Ganesha and Skanda. However, before proceeding to connect Mohan's tale to the larger cultural story, let me note that I have ignored the various versions of these myths in traditional texts and modern folklore—an undertaking which is rightly the preserve of mythologists and folklorists—and instead picked on their best-known, popular versions.

The popularity of Ganesha and Skanda as gods—psychologically representing two childhood positions of the Indian son—is certainly undeniable. Ganesha, the remover of obstacles and the god of all beginnings, is perhaps the most adored of the reputed 330 million Hindu gods. Iconically represented as a pot-bellied toddler with an elephant head and one missing tusk, he is represented proportionately as a small child when portrayed in the family group with his mother Parvati and father Shiva. His image, whether carved in stone or drawn up in a coloured print, is everywhere: in temples, homes, shops, roadside shrines, calendars. Ganesha's younger brother Skanda or Kartikeya, has his own following, especially in South India, where he is extremely popular and worshipped under the name of Murugan or Subramanya. In contrast to Ganesha, Skanda is a handsome child, a youth of slender body and heroic exploits who, in analytic parlance, may be said to occupy the phallic position.

Ganesha's myths tell us one part of Mohan's inner life while those of Skanda reveal yet another. Ganesha, in many myths, is solely his mother Parvati's creation. Desirous of child and lacking Shiva's cooperation in the venture, she created him out of the dirt and sweat of her body mixed with unguents. Like Mohan's fantasies of his femininity, Ganesha, too, is not only his mother's boy but contains her very essence. Mohan, even while indubitably male like Skanda, is immersed in the world of mothers which an Indian extended family creates for the child. Skanda, like Mohan, is the son of more than one mother: his father Shiva's seed, being too powerful, could not be borne by one woman and wandered from womb to womb before Skanda took birth. Mohan's ravenous consumption of sweets to restore feelings of well-being has parallels with Ganesha's appetite for modakas, the sweet wheat or rice balls which devotees offer to the god in large quantities, 'knowing' that the god is never satisfied, that his belly empties itself as fast as it is filled.[9] For, like the lean Mohan, the fat god's sweets are a lifeline to the mother's breast; his hunger for the mother's body, in spite of temporary appeasements, is ultimately doomed to remain unfulfilled. Mohan is further like Ganesha in that he, too, has emerged from infancy with an ample capacity for vital involvement with others.

In the dramatization of Mohan's dilemma in relation to the mother, brought to a head by developmental changes that push the child towards an exploration of the outer world while they also give him increasing intimations of his biological rock-bottom identity as a male, Ganesha and Skanda play the leading roles. In a version common to both south India and Sri Lanka the myth is as follows:

> A mango was floating down the stream and Uma (Parvati), the mother, said that whoever rides around the universe first will get the mango [in other versions, the promise is of *modakas* or wives). Skanda impulsively got on his golden peacock and went around the universe. But Ganesha, who rode the rat, had more wisdom. He thought: 'What could my mother have meant by this?' He then circumambulated his mother, worshipped her and said, 'I have gone around my universe.' Since Ganesha was right his mother gave him the mango. Skanda was furious when he arrived and demanded the mango. But before he could get it Ganesha bit the mango and broke one of his tusks.[10]

Here, Skanda and Ganesha are personifications of the two opposing wishes of the older child on the eve of the Oedipus complex. He is torn between a powerful push for independent and autonomous functioning and an equally strong pull towards surrender and re-immersion in the enveloping maternal fusion from which he has just emerged. Giving in to the pull of individuation and independence, Skanda becomes liable to one kind of punishment—exile from the mother's bountiful presence, and one kind of reward—the promise of functioning as an adult, virile man. Going back to the mother—and I would view Ganesha's eating of the mango as a return to and feeding at the breast, especially since we know that in Tamil Nadu the analogy between a mango and the breast is a matter of common awareness[11]—has the broken tusk, the loss of potential masculinity, as a consequence. Remaining an infant, Ganesha's reward, on the other hand, will be never to know the pangs of separation from the mother, never to feel the despair at her absence. That Ganesha's lot is considered superior to Skanda's is perhaps an indication of the Indian man's cultural preference in the dilemma of separation–individuation. He is at one with his mother in her wish not to have the son separate from her, individuate out of their shared anima.[12]

For Mohan, as we have seen, the Ganesha position is often longed for and sometimes returned to in fantasy. It does not, however, represent an enduring solution to the problem of maintaining phallic desire in the face of the overwhelming inner presence of the Great Mother. Enter Skanda. After he killed the demon Taraka who had been terrorizing the gods, the goddess became quite indulgent towards her son and told him to amuse himself as he pleased. Skanda became wayward, his lust rampant. He made love to the wives of the gods and the gods could not stop him. Upon their complaining to the goddess, she decided she would assume the form of whatever woman Skanda was about to seduce. Skanda summoned the wife of one god after another but in each saw his mother and became passionless. Finally thinking that 'the universe is filled with my mother' he decided to remain celibate for ever.

Mohan, too, we saw, became 'passionless' whenever the motherly woman he fancied in the bus turned to face him. However, instead of celibacy, he tried to hold on to desire by killing the sexual part of the mother, deadening the lower portion of her trunk, which threatened him with impotence. Furthermore, the imagined sexual overpoweringness of the mother, in the face of which the child feels hopelessly inadequate, with fears of being engulfed and swallowed by her dark depth, is not experienced by Mohan in the form of clear-cut fantasies but in a recurrent nightmare from which he wakes up screaming. Elsewhere, I have traced in detail the passage of the powerful, sexual mother through Hindu myths, folk beliefs, proverbs, symptoms, and the ritual worship of the goddess in her terrible and fierce forms.[13] Here, I shall only narrate one of the better-known myths of Devi, widely reproduced in her iconic representations in sculpture and painting, in order to convey through the myth's language of the concrete, of image and symbol, some of the quality of the child's awe and terror of this particular maternal image.

The demon Mahisasura had conquered all the three worlds. Falling in love with the goddess, he sent a message to make his desire known to her. Devi replied that she would accept as her husband only someone who defeated her in battle. Mahisasura entered the battlefield with a vast army and a huge quantity of fighting equipment. Devi came alone, mounted on her lion. The gods were surprised to see her without even an armour, riding naked to the combat. Dismounting, Devi started dancing and cutting off the heads of millions and millions of demons with her sword to the rhythm of her movement. Mahisasura, facing death, tried to run away by becoming an elephant. Devi cut off his trunk. The elephant became a buffalo and against its thick hide Devi's sword and spear were of no avail. Angered, Devi jumped on the buffalo's back and rode it to exhaustion. When the buffalo demon's power of resistance had collapsed, Devi plunged her spear into its ear and Mahisasura fell dead.

The myth is stark enough in its immediacy and needs no further gloss on the omnipotence and sexual energy of the goddess, expressed in the imagery of her dancing and riding naked, exhausting even the most powerful male to abject submission and ultimately death, decapitating (that is, castrating) millions of 'bad boys' with demonic desires, and so on. The only feature of the myth I would like to highlight, and which is absent both in Mohan's case vignette and in the myths narrated so far is that of the sword- and spear-wielding Devi as the phallic mother. In the Indian context, this fantasy seems more related to Chasseguet–Smirgel's[14] notion of the phallic mother being a denial of the adult vagina and the feelings of inadequacy it invokes rather than allowing its traditional interpretation as a denial of castration anxiety. In addition, I would see the image of the goddess as man–woman (or, for the matter, of Shiva as *ardhanarishwara*, half man–half woman) as incorporating the boy's wish to become a man without having to separate and sexually differentiate from the mother, to take on male sexual attributes while not letting go the female ones.

The myth continues that when Devi's frenzied dancing did not come to an end even after the killing of the buffalo demon, the gods became alarmed and asked Shiva for help. Shiva lay down on his back and when the goddess stepped on her husband, she hung out her tongue in shame and stopped. Like Mohan's gentle and somewhat withdrawn father who was the only one who could help in dissipating the impact of the nightmare, Shiva too enters the scene supine, yet a container for the great mother's energy and power.

In other words, the father may be unassuming and remote, yet powerful. First experienced as an ally and a protector (or even as a co-victim), the father emerges as a rival only later. The rivalry too, in popular Indian myths and most of the case histories, is not so much that of Oedipus, where the power of the myth derives from the son's guilt over a fantasized and eventually unconscious parricide. The Indian context stresses more the father's envy of what belongs to the son—including the mother—and thus the son's persecution anxiety as a primary motivation in the father–son relationship. It is thus charged with the fear of filicide and with the son's castration, by self or the father, as a solution to father–son competition: Shiva's beheading of Ganesha who on the express wish of his mother stood guard at her private chambers while she bathed, and the replacement of his head by that of an elephant and the legends of Bhishma and Puru, who renounced sexual functioning in order to keep the affections of their fathers intact, are some of the better known illustrations.[15] However, the fate of fathers and sons and families and daughters are different narratives ... stories yet to be told, texts still to be written.

The importance of the Oedipus complex in classical psychoanalysis lies not only in it being a dominant organizing pattern of a boy's object relations but also in it being the fulcrum of Freud's cultural theory. Freud considered the myth of Oedipus as a hegemonic narrative of all cultures at all times although enough evidence is now available to suggest that its dominance may be limited to some Western cultures at certain periods of their history. In other words, the Oedipus complex, in one variation or the other, may well be universal but not equally hegemonic across cultures. Similarly, I suggest the Ganesha complex, discussed in this essay together with its myth, is equally universal at a certain stage of the male child's development. It is a mythologem for relations between mother and child at the eve of Oedipus before any significant triangulation has taken place. The Ganesha complex, I have tried to show, is also the hegemonic developmental narrative of the male self in Hindu India. In another of its variations as the Ajase complex, it has also been postulated as the dominant narrative of the male self in Japan.

Culture and Human Development

Cultural ideas and ideals, manifested in their narrative form as myths, are the innermost experience of the self. One cannot therefore speak of an 'earlier' or 'deeper', of the self beyond cultural reach. As a 'depth psychology', psychoanalysis dives deep but in the same waters in which the cultural rivers, too, flow. Pre-eminently operating from within the heart of the Western Myth, enclosed in the *mahamaya* of Europe—from myths of ancient Greece to the 'illusions' of the Enlightenment—psychoanalysis has had little opportunity to observe from within, and with empathy, the deeper import of other cultures, myths in the workings of the self.

The questions relating to the 'how' of this process are bound up with the larger issue of the relationship between the inner and outer worlds which has been of perennial psychological and philosophical interest. It is certainly not my intention to discuss these questions at any length. I would only like to point out that apart from some notable exceptions, such as Erik Erikson[16] who both held aloft and significantly contributed to a vision of a 'psychoanalysis sophisticated enough to include the environment', the impact of culture on the development of a sense of identity—in the construction of the self, in modern parlance—has been generally underestimated. Freud's 'timetable' of culture entering the psychic structure relatively late in life as 'ideology' of the superego[17] has continued to be followed by other almanac makers of the psyche. Even Heinz Kohut, as Janis Long[18] has shown, does not quite follow the logical implications of his concept of 'selfobject'. These are, of course, the aspects of the other which are incorporated in the self and are experienced as part of one's own subjectivity. Kohut, too, follows Freud in talking of a 'culture selfobject' of later life,[19] derived in part from cultural ideas and ideals, which helps in maintaining the integrity and vitality of the individual self. Yet the idea of a selfobject which goes beyond the notion of a budding self's relatedness to the environment, to the environment's gradual transmutation into *becoming* the self implies that '*what* the parents respond to in a developing child, *how* they respond and what they present as idealizable from the earliest age'[20]—surely much of it a cultural matter—will be the raw material for the child's inner construction of the self. In other words, a caretaker's *knowing* of the child, a knowing in which affect and cognition are ideally fused, is in large part cultural and forms the basis of the child's own knowing of his or her self. The notion that the construction and experience of the self is greatly influenced by culture from the very beginning does not imply that there is no difference between individual faces and cultural masks, no boundary between inner and outer worlds. The tension between the two is what gives psychoanalysis and literature much of their narrative power. What I seek to emphasize here is that this boundary cannot be fixed either in time or psychic space. It is dynamic, mobile, and constantly subject to change.

Notes and References

1 Sinha, T.C., 1966, 'Psychoanalysis in India', in *Lumbini Park Silver Jubilee Souvenir*, Calcutta: Lumbini Park, p. 66.

2 Bose, G., 1950, 'The Genesis of Homosexuality', *Samiksa*, 4, p. 74.

3 Bose, G., 1948, 'A New Theory of Mental Life', *Samiksa*, 2, p. 158.

4 Bose, G., 1949, 'The Genesis and Adjustment of the Oedipus Wish', *Samiksa*, 3, pp. 222–10.

5 Spence, D.P., 1986, 'Narrative Smoothing and Clinical Wisdom', in T. Sarbin (ed.), *Narrative Psychology*, New York: Praeger.

6 Abraham, K., 1913, *Dreams and Myths: A Study in Race Psychology*, New York: Journal of Nervous and Mental Health Publishing Company.

7 Freud, S., 1908, 'Creative Writers and Daydreaming', *SE*, p. 152.

8 Obeyesekere, G., 1981, *Medusa's Hair*, Chicago: University of Chicago Press.

9 Courtright, P., 1986, *Ganesa*, New York: Oxford University Press, p. 114.

10 Obeyesekere, G., 1984, *The Cult of Pattini*, Chicago: University of Chicago Press, p. 471.

11 Egnor, M., 1984, '*The Ideology of Love in a Tamil Family*', Hobart & Smith College, unpublished mss.

12 Kakar, S., 1987, 'Psychoanalysis and Anthropology: A Renewed Alliance', *Contributions to Indian Sociology*, 21, pp. 85–8.

13 Kakar, S., 1978, *The Inner World: A Psychoanalytic Study of Childhood and Society in India*, Delhi and New York: Oxford University Press.

14 Chasseguet-Smirgel, J., 1964, 'Feminine Guilt and the Oedipus Complex', in J. Chasseguet-Smirgel (ed.), *Female Sexuality*, Ann Arbor: University of Michigan Press.

15 Kakar, S. and John M. Ross, 1987, *Tales of Love, Sex and Danger*, London: Unwin Hyman.

16 Erikson, E., 1950, *Childhood and Society*, New York: Norton.

17 Freud, S., 1922, 'New Introductory Lectures on Psychoanalysis', *SE*, p. 22.

18 Long, J., 1986, 'Culture, Self-object and the Cohesive Self ' unpublished paper presented at American Psychological Association Meeting.

19 Kohut, H., 1985, *Self Psychology and the Humanities*, New York: Norton.

20 Long, L., 'Culture, Self-object and the Cohesive Self '.

Culture in Psychoanalysis*

A Personal Journey

MY INTEREST IN THE ROLE of culture in psychoanalysis and psychology did not begin as an abstract intellectual exercise but as a matter of vital personal import. Without my quite realizing it at the time, it commenced when I started on my journey as a psychoanalyst more than thirty years ago, upon entering a five-day-a-week training session with a German analyst at the Sigmund-Freud-Institut in Frankfurt. At first, I registered the role of culture in my analysis as a series of niggling feelings of discomfort whose source remained incomprehensible for many months. Indeed, many years were to pass before I began to comprehend the cultural landscape of my mind in more than a rudimentary fashion.

I earned very little at the time and in spite of my frequent complaints on my poverty from the couch, I was disappointed when my analyst was prompt in presenting his bill at the end of the month and did not offer to reduce his fees. Without ever asking him directly, I let fall enough hints that he could be helpful in getting me a better paying job—for instance, as his assistant in the institute where he held an important administrative and teaching position. I felt betrayed and rejected when no practical assistance was forthcoming.

I did not have any problems in coming to my sessions on time but was resentful that my analyst was equally punctual in ending a session

* Revised version of an essay first published in *Social Analysis*, 50:2, 2006.

after exactly fifty minutes, sometimes when I had just got going and felt his involvement in my story had been equal to my own. After undergoing analysis for some months, I realized that my recurrent feelings of estrangement were not due to cultural differences in forms of politeness, manners of speech, attitudes towards time, or even differences in aesthetic sensibilities. (To me, at that time, Beethoven was just so much noise, while I doubt if my analyst even knew of the existence of Hindustani classical music, which so moved me.) The estrangement involved much deeper cultural layers of the self, which were an irreducible part of my subjectivity as, I suppose, they were a part of my analyst's. In other words, if during a session we sometimes suddenly became strangers to each other, it was because each of us found himself locked into a specific 'cultural identity', that was rarely conscious. In my case, this cultural identity was an 'Indian-ness' which I was to spend many years elucidating.[1]

A cultural Indian-ness or Indian identity is not an abstract concept, a subject of intellectual debate for academics, but something that informs the activities and concerns of daily life for a vast number of Indians while at the same time it guides them through the journey of life. How to behave towards superiors and subordinates in organizations, the kinds of food conducive to health and vitality, the web of duties and obligations in the family—all these are as much influenced by the cultural part of the mind as are ideas concerning the proper relationship between the sexes, or one's relationship to the Divine. Of course, for the individual Indian, this civilizational heritage may be modified or overlaid by the specific cultures of one's family, caste, class, or ethnic group. Yet, an underlying sense of Indian identity continues to persist, even into the third or fourth generation in the Indian Diasporas around the world, and not only when they gather together for a Diwali celebration or to watch a Bollywood movie.

At first glance, the notion of a singular Indian-ness—of an Indian identity—may seem far-fetched: How can one generalize about a billion people—Hindus, Muslims, Sikhs, Christians, and Jains—who speak fourteen major languages and are characterized by pronounced regional and linguistic identities? How can one postulate anything in common among a people divided not only by social class but also by India's signature system of caste, and with an ethnic diversity typical more of past empires than of modern nation-states? Yet, as attested to by foreign travellers throughout the ages, there is a unity or at least a harmony in this diversity that is often ignored or unseen because our modern eyes are more attuned to discern divergence and variance than resemblance. Indian-ness, then, is about similarities rather than the *surface* dazzle of differences among the inhabitants of this vast subcontinent, similarities produced by an overarching Indic, pre-eminently Hindu civilization that constitutes the 'cultural gene pool' of India's peoples.

This civilization has remained in constant ferment through the processes of assimilation, transformation, reassertion, and re-creation that came in the wake of its encounters with other civilizations and cultural forces, such as those unleashed by the advent of Islam in medieval times and European colonialism in the more recent past. The contemporary buffeting of Indic civilization by a West-centric globalization is only the latest in a long line of invigorating cultural encounters that can be called 'clashes' only from the narrowest of perspectives. Indic civilization is thus the common patrimony of all Indians, irrespective of their faith.

In a contentious polity, where various groups loudly clamour for recognition of their differences, the awareness of a common Indian-ness, the sense of 'unity within diversity', is generally absent. Like the Argentinian writer Jorg Luis Borges' remark on the absence of camels in the Koran because they were not exotic enough to the Arab to merit attention, the camel of Indian-ness is invisible or taken for granted by most of us. Our family resemblance begins to stand out in sharp relief only when it is compared to the profiles of peoples of other major civilizations or cultural clusters. A man, who is an Amritsari in Punjab, is a Punjabi in other parts of India and an Indian in Europe; the outer circle of his identity, his Indian-ness, is now salient for his self-definition as also for his recognition by others. This is why, in spite of persistent academic disapproval, people (including academics in their unguarded moments) continue to speak of 'the Indians', as they do of 'the Chinese', 'the Europeans', or 'the Americans', as a necessary and legitimate short-cut to a more complex reality.

What are some of the building blocks of this Indian-ness or Indian identity? Here, I will mention only some of the key ones: an ideology of family relationships in particular and relationships in general that derives from the institution of the joint family, a profoundly hierarchical view of social relations influenced by the institution of caste, an image of the human body and bodily processes that is based on the medical system of Ayurveda, a cultural imagination teeming with shared myths and legends that underscore a 'romantic' vision of human life and a relativistic, context-sensitive way of thinking.[2] Here, I can only give you a flavour of what I mean. Let me talk of relationships.

To begin with, let us take a specific relationship. In the universe of teacher–healers, I had slotted my analyst into a place normally reserved for a personal guru. From the beginning of the training analysis, it seems, I had pre-consciously envisioned our relationship in terms of a guru–disciple bond, a much more intimate affair than the contractual doctor–patient relationship governing my analyst's professional orientation. In *my* cultural model, he was the personification of the wise old sage benevolently directing a sincere and hardworking disciple who had abdicated the responsibility for his own welfare to the guru. My guru model also demanded that my analyst demonstrate his compassion, interest, warmth, and responsiveness much more openly than is usual or even possible in the psychoanalytic model guiding his therapeutic interventions. A handshake with a '*Guten Morgen*, Herr Kakar' at the beginning of the session and a handshake with an '*Auf Wiedersehen*, Herr Kakar' at the end of the session, even if accompanied by the beginnings of a smile, were not even starvation rations for someone who had adopted the analyst as his guru.

Our cultural orientations also attached varying importance to different family relationships. For instance, in my childhood, I had spent long periods of my young life in the extended families of my parents. Various uncles, aunts, and cousins had constituted a vital part of my growing up experience. To pay them desultory attention or to reduce them to parental figures in the analytic interpretations felt like a serious impoverishment of my inner world.

In practice, of course—and this is what makes psychoanalytic psychotherapy in non-Western societies possible—the cultural orientations of patients coming for psychoanalytic therapy are not diametrically opposite to those of the analyst. Most of non-Western patients seen by analysts in North America and Europe are 'assimilated' to the dominant culture of their host country to varying degrees, the contest between their original and new cultures not yet decisively tilted in favour of one or the other. Similarly, in non-Western countries, the clients for psychoanalytic therapy—like their analysts—are westernized to varying degrees. For instance, they tend to be more individualized in their experience of the self than the bulk of their more traditional countrymen.

As I said, I only wish to give a flavour of the deeper layers of what I have called Indian identity. I could go on, as I have done at other places, to highlight other fundamental differences and their consequences such as in the perception of what is masculine and what is feminine or the hierarchical vision of Indian eyes. However, I would like to get back to my personal journey and what happened in my own psychoanalysis. Was it destined to fail because we were both embedded in our cultural identities? What could my analyst have done? Did he need to acquire knowledge of my culture and, if so, what kind of knowledge? Would an anthropological, historical or philosophical grounding in Hindu culture have made him understand me better? Or was it a *psychoanalytical* knowledge of my culture that would have been more helpful? Psychoanalytic knowledge of a culture is not equivalent to its anthropological knowledge although there may be some overlap between the two. Psychoanalytic knowledge is primarily the knowledge of the culture's *imagination*, of its fantasy as encoded in its symbolic products—its myths and folktales, its popular art, literature and cinema.

Besides asking about the kind of knowledge, we also need to ask the question 'Which culture?' Would a psychoanalytic knowledge of Hindu culture have been sufficient in my case? Yes, I am a Hindu but also a Punjabi Khatri by birth. That is, my overarching Hindu culture has been mediated by my strong regional culture as a Punjabi and further by my Khatri caste. This Hindu Punjabi Khatri culture has been further modified by an agnostic father and a more traditional, believing mother, both of whom were also westernized to varying degrees. Is it not too much to expect any analyst to acquire this kind of prior cultural knowledge about his patients? On the other hand, is it OK for the analyst not to have *any* knowledge of his patient's cultural background? Or does the truth, as it often does, lie somewhere in the middle?

And now comes the surprise. My analyst was very good—sensitive, insightful, patient. And I discovered that as my analysis progressed, my feelings of estrangement that had given rise to all the questions on cultural differences became fewer and fewer. What was happening? Was the cultural part of my self becoming less salient as the analysis touched ever-deeper layers of the self, as many psychoanalysts have claimed?

George Devereaux, a psychoanalyst who was also an anthropologist and a pioneer in addressing the issue of culture in psychoanalytic therapy, claimed that in really deep psychoanalytic therapy, the analyst needed to know the patient's specific cultural background less fully ahead of time than in more superficial forms of psychotherapy. In his conception of psychoanalysis as a universal, a-cultural science, the personality disorders that were the object of psychoanalysis represented a partial regression of (cultural) man to (universal) *homo sapiens*. 'For this reason,' he writes, 'children and abnormal members of our society resemble their counterparts in other cultures far more than the normal members of our society resemble the normal members of other ethnic groups.'[3] A deep analysis would reveal the same universal fantasies and desires though, he allowed, the constellation of defense mechanisms could be culturally influenced.

In fact, for Devereaux, the most important (and harmful) influence exerted by culture on psychoanalytic therapy was not the analyst's indifference but his *interest* in cultural factors. He rightly pointed to the counter-transference danger of an analyst getting *too* interested in his analytic patient's culture. Sensitive to the analyst's interest, the patient would either gratify this interest by long discourses on his cultural practices or use these as red herrings to divert the analyst from probing deeper into his personal motivations. Freud is reputed to have sent a prospective patient, an Egyptologist, to another analyst because of Freud's own interest in Egyptology.

Most analysts have followed Devereaux's lead in maintaining that all those who seek help from a psychoanalyst have in common many fundamental and universal components in their personality structure. Together with the universality of the psychoanalytic method, these common factors sufficiently equip the analyst to understand and help his patient irrespective of the patient's cultural background, a view reiterated by a panel of the American Psychoanalytic Association more than forty years ago on the role of culture in psychoanalysis.[4] There are certainly difficulties such as the ones enumerated by Ticho[5] in treating patients of a different culture: a temporary impairment of the analyst's technical skills, empathy for the patient, diagnostic acumen, the stability of self and object representations, and the stirring up of counter-transference manifestations which may not be easily distinguishable from stereotypical reactions to the foreign culture. Generally, though, given the analyst's empathetic stance and the rules of analytic procedure, these difficulties are temporary and do not require a change in analytic technique. It is useful but not essential for the analyst to understand the patient's cultural heritage.

I believe that these conclusions on the role of culture in psychoanalytic therapy, which would seem to apply to my own experience, are superficially true but deeply mistaken. For what I did, and I believe most patients do, was to enthusiastically, if unconsciously, acculturate to the analyst's culture—in my case, both to his broader Western, north-European culture and to his particular Freudian psychoanalytic culture

My intense need to be 'understood' by the analyst, a need I shared with every patient, gave birth to an unconscious force that made me underplay those cultural parts of my self that I believed would be too foreign to the analyst's experience. Now, we know that every form of therapy is also an enculturation. As Fancher remarks:

> By the questions we ask, the things we empathize with, the themes we pick for our comment, the ways we conduct ourselves towards the patient, the language we use—by all these and a host of other ways—we communicate to the patient our notions of what is 'normal' and normative. Our interpretations of the origins of a patient's issues reveal in pure form our assumptions of what causes what, what is problematic about life, where the patient did not get what s/he needed, what should have been otherwise.[6]

As a patient in the throes of 'transference love', I was exquisitely attuned to the cues to my analyst's values, beliefs, and vision of the fulfilled life, which even the most non-intrusive of analysts cannot help but scatter during the therapeutic process. I was quick to pick up the cues that unconsciously shaped my reactions and responses accordingly, with their overriding goal to please and be pleasing in the eyes of the beloved. In the throes of this love, what I sought was closeness to the analyst, including the sharing of his culturally shaped interests, attitudes, and beliefs. This intense need to be close and to be understood, paradoxically by removing parts of the self from the analytic arena of understanding, was epitomized by the fact that I soon started dreaming in German, the language of my analyst, something I have not done before or after my analysis.

The analysis being conducted in German fostered the excision of parts of my self. One's native tongue, the language of one's childhood, is intimately linked with emotionally coloured sensory-motor experiences. Psychotherapy in a language that is not the patient's own is often in danger of leading to 'operational thinking', that is, verbal expressions lacking associational links with feelings, symbols, and memories.[7] However grammatically correct and rich in its vocabulary, the alien language suffers from emotional poverty, certainly as far as early memories are concerned. To give an example: there is often an impersonal tone characteristic of operational thinking when one of my bilingual patients reports significant experiences in English and much greater variations in affect when the same experience is described in Hindi, the patient's mother tongue. When in one of his sessions the patient reported, in English, that the previous night he had said to his wife, 'Let's have sex', his tone was detached, even slightly depressive.

When asked what exactly he had said in Hindi, the answer was, '*teri le loon* (I'll take yours)'. The much more concrete Hindi expression, demanding the use of the wife's vagina, objectifying the person, evoked in him not only greater feelings of an aggressive excitement (and shame while reporting it) but was also associated with fearful memories of childhood play when the same expression was directed at him by an older boy.

How should a Western psychoanalyst, then, approach the issue of cultural difference in his practice? The ideal situation would be that this difference exists only minimally, in the sense that the analyst has obtained a psychoanalytic knowledge of the patient's culture through a long immersion in its daily life and its myths, its folklore and literature, its language and its music—an absorption not through the bones, as in case of his patient, but through the head—and the heart. Anything less than this maximalist position has the danger of the analyst succumbing to the lure of cultural stereotyping in dealing with the particularities of the patient's experience. In cross-cultural therapeutic dyads, little knowledge is indeed a dangerous thing, collapsing important differences, assuming sameness when only similarities exist. What the analyst needs is not a detailed knowledge of the patient's culture but a serious questioning and awareness of the assumptions underlying his own, that is, the culture he was born into and the culture in which he has been professionally socialized as a psychoanalyst. In other words, what I am suggesting is that in absence of the possibility of obtaining a psychoanalytic knowledge of his patient's culture, the analyst needs to strive for a state of affairs where the patient's feelings of estrangement because of his cultural differences from the analyst are minimized and the patient does not, or only minimally cuts off the cultural part of the self from the therapeutic situation. This is possible only if the analyst can convey a cultural openness which comes from becoming aware of his own culture's fundamental propositions about human nature, human experience, the fulfilled human life, and then to acknowledge their relativity by seeing them as cultural products, embedded in a particular place and time. He needs to become sensitive to the hidden existence of what Kohut[8] called 'health and maturity moralities' of his particular analytical school. He needs to root out cultural judgements about what constitutes psychological maturity, gender-appropriate behaviour, and 'positive' or 'negative' resolutions of developmental conflicts and complexes that often appear in the garb of universally valid truths.

Given that ethnocentrism, the tendency to view alien cultures in terms of our own, and unresolved cultural chauvinism, are the patrimony of all human beings, including that of psychoanalysts, the acquisition of cultural openness is not an easy task. Cultural biases can lurk in the most unlikely places. For instance, psychoanalysts have traditionally accorded a high place to artistic creativity. To paint, sculpt, engage in literary and musical pursuits have not always and everywhere enjoyed the high prestige they do in modern Western societies. In other historical periods, many civilizations, including mine to this day, placed religious creativity at the top of their scale of desirable human endeavours. Psychoanalysts need to imagine that in such cultural settings, the following conclusion to a case report could be an example of a successful therapeutic outcome: 'The patient's visions increased markedly in quantity and quality and the devotional mood took hold of her for longer and longer periods of time.'

A therapist can evaluate his progress towards this openness by the increase in his feelings of curiosity and wonder when the cultural parts of the patient's self find their voice in therapy, when the temptation to pathologize the cultural part of his patient's behaviour decreases, when his own values no longer appear as normal and virtuous, and when his wish to instruct the patient in these values diminishes markedly.

What about the cultural dilemmas of a non-Western analyst, such as myself, practising a Western discipline in an Asian country, is a question I have often been asked. Psychoanalysis, we know, is informed by a vision of human experience that emphasizes man's individuality and his self-contained psyche. In the psychoanalytic vision, each of us lives in our own subjective world, pursuing pleasures and private fantasies, constructing a life and a fate that will vanish when our time is over. This view emphasizes the desirability of a reflective awareness of one's inner states, an insistence that our psyches harbour deeper secrets than we care to confess, the existence of an objective reality that can be known, and an essential complexity and a tragedy of life whereby many wishes are fated to remain unfulfilled. This vision is in contrast to my Hindu cultural heritage, which sees life not as a tragic but as a romantic quest that can extend over many births, with the goal and possibility of apprehending another, 'higher' level of reality beyond the shared, verifiable, empirical reality of our world, our bodies, and our emotions. At the beginning of my practice in India, I was acutely aware of the struggle within myself between my inherited Indian culture and the Freudian psychoanalytic culture that I had recently acquired and in which I had been professionally socialized. My romantic Indian vision of reality could not be reconciled with the ironic psychoanalytic vision, nor could the Indian view of the person and the sources of human strengths be reconciled with the Freudian view—now also mine—on the nature of the individual and his or her world. With Goethe's Faust, I could only say:

Your spirit only seeks a single quest
so never learns to know its brother
Two souls, alas, dwell in my breast
And one would gladly sunder from the other.

Some colleagues try to sunder the two souls by unreservedly identifying with their professional socialization, radically rejecting their Indian heritage. Many of them have migrated to Western countries to work as therapists, to all apparent purposes indistinguishable from their Western colleagues. Some who stay in India struggle to hold onto their professional identity by clinging to each psychoanalytic orthodoxy. Loath to be critical of received wisdom and exiled from Rome, they become more conservative than the pope. Others, like myself, live with the oppositions, taking comfort from the Indian view that every contradiction does not need a resolution, that contradictions can co-exist in the mind like substances in water that are in suspension without necessarily becoming a solution.

I think I resolved this dilemma as do some men in Indian families who, after marrying, are caught up in the conflict between their mothers and wives, each asking the husband/son to choose between them. Unable to make this choice, the men often react by becoming detached from both. I found that the only way I could keep my affection for psychoanalytic and Hindu cultures intact was by loving each less—not by cutting myself off from one or the other but by engaging more critically with each. The loss of a certain measure of innocence and enthusiasm is the price paid for this strategy, a price that may not be too high for preventing a closing of the mind and for keeping intact a curiosity that is not satisfied with easy answers.

In conclusion, I would say that I do not doubt the universals of human nature. What I am pleading for is much more sensitive and careful delineation of what these universals actually are. Culture is not something that is a 'later' accretion to the psyche (in contrast to the notion of 'earlier' layers) or a matter of 'surface', in contrast to some imagined 'depths'. The culture in which an infant grows up, modern neurosciences tell us, constitutes the software of the brain, much of it already in place by the end of childhood. Not that the brain, a social and cultural organ as much as a biological one, does not keep changing with interactions with the environment in later life. Like the proverbial river one never steps into twice, one never uses the same brain twice. Even if our genetic endowment were to determine 50 per cent of our psyche and early childhood experiences another 30 percent, there is still a remaining 20 per cent that changes through the rest of our lives. Yet, as the neurologist and philosopher Gerhard Roth observes, 'Irrespective of its genetic endowment, a human baby growing up in Africa, Europe or Japan will become an African, a European or a Japanese. And once someone has grown up in a particular culture and, let us say, is 20 years old, he will never acquire a full understanding of other cultures since the brain has passed through the narrow bottleneck of "culturalization".'[9] (My translation) As the anthropologist Clifford Geertz quipped on his fieldwork in Java, 'You are human only if you are a Javanese.'

Notes and References

1 Kakar, S., 1978, *The Inner World: Childhood and Society in India*, Delhi/New York: Oxford University Press; 1982, *Shamans, Mystics and Doctors*, New York: Knopf; 1987, 'Psychoanalysis and Non-western Cultures', *International Review of Psychoanalysis*, vol. 12, pp. 441–8; 1989, 'The Maternal–Feminine in Indian Psychoanalysis', *International Review of Psychoanalysis*, 16(3), pp. 355–62; 1994, 'Clinical Work and Cultural Imagination', *Psychoanalytic Quarterly*, vol. 64, pp. 265–81; Kakar, S. and K. Kakar, 2006, *The Indians: Portrait of a People*, Delhi: Penguin-Viking.

2 Kakar and Kakar, *The Indians*.

3 Devereaux, G., 1953, 'Cultural Factors in Psychoanalytic Therapy', *Journal of American Psychoanalysis*, vol. 1, p. 632.

4 Jackson, S., 1968, 'Panel on Aspects of Culture in Psychoanalytic Theory and Practice', *Journal of American Psychoanalytic Association*, vol. 16, pp. 651–70.

5 Ticho, G., 1971, 'Cultural Aspects of transference and Countertransference', *Bulletin of Menninger Clinic*, 35(5), pp. 313–26.

6 Fancher, R.T., 1993, 'Psychoanalysis as Culture', *Issues in Psychoanalytic Psychology*, 15(2), pp. 89–90.

7 Bash-Kahre, E., 1984, 'On Difficulties Arising in Transference and Countertransference when Analyst and Analysand have Different Socio-cultural Backgrounds', *International Review of Psychoanalysis*, pp. 61–7.

8 Kohut, H., 1979, 'The Two Analyses of Mr Z.', *International Journal of Psychoanalysis*, vol. 60, p. 12.

9 Roth, G., 2006, *Die Zeit*, 23 Feburary, p. 36.

Erotic Love

Gandhi and Women*

CONTINUING MY SEARCH for facets of the man–woman relationship in India, I turn to the autobiographical writings of one of the greatest men of the twentieth century. Although my task of psychoanalytic deconstruction, the activity of taking a text apart by bringing out its latent meanings, remains the same, Gandhi's fame and status as a culture hero makes this enterprise both easier and more difficult.

The task is easier in that the retrospective narrative enrichment engaged in by every autobiographer who consciously or otherwise selects and orders details of his life so as to create a coherent and satisfying story, explaining and indeed justifying his present situation for the particular audience he has in mind—is capable of correction and modification through the accounts of other actors involved in the hero's epic.[1] The inconsistencies and the omission of vital details which may otherwise mar the symmetry of the hero's unconscious myth about himself, are easier to detect in the case of a man like Gandhi who has attracted so much biographical attention, both contemporary and posthumous. I may, though, add here that Gandhi's autobiographical writings, *The Story of My Experiments with Truth* the foremost among them, are marked by a candour and honesty which, if not unique, are certainly rare in the annals of self narration. In his quasi-mystical preoccupation with 'truth',

* From *Intimate Relations: Exploring Indian Sexuality*, Delhi: Viking-Penguin, 1989; University of Chicago Press, 1990.

the blame for any distortions in the story of his self-revelation can be safely laid at the door of the narrator's unconscious purposes rather than ascribed to any deliberate efforts at omission or concealment.

The work of deconstruction is made more difficult as Gandhi is the foremost culture-hero of modern India. For an Indian child, the faces of Gandhi and other heroes like Nehru and Vivekananda are identical, with the masks crafted by the culture in order to provide ideals for emulation and identification. Every child in India has been exposed to stock narratives that celebrate their genius and greatness, the portraits utterly devoid of any normal human blemish such as envy, anger, lust, ordinariness, pettiness, or stupidity. The Indian analyst, also a child of his culture, is thus bound to have a special kind of 'counter-transference' towards the culture-hero as a biographical subject. In other words, the analytic stance of respectful empathy combined with critical detachment, difficult enough to maintain in normal circumstances, becomes especially so in the case of a man like Gandhi. His image is apt to merge with other idealized figures from the biographer's own past, who were loved and admired yet secretly rebelled against. The analytic stance must then be charted out between contradictory hagiographic and pathographic impulses that seek constantly to buffet it.

For the analyst, the story of a man's relationship with women inevitably begins ('and also ends', sceptics would add) with his mother. Yet we know the mother–son dyad to be the most elusive of all human relationships. Located in the life space before the birth of language, the effort to recapture the truth of the dyad through words alone can give but teasing intimations of the hallucinatory intensity of a period when the mother, after giving the son life, also gave him the world. With some exceptions, like that of Nabokov, a mother cannot speak to her son through memory alone.[2] *Her* truth lies in the conjunction, indeed confabulation of imagination, symbols, and reality through which she was earlier perceived and through which she may be later conjured, the latter being a rare artist's gift. For others, including Gandhi, the truth of the dyad we once built with our mothers is but fragmentarily glimpsed in various maternal proxies—from inanimate objects ('part' or 'transitional' objects in analytic parlance) which a child endows with her vital spirit, to the woman who will later attract and hold him. Like all mothers, Putlibai, whose favourite, Gandhi was by virtue of his being the youngest child, and whose special object of care and concern he remained because of his sickly constitution, is an abiding yet diffuse presence in her son's inner life, an intensely luminous being albeit lacking definition. We will discover her chimerical presence in Gandhi's relationships with various other women in whom she was temporarily reincarnated, his wife Kasturbai the foremost among them.

In his autobiography, written over a five-year period during his mid-fifties, Gandhi begins the account of his sexual preoccupations and struggles with his marriage at the age of thirteen. He had been betrothed to Kasturbai Nakanji, the daughter of a well-to-do merchant in his hometown of Porbandar, since they were both seven years old. Now, with the two children entering puberty, the families decided that the time for the nuptials had finally arrived.

In Kathiawar, on the west coast of India, the region where Gandhi grew up and where his father was the prime minister of a small princely state, such child marriages were the norm rather than the exception. Writing forty-three years after the event, Gandhi could still recall the details of the marriage festivities. His elder brother and a cousin were to be married at the same time in one big ceremony and young Mohandas was excited by the prospect of new clothes, sumptuous wedding feasts, and the evenings and nights full of music and dance. During the ceremony itself, whenever the couple was required to hold hands for a particular rite, Mohandas would secretly give Kasturbai's hand a squeeze which she, in turn, eagerly reciprocated.

The excitement of the wedding was marred by one jarring incident. On his way to the celebrations, Mohandas's father had a serious accident when the horse carriage he was travelling in overturned, and he arrived late for the ceremony, with bandages covering his arms and back. The young boy was much too excited by what was happening to him to pay attention to the injured father, a fact that the older man notes with shame: 'I was devoted to my father but I was equally devoted to sensuality. Here by sensuality I do not mean one organ but the whole realm of sensual enjoyment.'[3]

Looking back at his younger self, Gandhi feels that sex became an obsession with the adolescent Mohandas. At school, his thoughts were constantly with his wife, as he impatiently waited for the night to descend when he could go to her. He was also consumed by a raging jealousy. He wanted to know of every move his wife made in his absence and would forbid her to go out alone to the temple, on household errands, or to meet girlfriends. Kasturbai was not the sort of girl to accept such unreasonable restrictions and accusations based on unfounded jealousy with any degree of equanimity. Small in stature, she was an attractive girl with glossy black hair, large dark eyes set deep in an oval face, a well-formed mouth, and a determined chin. She was by no means a female creature subservient to male whims and could easily be self-willed and impatient with her young husband. They had violent quarrels, dissolved in the love-making of the night, only to re-emerge with the light of day.

Later in life, Gandhi, regretting his treatment of Kasturbai during the first 15 years of their married life, gave two causes for his jealousy. The first was the projection of his own turbulent sexual wishes and fantasies onto his wife—'I took out my anger at her for my own weakness'—while the second was the influence of Sheikh Mehtab, the intimate friend of his youth. Physically strong, fearless, and rakishly handsome, while Mohandas was none of these, Sheikh Mehtab has been portrayed by Gandhi as his evil genius, the tempter whose blandishments Mohandas was incapable of resisting. The breacher of taboos and values Mohandas held dear, Sheikh Mehtab introduced the vegetarian lad to the guilt-ridden pleasures of eating meat, and was the organizer of their joint visit to a brothel. Mehtab constantly fuelled Gandhi's suspicions with regard to Kasturbai's fidelity. Reading about their youthful transgressions a hundred years later, to us Mehtab does not appear especially evil. He is neither more nor less than an average representative of the world of male adolescence, with its phallic displays and the ethic of a devil-may-care bravery. For a thirteen-year-old (and from all accounts, including his own) 'mama's boy,' dealing with the sexual upsurge of adolescence at the same time as the demand for establishing an emotional intimacy with a strange girl, Sheikh Mehtab must have been a godsend. He provided Mohandas with the adolescent haven where young men can be both dismissive and fearful of women and heterosexual love, where in the vague homoeroticism of masculine banter and ceaseless activism, a youth can gradually come to terms with the femininity within and without him. Little wonder that, in spite of the family's strong disapproval and Mohandas's own conscious view of their relationship as one between a reformer and a rake, their friendship remained close and lasted for almost twenty years. During his sojourn in England, Gandhi sent Mehtab money from his meagre allowance, voluntarily sought him out again after his return to India and later took his friend with him when he sailed for South Africa.

Two circumstances, Gandhi writes, saved him from becoming an emotional and physical wreck during the initial phase of his marriage. The first was the custom among the Hindus, wisely aware of the consuming nature of adolescent passion, of separating the husband and wife for long periods during the first years of marriage. Kasturbai was often away on extended visits to her family and Gandhi estimates that in the first six years of their married life they could not have lived together for more than half of this period.

The second saving circumstance was Gandhi's highly developed sense of duty, both as a member of a large extended family, with an assigned role and definite tasks, and as a son who was especially conscientious and conscious of his obligation to an ageing and ailing father. After coming home from school, Gandhi would first spend time with his father, massaging his legs and attending to his other needs. Even when he was thus engaged, his mind wandered as he impatiently waited for the filial service to come to an end, his fantasies absorbed by the images of his girl–wife in another room of the house. As all readers of his autobiography know, the conflict between sexual desire and his sense of duty and devotion to the father was to load the marriage, especially its physical side, with an enormous burden of guilt. We shall briefly recapitulate the incident that has often been reproduced either as a cautionary moral tale or as a choice text for psychoanalytical exegesis.

Gandhi's father had been seriously ill and his younger brother had come to look after him, a task he shared with the son. One night around 10:30 or 11:00, while Gandhi was massaging his father's legs, his uncle told him to rest. Happily, Gandhi rushed off to the bedroom to wake up his pregnant wife for sexual intercourse. After a few minutes, a servant knocked at the bedroom door and informed the couple that the father had expired. Gandhi talks of his lifelong feeling of remorse that blind lust had deprived him of the chance of rendering some last service to his father and thus missing the patriarch's 'blessing' which was instead received by the uncle. 'This is the shame I hinted at in the last chapter,' he writes,

> my sexual obsession even at the time of service to my father. Till today I have not been able to wash away this dark stain. I cannot forget that though my devotion to my parents was boundless and I could have given up everything for them, my mind was not free of lust even at that critical moment. This was an unforgivable lack in my service to my father. This is why in spite of my faithfulness to one woman I have viewed myself as someone blinded by sexuality. It took me a long time to free myself of lust and I have had to undergo many ordeals before I could attain this freedom.
>
> Before I close this chapter of my double shame I also want to say that the child born to my wife did not survive for more than a couple of days. What other outcome could there have been?[4]

Sexual passion endangers all the generations, Gandhi seems to say, not only the parents to whom one is morally and filially obliged, but the children conceived in sexual union.

At the age of eighteen, Mohandas left his wife and family behind (a son had been recently born) as he sailed for England to study law. He faced a good deal of opposition to his plans from his family and his community, which propounded the orthodox view that a man could not remain a good Hindu if he went abroad. Gandhi could leave for England with his family's consent (the community was not so easily mollified and declared him an outcaste) only after he made a solemn vow to his mother to avoid scrupulously the three inflamers of passion, 'wine, women, and meat'—the anxious Hindu counterpart of the more cheerful 'wine, women, and song'—during his sojourn in that distant island.

Gandhi's account of his three-year stay in England is striking in many ways. V.S. Naipaul has pointed out Gandhi's intense self-absorption, which made him oblivious to all the externals of his surroundings.[5] Gandhi does not mention the climate or the seasons. He does not describe London's buildings and streets, nor touch upon its social, intellectual, and political life.

What he immerses himself in and passionately discovers are fringe groups and causes which the mainstream English society would have unhesitatingly labelled 'eccentric'. An active member of the London Vegetarian Society and the 'Esoteric Christian Union' (many years later in South Africa he would proudly identify himself as the agent for these Societies on his letterhead), he was also a fervent admirer of Annie Besant, the heir of the Russian mystic Madame Blavatsky, and a self-declared 'bride of Christ'.

Knowing that till very recently (and again in the future) the core of Gandhi's self absorption was his concern with his sexuality, the meagre space he devotes to the stirring of sexual desire is even more striking. In the full flush of youth, learning such English graces as dancing, and becoming somewhat of a dandy, this passionate young man—a (however reluctant) sensualist—tells us very little about how he dealt with his desires and their inevitable stimulation in a society where the sexes mingled much more freely that in his native Kathiawar. The only exception to this silence is an incident near the end of his stay, when Gandhi was attending a conference of vegetarians in Portsmouth and stayed with a friend at the house of a woman, 'not a prostitute but of easy, virtue'. At night, while the three of them were playing cards, there was much sexual banter in which Gandhi enthusiastically participated. Gandhi was ready, as he says, 'to descend from speech into action', when his friend reminded him of his vows.

I was embarrassed, I came to my senses. In my heart I was grateful to the friend. I remembered my vow to my mother. I was trembling when I reached my room. My heart was racing. My condition was that of a wild animal who has just escaped the hunter. I think this was the first occasion I was 'possessed by passion' for a woman not my wife and desired to 'make merry' with her.[6]

This is the only explicit event in which higher duty opposed and conquered sexual temptation that is reported in this part of Gandhi's autobiography. The earlier sexual preoccupation, I would surmise, went underground, to re-emerge in two different streams which on the surface seem quite unrelated to genital sexuality. One of these streams is Gandhi's increasing preoccupation with religious and spiritual matters. He tells us of his visit to theosophists, conversations with Christian clergymen, the reading of inspirational and religious literature. At times, Gandhi seems to be quite aware of the connection between his sexual struggles and his spiritual interests. Thus he notes down the following verses from the *Bhagavad Gita*:

If one
Ponders on objects of the senses there springs
Attraction; from attraction grows desire,
Desire flames to fierce passion, passion breeds
Recklessness; then the memory—all betrayed—
Lets noble purpose go, and saps the mind,
Till purpose, mind, and man are all undone.

'These verses,' he says, 'made a deep impression on my mind, and they still ring in my ears.'[7]

The other stream is his obsession with food, an obsession that was to remain with him for the rest of his life. Page after page, in dreary detail, we read about what Gandhi ate and what he did not, why he partook of certain foods and why he did not eat others, what one eminent vegetarian told him about eggs and what another, equally eminent, denied. The connection between sexuality and food is made quite explicit in Gandhi's later life when his ruminations about his celibacy would almost invariably be followed by an exhaustive discussion of the types of food that stimulate desire and others that dampen it. Again, we must remember that in the Indian consciousness, the symbolism of food is more closely or manifestly connected to sexuality than it is in the West. The words for eating and sexual enjoyment, as A.K. Ramanujan reminds us, have the same root, *bhuj*, in Sanskrit, and sexual intercourse is often spoken about as the mutual feeding of male and female.[8]

On his return to India, Gandhi was faced with the necessity of making a living as a lawyer, a task for which he found himself both professionally and personally ill-equipped. A section of his caste was still hostile to him, having never forgiven him for his defiance of its mandate not to go abroad. There were further difficulties in his adjustments to the norms and mores of life in an Indian extended family—and in the family's adjustments to the newly acquired habits and values of its somewhat Anglicized member. Today, with infinitely larger numbers of people moving across cultural boundaries and back again, the urbane Indian might indulgently smile at the tragicomic aspects of this reverse cultural shock. Tea and coffee, oatmeal porridge, and cocoa were introduced to the breakfast table of the Gandhi household. Boots, shoes—and smelly socks—were to be worn in the burning heat of Kathiawar. Indeed, as a colonial subject, his identification with the British overlord was so strong that when some years later he was to sail for South Africa, he insisted on his sons being dressed like English public school boys with Etonian collars and ties. Poor Kasturbai was to dress up as a British lady—corset, bustle, high lace collar, laced shoes, and all. Her vehement protests and perhaps the absurdity of it all made him finally relent, though Kasturbai still had to dress up as a Parsi lady, a member of the community most respected by the British.

The marriage was still tempestuous, his driven genital desire the cause of these storms. His stay in England had neither reduced the strength of Gandhi's jealousy nor put an end to the nagging suspicions about his wife's fidelity. At the egging of his old friend Sheikh Mehtab, Gandhi went so far as to break Kasturbai's bangles—to an Indian girl the dreaded symbol of widowhood—and to send her back to her parents' house. It took him a year before he consented to receive her back and over four years before his suspicion was stilled.[9] Purists can be cruel, especially to those dependent women who threaten to devour their virtue.

Economic, social, and familial conflicts, besides the perennial erotic one, seem to have spurred Gandhi's travels on the spiritual path. In this journey he now acquired a guide, Raichandra, a young jeweller. Raichandra was a man after Gandhi's own heart, more interested in *moksha* (the release from the cycles of birth and death which Hindus believe govern the wandering of the individual soul) than in diamonds. The two men met often to discuss spiritual topics and the depth of Raichandra's sincerity, purpose, and knowledge of Hindu thought and scriptures made a deep impression on Gandhi's mind. Of the three men, he says, who had to greatest influence on his life (the others were Tolstoy and Ruskin), Raichandra was the only one with whom he had a long personal association. Indeed, the young jeweller who talked so eloquently about moksha was the nearest Gandhi came to having a guru, and 'In my moments of inner crisis, it was Raichandra with whom I used to seek refuge.'[10]

Unfortunately, in spite of the vast amount written on his life (over 400 biographical items), and the wealth of material contained in the 90 volumes of Gandhi's collected works, we know very little of the subjects of these talks, the letters they exchanged, or the kind of guidance Gandhi sought for his inner turbulence. From the available references, scattered in Gandhi's writings, it is evident that a central concern of their earnest exchanges was the relationship of sexuality to 'salvation', the transformation of sexual potency into psychic and spiritual power—the core issue, in fact, of much of Hindu metaphysics and practice. Gandhi notes that the idea that 'milk gives birth to sexual passions is something which I first learnt from Raichandrabhai', and he ascribes to the jeweller the predominant role in his decision to become a celibate.[11]

In 1893, at the age of twenty-four Gandhi left for South Africa where he had been engaged as a lawyer by an Indian businessman. With brief interruptions for home visits, he was to stay there for the next twenty-two years.

Gandhi's years in South Africa, especially from 1900 to 1910, roughly spanning the fourth decade of his life, were crucial for the formation of Gandhi's historical persona. During these years Gandhi remade himself in that final image which is now evoked by his name. The first great nonviolent political campaigns for the rights of Indians living in South Africa, which introduced and refined the instrument of *Satyagraha* (literally, insistence on truth), took place during this period, at the end of which it would become well-known in many parts of the world. Equally important for our purposes is the fact that it was also during these years that he defined for himself the kind of personal life he would lead, and developed his ideas on the desired relationship between the sexes which would form the foundation for his own marriage with Kasturbai.

Founding and living in communes with disciples and seekers who shared his vision, radically experimenting with food and alternative systems of healing such as nature cure, generally embracing an ascetic lifestyle, the cornerstone of his personal life was *brahmacharya* or celibacy. Indeed brahmacharya was one leg of a tripod of which the other two were nonviolence (*ahimsa*) and truth (*satya*), which he adopted as the conscious basis for his adult identity and about which he would later write: 'Nonviolence came to me after a strenuous struggle, brahmacharya I am still struggling for, but truth has always come naturally to me.'[12]

The decision for sexual abstinence was taken in 1901, the year in which Raichandra died and in which Gandhi had just become a father for the fourth time (Devdas, the youngest son, was born in 1900). Both these circumstances must have contributed to Gandhi's resolve to renounce sexuality. The birth of the son, as we know from the account of the fateful night of the father's death and the newborn who did not survive because of *his father's* accursed lust, was a reminder of Gandhi's despised genital desires and therefore a stigma. To give them up was an offering made at the altar of Raichandra's (and, we would conjecture, his father's) departed soul. Kasturbai had not been consulted and Gandhi confesses that for the first few years he was only 'more or less successful' in his practice of self restraint.[13] Gandhi had left for India with his family in November 1901 and returned to South Africa the next year after promising his wife that she would soon follow. Yet, once he was back in South Africa, Gandhi was reluctant to have Kasturbai join him. Paramount in his decision must have been the fact that his resolve to abstain from sexual intercourse was still fragile. The monetary argument he advances in the letters to his relatives, where he asks their help in persuading his wife to remain behind for two to three years, namely, that the savings he could make in South Africa would enable her and the children to lead an easy life in India,[14] neither jibes with the realities of running a household alone nor with Gandhi's character and temperament. Only a few months earlier, while leaving for India, he had gifted all the gold and diamond jewellery presented to him by a grateful Indian community to a trust, maintaining, 'I feel neither I nor my family can make any personal use of the costly present', and that what he valued was their affection and not money.[15]

Gandhi finally took the vow to observe complete celibacy in 1906 when he was thirty-seven years old, on the eve of his first nonviolent political campaign in South Africa. The preceding five years of attempted abstinence he felt, had only been a preparation for what would amount to a total and irrevocable renunciation of sexuality. The example of Tolstoy further deepened his resolve. As he writes in 1905, 'He (Tolstoy) used to enjoy all pleasures of the world, kept mistresses, drank and was strongly addicted to smoking. ... He has given up all his vices, eats very simple food and has it in him no longer to hurt any living creature by thought, word or deed.'[16] Tolstoy's ideas on chastity, not only for the unmarried but also for the married, outlined in the *Kreuzer Sonata* (1889), were combined with the Hindu notions on brahmacharya to form Gandhi's own vision of the 'right' relationship between men and women. More than a personal code of conduct, these ideas regulated the life of all those who lived with him in his various communes (*ashrams*) in South Africa and India. Briefly summarized in his own words, this doctrine on the relationship between a couple holds that

The very purpose of marriage is restraint and sublimation of the sexual passion. Marriage for the satisfaction of sexual appetite is *vyabhichara*, concupisence … if they come together merely to have a fond embrace they are nearest the devil.

The only rule that can be laid down in such instances (if a child is not conceived) is that coitus may be permitted once at the end of the monthly period till conception is established. If its object is achieved it must be abjured forthwith.

There is not doubt that much of the sensuality of our nature, whether male or female, is due to the superstition, having a religious sanction, that married people are bound to share the same bed and the same room. But every husband and wife can make a fixed resolution from today never to share the same room or same bed at night, and to avoid sexual contact, except for one supreme purpose which it is intended for in both man and beast.[17]

Whatever its other consequences, there is little doubt that Gandhi's vow of celibacy distinctly improved his marriage, perhaps because poor Kasturbai was no longer perceived as a seductive siren responsible for his lapses from a longed-for ideal of purity. Ever since they had been in South Africa, there was much bickering and quarrelling between the two. They had fought over her desire to keep her ornaments while Gandhi sought to convince her of the virtues of non-possession. There was a major explosion, in which Gandhi almost turned her out of the house, over his wish that she clean up after an untouchable Christian visitor, a task abhorrent to a traditional Hindu woman with her deeply ingrained taboos about pollution. There was a running battle between the couple over their eldest son Harilal's wish that he grow up like other boys of his age and be allowed to avail of formal schooling. Gandhi's radical views on education would not allow the son to be sent to school, while Kasturbai was obstinate in the advocacy of her firstborn's cause.

From all accounts, before the vow of brahmacharya, Gandhi was an autocrat with his wife, 'completely steel', as he tried to bend her to his will and get her to embrace what must have appeared to her as eccentric notions that endangered the present and future welfare of the family.

After 1906, their relationship improved steadily and Gandhi could write with some justification that 'I could not steal into my wife's heart until I decided to treat her differently than I used to do, and so I restored to her all her rights by dispossessing myself of any so-called rights as her husband.'[18] In their later years, though there were occasional disagreements, generally with respect to the children and Kasturbai's discomfort with the many women in the various ashrams who jostled each other to come closer to Gandhi, the marriage was marked by deep intimacy and a quiet love which impressed everyone who witnessed the old couple together.

For Gandhi, celibacy was not only the sine qua non for moksha, but also the mainspring of his political activities. It is from the repudiation, the ashes of sexual desire, that the weapon of nonviolence which he used so effectively in his political struggle against the racial oppression of the South African white rulers and later against the British Empire, was phoenix-like born. As Gandhi puts it:

> *Ahimsa* (nonviolence) means Universal Love. If a man gives his love to one woman, or a woman to one man, what is there left for the world besides? It simply means, 'We two first, and the devil take all the rest of them.' As a faithful wife must be prepared to sacrifice her all for the sake of her husband, and a faithful husband for the sake of his wife, it is clear that such persons cannot rise to the height of Universal Love, or look upon all mankind as kith and kin. For they have created a boundary wall round their love. The larger their family, the farther are they from Universal Love. Hence one who would obey the law of *ahimsa* cannot marry, not to speak of gratification outside the marital bond.[19]

As for those who are already married, 'If the married couple can think of each other as brother and sister, they are freed for universal service. The very thought that all women in the world are his sisters, mothers and daughters will at once enable a man to snap his chains.'[20]

The truth of Gandhi's assertion that sexual love limits rather than expands personal concerns and that the narrow role of a husband is antithetical to the larger identity of one who would husband the world is not at issue here. Our intention for the moment is to elucidate Gandhi's conflict in the way he viewed it—in this case, the imperatives of desire straining against the higher purpose of unfettered service to community. Yet another of his pansexualist formulations of thc conflict has it that the gratification of sexual passion vies with a man's obligation to enhance personal vitality and psychic power. 'A man who is unchaste loses stamina, becomes emasculated and cowardly,'[21] is a sentiment often echoed in his writings as is the reiteration that his capacity to work in the political arena was a result of the psychic power gained through celibacy. Still another, later formulation is put in religious and spiritual terms—sexuality compromises his aspiration to become 'God's eunuch'. Reminiscent of Christ's metaphors of innocent childhood to describe would-be entrants to the kingdom of heaven and Prophet Mohammed's welcoming of 'those made eunuchs', not through an operation but through prayer to God, Gandhi too would see sexual renunciation as a precondition for self realization and, Moses-like, for seeing God 'face to face'.

Like his communes, which are a combination of the ashrama of the ancient sages described in the Hindu epics and the Trappist monastery in South Africa which so impressed him on a visit, Gandhi's views on the importance and merits of celibacy too seem to be derived from a mixture of Hindu and Christian religious traditions. Where Gandhi proceeded to give these views a special twist, going much beyond the cursory juxtaposition of sexuality and eating made in his culture, was in emphasizing, above all, the relation of food to the observance of celibacy. Experiments with food, to find that elusive right combination which would keep the libido effectively dammed, continued right through to the end of his life. In South Africa, as reported by an admiring yet detached disciple, there were months of cooking without salt or any condiments. Another period witnesses the absence of sugar, dates, and currants being added for sweetening purposes. This was followed by a period of 'unfired' food served with olive oil. Food values were most earnestly discussed and their effect upon the human body and its moral qualities solemnly examined. For a time, a dish of raw chopped onions, as a blood purifier, regularly formed part of the dinner meal … Ultimately Mr Gandhi came to the conclusion that onions were bad for the passions, and so onions were cut out. Milk, too, Mr Gandhi said, affected the 'passion' side of human life and thereafter milk was abjured likewise. 'We talk about food quite as much as gourmands do,' I said on one occasion to Mr Gandhi. 'I am sure we talk about food more than most people, we seem to be always thinking of the things we either may or may not eat. Sometimes, I think it would be better if we just ate anything and did not think about it at all.'[22] However, for Gandhi food was a deathly serious business.

Control of palate is very closely connected with the observance of *brahmacharya* (celibacy). I have found from experience that the observance of celibacy becomes comparatively easy, if one acquires mastery over the palate. This does not figure among the observances of time-honoured recognition. Could it be because even great sages found it difficult to achieve. Food has to be taken as we take medicine, without thinking whether it is tasty or otherwise, and only in quantities limited to the needs of the body. … And one who thus gives up a multitude of eatables will acquire self control in the natural course of things.[23]

The above passage is reminiscent of St Augustine who, too, would take food as physic, strive daily against concupiscence in eating and drinking, and assert that 'the bridle of the throat then is to be held attempted between slackness and stiffness'.[24] St Augustine's attitude towards food, though, is part of his attempt to gain a general freedom from the grip of sensuality, including 'the delights of the ear (that) had more firmly entangled and subdued me'.[25] Augustine treats imbibition as he does all sensory input. Gandhi, on the other hand, makes of food a primary regulator of the genital impulses. 'A man of heightened sexual passion,' he writes, 'is also greedy of the palate. This was also my condition. To gain control over the organs of both generation and taste has been difficult for me.'[26]

A radical cure for his epicurean disease is, of course, fasting, and Gandhi was its enthusiastic proponent. 'As an external aid to brahmacharya, fasting is as necessary as selection and restriction of diet. So overpowering are the senses that they can be kept under control only when they are completely hedged in on all sides, from above and from beneath.'[27] Remembering Gandhi's great fasts during his political struggles, we can see how fasting for him would have another, more personal meaning as a protector of his cherished celibacy and thus an assurance against the waning of psychic, and, with it, political power.

Battle, weapons, victory, and defeat are a part of Gandhi's image in his account of a life-long conflict with the dark god of desire, the only opponent he did not engage non-violently nor could ever completely subdue. The metaphors that pervade the descriptions of this passionate conflict are of 'invasions by an insidious enemy' who needs to be implacably 'repulsed'; while the perilous struggle is like 'walking on a sword's edge'. The god himself (though Gandhi would not have given Kama, the god of love, the exalted status accorded him in much of Hindu mythology) is the 'serpent which I know will bite me', 'the scorpion of passion', whose destruction, annihilation, conflagration, is a supreme aim of his spiritual strivings. In sharp contrast to all his other opponents whose humanity he was always scrupulous to respect, the god of desire was the only antagonist with whom Gandhi could not compromise and whose humanity (not to speak of his divinity) he always denied.

For Gandhi, defeats in this war were occasions for bitter self-reproach and a public confession of his humiliation, while the victories were a matter of joy, 'fresh beauty', and an increase in vigour and self confidence that brought him nearer to the moksha he so longed for. Whatever may be his values to the contrary, a sympathetic reader, conscious of Gandhi's greatness and his prophetic insights into many of the dilemmas of modem existence, cannot fail to be moved by the dimensions of Gandhi's personal struggle—heroic in its proportion, startling in its intensity, interminable in its duration. By the time Gandhi concludes his autobiography with the words:

> To conquer the subtle passions seems to me to be far harder than the conquest of the world by the force of arms. Ever since my return to India I have had experiences of the passions hidden within me. They have made me feel ashamed though I have not lost courage. My experiments with truth have given, and continue to give, great joy. But I know that I must traverse a perilous path. I must reduce myself to zero,[28]

No reader can doubt his passionate sincerity and honesty. His is not the reflexive, indeed passionless moralism of the more ordinary religionist.

How did Gandhi himself experience sexual desire, the temptations, and the limits of the flesh? To know this, it is important that we listen closely to Gandhi's voice describing his conflicts in the language in which he spoke of them—Gujarati, his mother tongue. Given the tendency towards hagiolatry among the followers of a great man, their translations, especially of the Master's sexual conflicts, are apt to distort the authentic voice of the man behind the saint. The English translation of Gandhi's autobiography by his faithful secretary, Mahadev Desai, in spite of the benefit of Gandhi's own revision, suffers seriously from this defect, and any interpretations based on this translation are in danger of missing Gandhi's own experience. Take, for instance, one famous incident from Gandhi's youth, of the schoolboy Gandhi visiting a prostitute for the first time in the company of his Muslim friend and constant tempter, Sheikh Mehtab. The original Gujarati version describes the incident as follows:

> I entered the house but he who is to be saved by God remains pure even if he wants to fall. I became almost blind in that room. I could not speak. Struck dumb by embarrassment, I sat down on the cot with the woman but could not utter a single word. The woman was furious, gave me a couple of choice abuses and showed me to the door [my translation].[29]

The English translation, however, is much less matter-of-fact. It is full of Augustinianisms in which young Gandhi goes into a 'den of vice' and tarries in the 'jaws of sin.' These are absent in the original. By adding adjectives such as 'evil' and 'animal' before 'passions', the translation seems to be judging them in a Christian theological sense that is missing in Gandhi's own account. St Augustine, for instance—with whose *Confessions* Gandhi's *Experiments* has much in common—was rent asunder because of the 'sin that dwelt in me', by 'the punishment of a sin more freely committed, in that I was a son of Adam'.[30] Gandhi, in contrast, uses two words, *vishaya* and vikara, for lust and passion respectively. The root of vishaya is from poison, and that is how he regards sexuality—as poisonous, for instance, when he talks of it in conjunction with serpents and scorpions. The literal meaning of *vikara*, or passion, is 'distortion,' and that is how passions are traditionally seen in the Hindu view, waves of mind that distort the clear waters of the soul. For Gandhi, then, lust is not sinful but poisonous, contaminating the elixir of immortality. It is dangerous in and of itself, 'destructuralizing' in psychoanalytic language, rather than merely immoral, at odds, that is, with certain social or moral injunctions. To be passionate is not to fall from a state of grace, but to suffer a distortion of truth. In contrast to the English version, which turns his very Hindu conflict into a Christian one, Gandhi's struggle with sexuality is not essentially a conflict between sin and morality, but rather one between psychic death and immortality, on which the moral quandary is superimposed.

We can, of course, never be quite certain whether Gandhi was a man with a gigantic erotic temperament or merely the possessor of an overweening conscience that magnified each departure from an unattainable ideal of purity as a momentous lapse. Nor is it possible, for that matter, to evaluate the paradoxical impact of his scruples in intensifying the very desires they opposed. Both fuelled each other, the lid of self-control compressing and heating up the contents of the cauldron of desire, in Freud's famous metaphor, their growing intensity requiring ever greater efforts at confinement.

Gandhi himself, speaking at the birth centenary of Tolstoy in 1928, warns us to refrain from judgements. While talking of the import of such struggles in the lives of great *homo religiosi*, he seems to be asking for empathy rather than facile categorization:

> The seeming contradictions in Tolstoy's life are no blot on him or sign of his failure. They signify the failure of the observer. ... Only the man himself knows how much he struggles in the depth of his heart or what victories he wins in the war between Rama and Ravana.* The spectator certainly cannot know that.[31]

In judging a great man, Gandhi goes on to say, and here he seems to be talking as much of himself as Tolstoy,

> God is witness to the battles he may have fought in his heart and the victories he may have won. These are the only evidence of his failures and successes ... If anyone pointed out a weakness in Tolstoy though there could hardly be an occasion for anyone to do so for he was pitiless in his self-examination, he would

*The good and evil protagonists of the Indian epic, *Ramayana*.

magnify that weakness to fearful proportions. He would have seen his lapse and atoned for it in the manner he thought most appropriate before anyone had pointed it out to him.[32]

This is a warning we must take seriously but do not really need. Our intention is not to 'analyse' Gandhi's conflict in any reductionist sense but to seek to understand it in all its passion—and obscurity. Gandhi's agony is ours as well, after all, an inevitable by-product of the long human journey from infancy to adulthood. We all wage wars on our wants.

A passionate man who suffered his passions as poisonous of his inner self and a sensualist who felt his sensuality distorted his inner purpose, Gandhi's struggle with what he took to be the god of desire was not unremitting. There were long periods in his adulthood when his sensuality was integrated with the rest of his being. Old movie clips and reminiscences of those who knew him in person attest to some of this acceptable sensuality. It found expression in the vigorous grace of his locomotion; the twinkle in his eye and the brilliance of his smile; the attention he paid to his dress—even if the dress was a freshly laundered, spotless loincloth; the care he directed to the preparation and eating of his simple food; the delight with which he sang and listened to devotional songs; and the pleasure he took in the daily oil massage of his body. The Christian St Augustine would have been altogether shocked. Here, then, the Indian ascetic's path diverges from that trod by the more austere and self-punishing western monk. Here, too, from Gandhi's sensuous gaiety, stems his ability to rivet masses of men not by pronouncement in scripture but by his very presence.

In Gandhi's periods of despair, occasioned by real-life disappointments and setbacks in the socio-political campaigns to which he had committed his life, the integration of his sensuality and spirituality would be threatened and again we find him obsessively agonizing over the problem of genital desire. Once more he struggled against the re-emergence of an old antagonist whom he sought to defeat by public confessions of *his* defeats.

One such period spans the years between 1925 and 1928, after his release from jail when he was often depressed, believing that the Indian religious and political divisions were too deep for the country to respond to his leadership and that Indians were not yet ready for his kind of nonviolent civil disobedience. There was a breakdown with a serious condition of hypertension and doctors had advised him long rest. Interestingly, this is also the period in which he wrote his confessional autobiography, where he despondently confides, 'Even when I am past 56 years, I realize how hard a thing it (celibacy) is. Every day I realize more and more that it is like walking on the sword's edge, and I can see every moment the necessity of continued vigilance.'[33] His ideals and goals failing him, Gandhi finds sublime purpose and intent crumbling, exposing desires held in abeyance. These then become pre-potent. The psychoanalyst would speak in this instance of the disintegration of 'sublimations'—conversions of base wishes into socially sanctioned aspirations—and the lonely, painful regression which ensues.

In the copious correspondence of the years 1927 and 1928, the two longest and the most personally involved letters are neither addressed to his close political co-workers and leaders of future free India such as Nehru, Patel or Rajagopalachari, nor do they deal with vital political or social issues. The addressees are two unknown young men, and the subject of the letters is the convolutions of Gandhi's instinctual promptings. Responding to Balakrishna Bhave, who had expressed doubts about the propriety of Gandhi placing his hands on the shoulders of young girls while walking, Gandhi conducts a characteristic, obsessive search for any hidden eroticism in his action.[34] The other letter, to Harjivan Kotak, deserves to be quoted at some length since it details Gandhi's poignant struggle, his distress at the threatened breakdown of the psycho-sensual synthesis.

When the mind is disturbed by impure thoughts, instead of trying to drive them out one should occupy it in some work, that is, engage it in reading or in some bodily labour which requires mental attention too. Never let the eyes follow their inclination. If they fall on a woman, withdraw them immediately. It is scarcely necessary for anyone to look straight at a man's or woman's face. This is the reason why *brahmacharis*, and others too, are enjoined to walk with their eyes lowered. If we are sitting, we should keep them steady in one direction. This is an external remedy, but a most valuable one. You may undertake a fast if and when you find one necessary. … You should not be afraid even if you get involuntary discharges during a fast. *Vaids* (traditional doctors) say that, even when impure desires are absent, such discharges may occur because of pressure in the bowels. But, instead of believing that, it helps us more to believe that they occur because of impure desires. We are not always conscious of such desires. I had involuntary discharges twice during the last two weeks. I cannot recall any dream. I never practised masturbation. One cause of these discharges is of course my physical weakness but I also know that there are impure desires deep down in me. I am able to keep out such thoughts during waking hours. But what is present in the body like some hidden poison, always makes its way, even forcibly sometimes. I feel unhappy about this, but am not nervously afraid. I am always vigilant. I can suppress the enemy but have not been able to expel him altogether. If I am truthful, I shall succeed in doing that too. The enemy will not be able to endure the power of truth. If you are in the same condition as I am, learn from my experience. In its essence, desire for sex-pleasure is equally impure, whether its object is one's wife or some other woman. Its results differ. At the moment, we are thinking of the enemy in his essential nature. Understand, therefore, that so far as one's wife is concerned you are not likely to find anyone as lustful as I was. That is why I have described my pitiable condition to you and tried to give you courage.[35]

A 'hidden power', an 'enemy to be expelled'—in such circumstances the body becomes a strange land inhabited by demons of feeling and impulse divided from the self. With setbacks in unity of intent, there is a further fragmenting of the self. The moral dilemma stirs conflicts of a primeval order, when early 'introjects'—those presences bound to desire out of which we construct our primary self—are awakened, taste blood or better, poison, and threaten our identity—our sense of wholeness, continuity, and sameness.

Another emotionally vulnerable period comprises roughly eighteen months from the middle of 1935 onwards, when Gandhi was almost sixty-six years old. Marked by a 'nervous breakdown', when his blood pressure went dangerously out of control, Gandhi was advised complete rest for some months by his doctors. He attributed this breakdown to overwork and especially mental exhaustion brought on by the intensity of his involvement and emotional reactions to the personal problems of his co-workers. He considered these as important as those pertaining to the country's independence, regretting only that he had not reached the Hindu ideal, as outlined in the *Gita*, of detachment from emotions. Gandhi used this enforced rest for introspection and decided to give up his practice of walking with his hands on the shoulders of young girls. In 'A Renunciation', an article he wrote for his newspaper during this time, he traced the history of this particular practice, reiterated the purity of his paternal intentions towards the girls involved, acknowledged that he was not unaware of the dangers of the liberty he was taking, and based his renunciation on the grounds of setting a good example to the younger generation.[36]

What is more significant is that in the very first article he was allowed to write by his doctors, Gandhi, meditating on the causes of his ill-health, comes back to the question of his celibacy. He mentions an encounter with a woman during the period of convalescence in Bombay, which not only disturbed him greatly but made him despise himself. In a letter to Prema Kantak, a disciple and confidante in his Sabarmati ashram, he elaborates on this incident further.

I have always had the shedding of semen in dreams. In South Africa the interval between two ejaculations may have been in years. I do not remember it fully. Here the time difference is in months. I have mentioned these ejaculations in a couple of my articles. If my *brahmacharya* had been without this shedding of semen then I would have been able to present many more things to the world. But someone who from the age of 15 to 30 has enjoyed sexuality (*vishya-bhog*)-even if it was only with his wife—whether such a man can conserve his semen after becoming a *brahmachari* seems impossible to me. Someone whose power of storing the semen has been weakened daily for 15 years cannot hope to regain this power all at once. That is why I regard myself as an incomplete *brahmachari*. But where there are no trees, there are thorn bushes. This shortcoming of mine is known to the world.

The experience which tortured me in Bombay was strange and painful. All my ejaculations have taken place in dreams; they did not trouble me. But Bombay's experience was in the waking state. I did not have any inclination to fulfil that desire. My body was under control. But in spite of my trying, the sense organ remained awake. This experience was new and unbecoming. I have narrated its cause.* After removing this cause the wakefulness of the sense organ subsided, that is, it subsided in the waking state.

In spite of my shortcoming, one thing has been easily possible for me, namely that thousands of women have remained safe with me. There were many occasions in my life when certain women, in spite of their sexual desire, were saved or rather I was saved by God. I acknowledge it one hundred percent that this was God's doing. That is why I take no pride in it. I pray daily to God that such a situation should last till the end of my life.

To reach the level of Shukadeva is my goal.+ I have not been able to achieve it. Otherwise in spite of the generation of semen I would be impotent and the shedding will become impossible.

The thoughts I have expressed recently about *brahmacharya* are not new. This does not mean that the ideal will be reached by the whole world or even by thousands of men and women in my lifetime. It may take thousands of years, but *brahmacharya* is true, attainable and must be realized.

* By remaining inactive and eating well, passions are born in the body.

+ Son of Vyasa, Shukadeva is the mythical reciter of the *Bhagavatapurana*. In spite of having married and lived the life of a householder (like Gandhi, he was the father of four sons) in later life he succeeded in conquering his senses to an extent that he rose up to the Heavens and shone there like a second sun.

Man has still to go a long way. His character is still that of a beast. Only the form is human. It seems that violence is all around us. In spite of this, just as there is no doubt about truth and nonviolence similarly there is no doubt about *brahmacharya.*

Those who keep on burning despite their efforts are not trying hard enough. Nurturing passion in their minds they only want that no shedding of semen take place and avoid women. The second chapter of *Gita* applies to such people.

What I am doing at the moment is purification of thought. Modern thought regards *brahmacharya* as wrong conduct. Using artificial methods of birth control it wants to satisfy sexual passion. My soul rebels against this. Sexual desire will remain in the world, but the world's honour depends on *brahmacharya* and will continue to do so.[37]

Further self-mortification was one of his responses to what he regarded as an unforgivable 'lapse'. Even the ascetic regimen of the ashram now seemed luxurious. Leaving Kasturbai to look after its inmates, he went off to live in a one-room hut in a remote and poverty-stricken, untouchable village. Though he wished to be alone—a wish that for a man in his position was impossible of fulfilment—he soon became the focus of a new community.

Another dark period covers the last two years of Gandhi's life. The scene is India on the eve of Independence in 1947. A Muslim Pakistan is soon to be carved out of the country, much against Gandhi's wishes. His dream of Hindus and Muslims living amicably in a single unified state seems to be shattered beyond hope. Gandhi would even postpone Independence if the partition of the country could be averted, but his voice does not resonate quite so powerfully in the councils where the transfer of power is being negotiated. The air hangs heavy with clouds of looming violence. Hindus and Muslims warily eye each other as potential murderers … or eventual victims. The killings have already started in the crowded back-alleys of Calcutta and in the verdant expanses of rural Bengal, where the 78-year-old Mahatma is wearily trudging from one village to another, trying to stem the rushing tide of arson, rape, and murder that will soon engulf many other parts of the country. The few close associates who accompany him on this mission of peace are a witness to his despair and helpless listeners to the anguished cries of '*Kya karun, kya karun*? (What should I do? What should I do?)' heard from his room in the middle of the night.[38] 'I find myself in the midst of exaggeration and falsity,' he writes, 'I am unable to discover the truth. There is terrible mutual distrust. Oldest friendships have snapped. Truth and *Ahimsa* (nonviolence) by which I swear and which have to my knowledge sustained me for 60 years, seem to fail to show the attributes I ascribed to them.'[39]

For an explanation of his 'failures' and sense of despair, Gandhi would characteristically probe for shortcomings in his abstinence, seeking to determine whether the god of desire had perhaps triumphed in some obscure recess of his mind, depriving him of his powers. Thus in the midst of human devastation and political uncertainty, Gandhi wrote a series of five articles on celibacy in his weekly newspaper, puzzling his readers who, as his temporary personal secretary, N.K. Bose, puts it, 'did not know why such a series suddenly appeared in the midst of intensely political articles'.[40]

But more striking than this public evidence of his preoccupation were his private experiments wherein the aged Mahatma pathetically sought to reassure himself of the strength of his celibacy. These experiments have shocked many and have come to be known as 'having naked young women sleep with him when he was old', although their intent and outcome were far removed from the familiar connotations of that suggestive phrase. In the more or less public sleeping arrangements of his entourage while it rested in a village for the night, Gandhi would ask one or another of his few close women associates (his 19-year-old granddaughter among them) to share his bed and then try to ascertain in the morning whether any trace of sexual feeling had been evoked, either in himself or in his companion.[41] In spite of criticism by some of his close co-workers, Gandhi defended these experiments, denying the accusation that they could have ill effects on the women involved. Instead, he viewed them as an integral part of the *Yagna* he was performing—the Hindu sacrifice to the gods—whose only purpose was a restoration of personal psychic potency that would help him to regain control over political events and men, a control which seemed to be so fatally slipping away. Again he exploits his desires (and, admittedly, women) for the sake of his cause—the prideful vice of an uncompromisingly virtuous man.

Two Women

In his middle and later years, a number of young women, attracted by Gandhi's public image as the Mahatma, his cause, or his fame, sought his proximity and eventually shared his ashram life. These women, who in many cases had left their well-appointed middle- and upper-class homes to take upon themselves the rigours of an ascetic lifestyle, were all else but conventional. Some of them were not only 'highstrung' but can fairly be described as suffering from emotional crises of considerable magnitude. Like their counterparts today who seek out well-known gurus, these women too were looking for the therapist in Gandhi as much as the Mahatma or the leader embodying Indian national aspirations. If toning down the intensity of a crippling emotional disturbance and awakening latent productive and creative powers that neither the individual nor the community 'knows' he or she possesses is the mark of a good therapist then, as we shall see later, Gandhi was an exceptional one. From women who were a little more than emotional wrecks, he fashioned energetic leaders directing major institutions engaged in the task of social innovation and actively participating in the country's Independence movement.

Gandhi's relationships with these women are fascinating in many ways. First, one is struck by the trouble he took in maintaining a relationship once he had admitted the woman to a degree of intimacy. Irrespective of his public commitments or the course of political events, he was punctilious in writing (and expecting) regular weekly letters to each one of his chosen women followers when they were separated during his frequent visits to other parts of the country or his lengthy spells of imprisonment. Cumulatively, these letters build up a portrait of the Mahatma which reveals his innermost struggles, particularly during the periods of heightened emotional vulnerability, and the role played therein by Woman, as embodied in the collectivity of his chosen female followers.

At their best, the letters are intensely human, full of wisdom about life and purpose. Even at times of stress, they are invariably caring as Gandhi encourages the women's questions, advises them on their intimate problems, and cheerfully dispenses his favourite dietary prescriptions for every kind of ailment. As he writes to one of them: 'Your diagnosis is a correct one. The pleasure I get out of solving the *ashram's* problems, and within the *ashram* those of the sisters, is much greater than that of resolving India's dilemmas.'[42]

The second striking characteristic of these letters is what appears to be Gandhi's unwitting effort simultaneously to increase the intimacy with the correspondent and to withdraw if the woman wished for a nearness that crossed the invisible line he had drawn for both of them. The woman's consequent hurt or withdrawal is never allowed to reach a point of breakdown in the relationship. Gandhi employed his considerable charm and powers of persuasion to draw her close again, the hapless woman oscillating around a point between intimacy and estrangement, nearness and distance. The emotions aroused, not only in the women (who were also in close contact with each other) but to some degree in Gandhi, simmered in the hothouse ashram atmosphere to produce frequent explosions. In accordance with our narrative intent, let us look at the stories of two of these women, making of them brief tales rather than the novel each one of them richly deserves.

Prema Kantak belonged to a middle-class family from a small town in Maharashtra. She was still a schoolgirl when she heard about Gandhi and the wonderful work he had done for the cause of Indians in South Africa. An only daughter among five sons, she was a favourite of her father and enjoyed more than the usual freedom for a girl of her class and times.

As Prema grew into youth, she was gripped by the fervour of nationalist politics and agonized over personal spiritual questions, interests which Gandhi too combined in his person. Had he not maintained that 'politics without religion is dangerous?'

Her first encounter with the great man took place when Gandhi came to address students of her college at Poona. After the talk, she remembers going up to the platform where he was sitting so as to touch his feet in the traditional Indian gesture of respect. Since Gandhi was sitting cross-legged, his feet were tucked under his body. Prema reports:

> Without any mental reservations I touched his knee with my finger and saluted him. With a start he turned to look at me, reciprocated the greetings and looked away. If he but knew that by touching him my heart had blossomed forth with incomparable pride! With the pure touch an electric current ran through my body and I walked home lost in a world of bliss![43]

Sensitive and emotional, intelligent and idealistic, Prema refused to follow the traditional life plan of an Indian girl and get married, perhaps also because of a problematic (most analysts would say 'classically hysterical') attitude towards sexuality. 'Once, when I was 16, I was reading the *Bhagavata*,' she writes, 'when I came to the conversation between Kapila and Devahuti,* I learnt how babies come into world. I remember that my hair stood up on end. I visualized my own conception and was seized with disgust towards my parents and my body! My life seemed dirty! This disgust remained with me for many years.'[44] After a bitter quarrel between the daughter and her beloved father, Prema left home to live in a women's hostel. She earned her livelihood by tutoring children while she continued her studies towards a Master's degree.

Prema's fascination for Gandhi and her decision to go and live with him in the *ashram* is quite understandable. In the very nature of the ashram life and its ideals, there is a promised protection from disgusting sexuality.

*Kapila is the legendary expounder of the Samkhya system of Hindu philosophy. Devahuti is Kapila's mother.

In her wishful imagination Gandhi looms up as the ideal parent who will soothe the hurt caused by the disappointment in the real-life one. He is also the admired mentor for Prema's political and spiritual interests, who is capable of comprehending the deeper needs of her soul.

At the age of twenty-three, then, bubbling with innocent enthusiasm, Prema found herself in Ahmedabad in the Mahatma's presence. As was his wont, at first Gandhi discouraged her. He described to her in detail the hard physical work, the chores of cutting vegetables, grinding grain, cooking meals, cleaning utensils and toilets which awaited her if she adopted the ashram life. Prema, exultant in her youthful vitality and idealism, dismissed his cautions as trifles. 'I want to do something tremendous!', she exclaimed on one of her very first nights in the ashram. With wry humour, Gandhi tried to temper her exuberance without crushing her spirit. 'The only tremendous thing you can do just now is go to sleep,' he said.[45]

At the start of her stay, when Gandhi was out of town for a few days, Prema had the following dream. She is a little girl reclining in Gandhi's lap. From his breast, a stream of sweet, good milk is flowing straight into her mouth. Prema is drinking the milk and the Mahatma is saying, 'Drink, drink, drink more.' Prema is replete but the milk continues to flow and Gandhi keeps insisting that she drink more. Prema's clothes and body are thoroughly soaked in milk but the stream is unending. She wakes up in alarm.[46]

On narrating her dream to Gandhi and asking for an interpretation, Gandhi replied, 'Dreams can have the quality of purity (*sattvik*) or of passion (*rajasik*). Your dream is a pure one. It means that you feel protected with me.'[47] From the orthodox Freudian view, the interpretation cannot be faulted. An instinctive psychoanalyst, Gandhi provides reassurance to the patient and encourages her to give him her trust at this stage of their relationship. Unwittingly following the technical rule of proceeding from the surface to the depths, his interpretation could have been as easily made by an analyst who, for the time being, would have kept his hypotheses on the deeper imports of the dream images—of the symbolic equivalence of milk and semen, Prema's greedy voraciousness, her possible fantasy regarding the persecuting breast and so on—quietly to himself.

In the ashram, the competition among women for Gandhi's attention was as fierce as it is in any guru's establishment today. When he went for his evening constitutional, Gandhi would walk with his hands around the shoulders of the ashram girls. There was intense jealousy among them as each kept a hawk's eye for any undue favouritism—the number of times a girl was singled out for the mark of this favour, the duration of time a girl had Bapu's hands on her shoulder and so on. At first Prema felt aggrieved when other girls teased her, 'Prema-*ben*, Bapuji does not put his hands on *your* shoulders!' 'Why should he? I am not like you to push myself forward!' Prema would reply spiritedly. 'No, he never will. The *ashram* rule is that he can keep his hands only on the shoulders of girls who are younger than 16.'[48]

Prema felt her deprivation acutely and approached Gandhi who asked her to get the ashram superintendent's permission if she wanted him to treat her like the younger girls. Prema's pride was hurt and she responded angrily, 'Why should I hanker after your hand so much that I have to go and get permission?' and stalked off. One night, however, Gandhi had gone to the toilet since he was suffering from diarrhoea because of one of his food experiments. He had fainted from weakness and Prema, who had heard him fall, reached his side. Gandhi walked back leaning his body against her for support and she even lifted him onto the bed. From that night onwards she often accompanied him on his evening walk, with his hand on her shoulder, while she, I imagine, looked around her with the pride of the chosen one, a victor in the secret struggle among the women. In her elation at being closer to him, she tells us, she once kissed his hands saying. 'The hand that has shaken the British throne is resting on my shoulders! What a matter of pride!' Gandhi had laughed, 'Yes, how proud we all are!' and, clowning, he threw out his chest and strutted about in imitation of a stage emperor.[49]

In 1933, when she was twenty-seven years old, Gandhi begged Prema to give him as *bhiksha* (meritorious alms) a lifelong vow of celibacy. Prema wrote back that there was no difficulty in her compliance with his wish as celibacy was in any case her ideal. In unreflected arrogance she added, 'I may sleep with any man on the same bed during the whole night and get up in the morning as innocent as a child.' Touched on a sore spot, Gandhi reprimanded her on a pride unbecoming a celibate. From mythology he gave examples of those whose pride in their celibacy had gone before a grievous fall. She was no goddess (*devi*), he said, since she still had her periods. For Gandhi believed that in a really celibate woman menstruation stopped completely, the monthly period being but a stigmata of vikara, of the sexual distortions of a woman's soul.[50]

Gradually, Prema was trusted with greater and greater responsibilities in running the ashram, though her constant struggle, like those of most other women, was for an intimate closeness with Gandhi. He would try to turn her thoughts towards the ashram community, instruct her to regard herself as belonging to the community and vice versa. 'You are dear to me, that is why "your" ashram is dear to me. Love wants an anchor, love needs touch. It is human nature that not only the mind needs an anchor but also the body and the sense organs,' she would argue back.[51] He would ask her to sublimate her emotions, affectionately call her hysterical, explaining that by hysterical he meant someone under an excessive sway of emotions. He would berate her for her lapses and then coax and cajole her back if she showed any signs of withdrawal. Prema felt that the 'Old Beloved,' her affectionate name for him, had ensnared her. Gandhi replied,

> I do not want to snare anyone in my net. If everyone becomes a puppet of mine then what will happen to me? I regard such efforts as worthless. But even if I try to trap someone you shouldn't lose your self confidence. Your letters prove that you are on guard. Yes, it is true that you have always been fearful of being caught in my net. That is a bad sign. If you have decided (to throw in your lot with me) then why the fear? Or perhaps it is possible that we mean different things by the word 'ensnare'?[52]

Feeling trapped—by the frustration of her own unconscious wishes in relation to Gandhi, the analyst would say—Prema sought to detach herself from him. She fought with him on what in retrospect seem minor issues. Remaining a devoted follower of Gandhi and his ideals, she was aware of a degree of estrangement from the Mahatma. Prema finally went back to Maharashtra in 1939 and set up an ashram in a small village. It was devoted to the fulfilment of Gandhi's social agenda—uplift of the poor and the untouchables, education of women, increasing the self sufficiency of the village community, and so on. Like the portentous dream after their initial meeting, the separation too is the occasion for a significant dream. In this dream, Prema is alone on a vast plain which meets the sky at the horizon. She is sitting in a chair in the middle of this plain with green grass all around her. Behind the chair, she senses the presence of a man. She cannot see him but has no doubt that the man is her protector and her companion. Suddenly four or five beautiful, well-dressed boys come running up to her with bouquets of flowers in their hands. She begins to talk to the boys. More and more children now appear with bouquets. From the sky, flowers begin to rain down upon her. She wakes up with a start. After waking up, when she thinks of the dream, she is convinced that the man standing behind her is Gandhi and that his blessings will always remain with her.[53]

As I reflect on the dream and its context, I cannot help musing (which is less an interpretation of the dream than my associations to it) that perhaps the dream fulfils some of Prema's contradictory wishes. Once again restored to the centre of her world with Gandhi, from which she has been recently excluded, she is the celibate devi of Hindu mythology on whom gods shower flowers from heaven as a sign of their approbation and homage. On the other hand, she has also become the life-companion of the Mahatma, bearing him not only the four sons Kasturbai had borne but many, many more adoring and adorable children.

Since it was the man rather than what he stood for who was the focus of her emotional life, Prema gradually drifted back to her earlier spiritual interests after Gandhi's death. As she consorted with yogis and mystics, the memory of the Mahatma and the years she had spent with him would become locked up in a comer of her mind, to be occasionally opened and savoured privately, a secret solace in times of distress.

In many ways, Madeline Slade was one of the more unusual members of Gandhi's female entourage. Daughter of an admiral in the British Navy who had been a commander of the East Indies Squadron, she was a part of the British ruling establishment, which both despised and feared Gandhi as an implacable foe. Brought up in the freedom of an upper-class English home of the era, Madeline had been dissatisfied and unhappy for years, and tells us that everything had been dark and futile till she discovered Gandhi and left for India when she was in her early thirties.[54] A great admirer of Beethoven—she had thought of devoting her life to the study of his life and music—her plans underwent a drastic change after she read Romain Rolland's book on Gandhi (*Mahatma Gandhi*, 1924). Not wishing to act hastily, she first prepared herself for the ordeal of ashram life in India. Madeline went about this task with her usual single-minded determination. She learned spinning and sitting cross-legged on the floor; she became a teetotaller and a vegetarian and learned Urdu. She then wrote to Gandhi expressing her wish and received a cordial reply inviting her to join him.

A tall, strapping woman, handsome rather than pretty, Madeline took avidly to the ascetic part of the ashram life. She clung to Gandhi with a ferocity which he found very unsettling, perhaps also because of the feelings which her strong need for his physical proximity in turn aroused in him. During the twenty-four years of their association, Gandhi would repeatedly send her away to live and work in other ashrams in distant parts of the country. She would have nervous breakdowns as a consequence of these separations and 'struggles of the heart' (as she called them) or 'spiritual agony' (as Gandhi put it), impetuously rush back to wherever Gandhi was only to be again banished from his presence. He tried to redirect her from her single-minded concentration on him as a person to the cause they both served.

The parting today was sad, because I saw that I pained you. I want you to be a perfect woman. I want you to shed all angularities. …

Do throw off the nervousness. You must not cling to me as in this body. The spirit without the body is ever with you. And that is more than the feeble embodied imprisoned spirit with all the limitations that flesh is heir to. The spirit without the flesh is perfect, and that is all we need. This can be felt only when we practise detachment. This you must now try to achieve.

This is how I should grow if I were you. But you should grow along your own lines. You will, therefore, reject all I have said in this, that does not appeal to your heart or your head. You must retain your individuality at all cost. Resist me when you must. For I may judge you wrongly in spite of all my love for you. I do not want you to impute infallibility to me.[55]

Madeline, now appropriately renamed Mira by Gandhi after the sixteenth century Indian woman–saint whose infatuation with Krishna was not much greater than Madeline's own yearning for the Mahatma, was however a battlefield of forces stronger than those amenable to reason. She was like the women described by the psychoanalyst Ralph Greenson, who come to analysis not to seek insight but to enjoy the physical proximity of the analyst.[56] Such patients relate a history of achievement and an adequate social life but an unsatisfactory love life characterized by wishes for incorporation, possession, and fusion. Gandhi's attitude to Mira, like that of the analyst with the patient, combined sympathetic listening with the frustration of wishes for gratification—a certain recipe, the mandrake root, for intensifying and unearthing ever more fresh capacities for love in her.[57] It further enhanced what analysts would call her transference to the Mahatma, a type of intense love felt for people who fulfil a role in our lives equivalent to the one fulfilled by parents in our childhood.

The presumption that their relationship was not quite one-sided and that Mira too evoked complex 'counter-transference' reactions in Gandhi is amply supported by his letters to her. Once, in 1927, when Mira had rushed to Gandhi's side on hearing that he was under severe strain, and had promptly been sent back, Gandhi wrote to her:

I could not restrain myself from sending you a love message on reaching here. I felt very sad after letting you go. I have been very severe with you, but I could not do otherwise. I had to perform an operation and I steadied myself for it. Now let us hope all would go on smoothly, and that all the weakness is gone.[58]

The letter was followed the next day with a post card: 'This is merely to tell you I can't dismiss you from my mind. Every surgeon has a soothing ointment after a severe operation. This is my ointment. …'[59] Two days later, yet another letter followed:

I have never been so anxious as this time to hear from you, for I sent you away too quickly after a serious operation. You haunted me in my sleep last night and were reported by friends to whom you had been sent, to be delirious, but without any danger. They said, 'You need not be anxious. We are doing all that is humanly possible.' And with this I woke up troubled in mind and prayed that you may be free from all harm. …[60]

From prison, where he was safe from her importunate physicality, Gandhi could express his feelings for her more freely. While translating a book of Indian hymns into English for her, he wrote: 'In translating the hymns for you I am giving myself much joy. Have I not expressed my love, often in storms than in gentle soothing showers of affection? The memory of these storms adds to the pleasure of this exclusive translation for you.'[61] As with his other women, Gandhi could not let Mira get away further than the distance he unconsciously held to be the optimal for his own feelings of well-being.

Like the child on his first explorations of the world who does not venture further from the mother than the length of an invisible string with which he seems attached to her, Gandhi too would become anxious at any break that threatened to become permanent and would seek to draw the woman closer to him.

Chi. Mira,
You are on the brain. I look about me, and miss you. I open the *charkha* (spinning wheel) and miss you. So on and so forth. But what is the use? You have done the right thing. You have left your home, your people and all that people prize most, not to serve me personally but to serve the cause I stand for. All the time you were squandering your love on me personally, I felt guilty of misappropriation. And I exploded on the slightest pretext. Now that you are not with me, my anger turns itself upon me for having given you all those terrible scoldings. But I was on a bed of hot ashes all the while I was accepting your service. You will truly serve me by joyously serving the cause. Cheer, cheer, no more of idle.

To this, Mira added the commentary, 'The struggle was terrible. I too was on a bed of hot ashes because I could feel that Bapu was. This was one of the occasions when, somehow or other, I managed to tear myself away.'[62]

In 1936, when Gandhi was recovering from his breakdown and had decided to leave Sabarmati to go and live by himself in a remote village, Mira thought she finally had a chance to fulfil her deepest longing, to live with Bapu in the countryside. Gandhi, however, was adamant. He would stay in the village Mira lived in only if she herself shifted to a neighbouring one. She writes,

> 'This nearly broke my heart, but somehow I managed to carry on, and when Bapu finally decided to come and live in Seagaon, I buried my sorrow in the joy of preparing for him his cottage and cowshed. For myself I built a little cottage a mile away on the ridge of Varoda village, and within a week of Bapu's coming to live in Seagaon I departed for the hut on the hill where I lived alone with my little horse as my companion.[63]

Even this relative nearness was not to last long as political events inexorably pulled Gandhi away on his travels.

In 1948, at the time of Gandhi's death, Mira was living in her own ashram near Rishikesh in the foothills of the Himalayas, devoting herself to the care of cattle in the nearby villages. Starting one ashram after another, deeper and deeper into the Himalayas, she was to live in India till 1958 after she decided to return to Europe, almost thirty-five years after she had first left home in search of Gandhi. I visited her with a friend in 1964, in the forests above Baden near Vienna where she now made her home in an isolated farmhouse with a dog and an old Indian servant from Rishikesh. Gracious but reserved, she offered us tea and biscuits and perfunctorily inquired about current events in India. She refused to talk about Gandhi, claiming that he did not interest her any longer. What animated her exclusively and what she enthusiastically talked about was Beethoven whom she saw as the highest manifestation of the human spirit. He had been her first love before she read Romain Rolland's book on Gandhi that was to change her life. Working on a biography of Beethoven and with his music as her dearest companion she had come back to the composer after a thirty-five-year detour with Gandhi. Somewhat disappointed, we left her to her new love. Walking towards our car parked a few hundred yards away from the farmhouse, we saw the servant come running up to us, desperation writ large on his lined face: 'Sahib, I don't want to live here. I want to go home. Please take me home.' I mumbled our apologies for being unable to help and left him standing on the grassy meadow, peering after us in the mild afternoon sun as we drove away.

To place Gandhi's sexual preoccupations in their cultural context, we should remember that sexuality, whether in the erotic flourishes of

Indian art and in the Dionysian rituals of its popular religion, or in the dramatic combat with ascetic longings of yogis who seek to conquer and transform it into spiritual power, has been a perennial preoccupation of Hindu culture. In this resides the reason, puzzling to many non-Indians, why in spite of the surface resemblances between Jungian concepts and Indian thought, it is Freud rather than Jung who fascinates the Indian mind. Many modern Indian mystics feel compelled, in fact, to discuss Freud's assumptions and conclusions about the vagaries and transfigurations of libido while they pass over Jung's work with benign indifference. Indian spirituality is pre-eminently a theory of 'sublimation.'

Indian 'mysticism' is typically intended to be an intensely practical affair, concerned with an alchemy of the libido that would convert it from a giver of death to a bestower of immortality. It is the sexual fire that stokes the alchemical transformation wherein the cooking pot is the body and the cooking oil is a distillation from sexual fluids. The strength of this traditional aspiration to sublimate sexuality into spirituality, semen into the elixir *soma,* varies in different regions with different castes. Yet though only small sections of Indian society may act on this aspiration, it is a well-known theory subscribed to by most Hindus, including non-literate villagers. In its most popular form, the Hindu theory of sublimation goes something like this.

Physical strength and mental power have their source in *virya*, a word that stands for both sexual energy and semen. Virya, in fact, is identical with the essence of maleness. Virya can either move downward in sexual intercourse, where it is emitted in its gross physical form as semen, or it can move upward through the spinal chord and into the brain, in its subtle form known as *ojas.* Hindus regard the downward movement of sexual energy and its emission as semen as enervating, a debilitating waste of vitality and essential energy. Of all emotions, it is said, lust throws the physical system into the greatest chaos, with every violent passion destroying millions of red blood cells. Indian metaphysical physiology maintains that food is converted into semen in a 30-day period by successive transformations (and refinements) through blood, flesh, fat, bone, and marrow till semen is distilled-40 drops of blood producing one drop of semen. Each ejaculation involves a loss of half an ounce of semen, which is equivalent to the vitality produced by the consumption of 60 pounds of food.

In another similar calculation with pedagogic intent, each act of copulation is equivalent to an energy expenditure of 24 hours of concentrated mental activity or 72 hours of hard physical labour.[64] Gandhi is merely reiterating these popular ideas when he says that

Once the idea, that the only and grand function of the sexual organ is generation, possesses men and women, union for any other purpose they will hold as criminal waste of the vital fluid, and consequent excitement caused to men and women as an equally criminal waste of precious energy. It is now easy to understand why the scientists of old have put such great value upon its strong transmutation into the highest form of energy for the benefit of society.[65]

If, on the other hand, semen is retained, converted into ojas and moved upwards by the observance of *brahmacharya*, it becomes a source of spiritual life rather than cause of physical decay. Longevity, creativity, physical and mental vitality are enhanced by the conservation of semen; memory, will power, inspiration—scientific and artistic—all derive from the observation of brahmacharya. In fact, if unbroken (*akhanda*) brahmacharya in thought, word, and deed can be observed for twelve years, the aspirant will obtain moksha spontaneously.

These ideas on semen and celibacy, I have emphasized above, are a legacy of Indian culture and are shared, so to speak, by Hindu saints and sinners alike. Indeed, the very first published case history in Indian psychoanalytic literature sounds like a parody of Gandhi.

The patient is a married young man and is the father of several children. He is of religious bent and his ideal in life is to attain what has been called in Hindu literature *Jivanmukti*, i.e., a state of liberation from worldly bondages and a perfect freedom from all sorts of passions whether bodily or mental. The possibility of the existence of such a state and of its attainment is never doubted by the patient as he says he has implicit faith in the Hindu scriptures which assert that the realization of *brahma* or supreme entity, results in such a liberation. (He believes) … that the only thing he has to do is to abstain from sex of all sorts and liberation will come to him as a sort of reward. … Since one pleasure leads to another it is desirable to shun all pleasures in life lest they should lead to sex. The patient is against forming any attachment whether it be with his wife or children or friend or any inanimate object. He is terribly upset sometimes when he finds that in spite of his ideal of no-attachment and no-sex, lascivious thoughts of the most vulgar nature and uncontrollable feelings of love and attraction arise in his mind. … In spite of his deep reverence for Hindu gods and goddesses filthy sexual ideas of an obsessional nature come into his mind when he bows before these images.[66]

The 'raising of the seed upwards,' then, is a strikingly familiar image in the Indian psycho-philosophical schools of self realization commonly clumped under the misleading label of 'mysticism.' As Wendy O'Flaherty remarks: 'So pervasive is the concept of semen being raised up to the head that popular versions of the philosophy believe that semen originates there.'[67] The concept is even present in the *Kamasutra*, the textbook of eroticism and presumably a subverter of ascetic ideals, where the successful lover is not someone who is overly passionate but one who has controlled, stilled his senses through brahmacharya and meditation.[68] Indian mythology, too, is replete with stories in which the gods, threatened by a human being who is progressing towards immortality by accruing immense capacities through celibacy and meditation, send a heavenly nymph to seduce the ascetic (even the trickling down of a single drop of sexual fluid counting as a fatal lapse), and thereby reduce him to the common human, carnal denominator.

Of course, given the horrific imagery of sexuality as cataclysmic depletion, no people can procreate with any sense of joyful abandon unless they develop a good deal of scepticism, if not an open defiance, in relation to the sexual prescription and ideals of the 'cultural superego.' The relief at seeing the ascetic's pretensions humbled by the opulent charms of a heavenly seductress is not only that of the gods but is equally shared by the mortals who listen to the myth or see it enacted in popular dance and folk drama. The ideals of celibacy are then simultaneously subscribed to and scoffed at. Whereas, on the one hand, there are a number of sages in the Indian tradition (Gandhi is only the latest one to join this august assemblage), who are admired for their successful celibacy and the powers it brought them, there are, on the other hand, also innumerable folktales detailing the misadventures of randy ascetics. In the more dignified myths, even the Creator is unable to sustain his chastity and is laid low by carnality.

The heavenly nymph Mohini fell in love with the Lord of Creation, Brahma. After gaining the assistance of Kama, the god of love, she went to Brahma and danced before him, revealing her body to him in order to entice him, but Brahma remained without passion. Then Kama struck Brahma with an arrow. Brahma wavered and felt desire, but after a moment he gained control. Brahma said to Mohini, go away, Mother, your efforts are wasted here. I know your intention, and I am not suitable for your work. The scripture says, 'Ascetics must avoid all women, especially prostitutes.' I am incapable of doing anything that the Vedas consider despicable. You are a sophisticated woman, look for a sophisticated young man, suitable for your work, and there will be virtue in your union. But I am an old man, an ascetic Brahmin; what pleasure can I find in a prostitute? Mohini laughed and said to him, 'A man who refuses to make love to a woman who is tortured by desire—he is an eunuch. Whether a man be a householder or ascetic or lover, he must not spurn a woman who approaches him, or he will go to Hell. Come now and make love to me in some private place,' and as she said this she pulled at Brahma's garment. Then the sages bowed to Brahma, 'How is it that Mohini, the best of celestial prostitutes, is in your presence?' Brahma said, to conceal his shame, 'She danced and sang for a long time and then when she was tired she came here like a young girl to her father.' But the sages laughed for they knew the whole secret, and Brahma laughed too.[69]

The piece of gossip that Gandhi 'slept with naked women in his old age' has therefore resounding echoes in the Indian cultural tradition. It arouses complex emotions in both the purveyor or and the listener, namely a malicious relief together with an aching disappointment that he may indeed have done so.

The ultimate if ironic refinement of celibacy is found in the Tantric version, where the aspirant is trained and enjoined to perform the sexual act itself without desire and the 'spilling of the seed,' thus divorcing the sexual impulse from human physiology and any conscious or unconscious mental representation of it. The impulse, it is believed, stirs up the semen in this ritual (and unbelievably passionless) sexual act and evokes energetic forces that can be re-channelled upwards. This and other Tantric techniques were familiar to Gandhi, whose own deeply held religious persuasion, Vaishnavism, was pervaded by many such Tantric notions. On the one hand, as we have seen, Gandhi often sounds like Chaitanya, the fifteenth century 'father' of north Indian Vaishnavism, who rejected a disciple for paying attention to a woman, saying: 'I can never again look upon the face of an ascetic who associates with women. The senses are hard to control, and seek to fix themselves on worldly things. Even the wooden image of a woman has the power to steal the mind of a sage. ...[70] On the other hand, however, Gandhi in his sexual experiments seems to be following the examples set by other famous Vaishnavas like Ramananda and Viswanatha. Ramananda, Chaitanya's follower and companion, used to take two beautiful young temple prostitutes into a lonely garden where he would oil their bodies, bathe, and dress them while himself remaining 'unaffected.'[71] The philosopher Viswanatha, it is said, went to lie with his young wife at the command of his guru: 'He lay with her on the bed, but Viswanatha was transformed, and he did not touch her, as it had been his custom to do. He lay with his wife according to the instructions of his guru ... and thus he controlled his senses.'[72]

There are germs of truth in the signal importance Indian cultural tradition attaches to sexuality. The notion, arising from this emphasis, that sexual urges amount to a creative fire—not only for procreation but, equally, in self creation—is indeed compelling. Further, a tradition that does not reduce sexual love to copulation but seeks to elevate it into a celebration, even a ritual that touches the partners with a sense of the sacred, and where orgasm is experienced as 'a symbolic blessing of man by his ancestors and by the nature of things,' is certainly sympathetic.[73] My concern here has to do with the concomitant strong anxiety in India surrounding the ideas of the 'squandering of the sperm' and 'biological self sacrifice.' Such ideas and the fantasies they betray cannot help but heighten an ambivalence towards women that verges on misogyny and phobic avoidance. As for self realization through renunciation of sexual love, I would tend to side with Thomas Mann when he observes:

> It is undeniable that human dignity realizes itself in the two sexes, male and female; so that when one is neither one nor the other, one stands outside the human pale and whence then can human dignity come? Efforts to sustain it are worthy of respect, for they deal with the spiritual, and thus, let us admit in honour, with the preeminently human. But truth demands the hard confession that thought and the spirit come badly off, in the long run, against nature. How little can the precepts of civilization avail against the dark, deep, silent knowledge of the flesh! How little it lets itself be taken in by the spirit![74]

How would Freud, who in his mid-life also chose to become celibate, have regarded Gandhi's celibacy and its intended efficacy? In general, Freud was understandably sceptical about the possibility that sexual abstinence could help to build energetic men of action, original thinkers, or bold reformers. Yet he also saw such attempts at the sublimation of 'genital libido' in relative terms:

> The relationship between the amount of sublimation possible and the amount of sexual activity necessary naturally varies very much from person to person and even from one calling to another. An abstinent artist is hardly conceivable; but an abstinent young savant is certainly no rarity. The latter can, by his self restraint, liberate forces for his studies; while the former probably finds his artistic achievements powerfully stimulated by his sexual experience.[75]

It is quite conceivable that Freud would have conceded the possibility of successful celibacy to a few extraordinary people of genuine originality with a self-abnegating sense of mission or transcendent purpose. In other words, he would have agreed with the Latin dictum that 'what is allowed to Jove is forbidden to the ox'. The psychoanalytic question is, then, not of sublimation but why Gandhi found phallic desire so offensive that he must, so to speak, tear it out by the very roots.

Some of Gandhi's uneasiness with phallic desire has to do with his feeling that genital love is an accursed and distasteful prerogative of the father. In his autobiography, in spite of expressing many admirable filial sentiments, Gandhi suspects his father of being 'oversexed' since he married for the fourth time when he was over forty and Putlibai, Gandhi's mother, was only eighteen. In his fantasy, we would suggest, Gandhi saw his young mother as the innocent victim of a powerful old male's lust to which the child could only be an anguished and helpless spectator, unable to save the beloved caretaker from the violation of her person and the violence done to her body. In later life, Gandhi would embrace the cause wherein the marriage of old men with young girls was adamantly opposed with great zeal. He wrote articles with such titles as 'Marriage of Old and Young or Debauchery?' and exhorted his correspondents who reported such incidents to fight this practice. The older men he respected and took as his models were those who shared his revulsion with genital sexuality. These were the men who (like Tolstoy and Raichandra) had sought to transform sexual passion into a more universal religious quest or (like Ruskin) into a moral and aesthetic fervour.

If phallic desire was the violent and tumultuous 'way of the fathers,' genital abstinence, its surrender, provided the tranquil, peaceful path back to the mother. Here Gandhi was not unlike St Augustine, who, too, inwardly beheld celibacy garbed in soothing, maternal imagery:

> … there appeared unto me the chaste dignity of Continence, serene, yet not relaxedly gay, honestly alluring me to come and doubt not; and stretching forth to receive and embrace me, her holy hands full of multitudes of good examples; there were so many young men and maidens here, a multitude of youth and every age, grave widows and aged virgins; and Continence herself in all, not barren, but a fruitful mother of children of joys …[76]

More specifically, the psychobiographical evidence we have reviewed above is compelling that Gandhi's relationships with women are dominated by the unconscious fantasy of maintaining an idealized relationship with the maternal body. This wished-for oneness with the mother is suffused with nurturance and gratitude, mutual adoration and affirmation, without a trace of desire which divides and bifurcates. Replete with wishes for fusion and elimination of differences and limits, Gandhi 'perceived' sexual desire, *both* of the mother and the child, as the single biggest obstacle to the preservation of this illusion. Many of his attitudes, beliefs, and actions with regard to women can then be understood as defensive manoeuvres against the possibility of this perception rising to surface awareness.

Since the mother is a woman, a first step in the defensive operations is to believe that women are not, or only minimally, sexual beings. 'I do not believe that woman is prey to sexual desire to the same extent as man. It is easier for her than for man to exercise self-restraint,'[77] is an opinion often repeated in his writings. Reflecting on his own experiences with Kasturbai, he asserts that 'There was never want of restraint on the part of my wife. Very often she would show restraint, but she rarely resisted me, although she showed disinclination very often.'[78] Whereas he associates male sexuality with unheeding, lustful violence, female sexuality, where it exists, is a passive, suffering acceptance of the male onslaught. This, we must again remember, is only at the conscious level. Unconsciously, his perception of masculine violence and feminine passivity seem to be reversed, as evident in the imagery of the descriptions of his few erotic encounters with women. In his very first adolescent confrontation, he is struck 'dumb and blind,' while the woman is confident and aggressive; in England, he is trembling like a frightened wild animal who has just escaped the (woman) hunter.

The solution to the root problem between the sexes is then, not a removal of the social and legal inequalities suffered by women—though Gandhi was an enthusiastic champion of women's rights—but a thoroughgoing desexualization of the male–female relationship, in which women must take the lead. 'If they will only learn to say "no" to their husbands when they approach them carnally. … If a wife says to her husband: "No, I do not want it," he will make no trouble. But she has not been taught. … I want women to learn the primary right of resistance.'[79]

Besides de-sexing the woman, another step in the denial of her desire is her idealization (especially of the Indian woman) as nearer to a purer divine state and thus an object of worship and adoration. That is why a woman does not need to renounce the world in the last stage of life to contemplate God, as is prescribed for the man in the ideal Hindu life cycle. 'She sees Him always. She has no need of any other school to prepare her for Heaven than marriage to a man and care of her children.'[80] Woman is also

the incarnation of *Ahimsa. Ahimsa* means infinite love, which, again means infinite capacity for suffering. Who but woman, the mother of man shows this capacity in the largest measure? Let her transfer that love to the whole of humanity, let her forget she ever was, or can be, the object of man's lust. And she will occupy her proud position by the side of the man as his mother, maker and silent leader.[81]

Primarily seeing the mother in the woman and idealizing motherhood is yet another way of denying feminine eroticism. When Millie Polak, a female associate in the Phoenix ashram in South Africa, questioned his idealization of motherhood, saying that being a mother does not make a woman wise, Gandhi extolled mother-love as one of the finest aspects of love in human life. His imagery of motherhood is of infants suckling on breasts with inexhaustible supplies of milk. For example, in a letter explaining why the *Gita*, the sacred book of the Hindus, is called Mother, he rhapsodizes,

It has been likened to the sacred cow, the giver of all desires (sic!). Hence Mother. Well, that immortal Mother gives all the milk we need for spiritual sustenance, if we would but approach her as babies seeking and sucking it from her. She is capable of yielding milk to her millions of babies from her exhaustless udder.

In doing the Harijan (untouchable) work in the midst of calumny, misrepresentations and apparent disappointments, her lap comforts me and keeps me from falling into the Slough of Despond.[82]

Whereas desexualizing, idealizing, and perceiving only the 'milky' mother in the woman is one part of his defensive bulwark which helped in preserving the illusion of unity with the maternal body intact, the other part consists of efforts at renouncing the gift of sexual desire, abjuring his own masculinity. Here we must note that the Hindu Vaishnava culture, in which Gandhi grew up and in which he remained deeply rooted, not only provides a sanction for man's feminine strivings, but raises these strivings to the level of a religious-spiritual quest. In devotional Vaishnavism, Lord Krishna alone is the male and all devotees, irrespective of their sex, are female. Gandhi's statement that he had mentally become a woman or that he envied women—and that there is as much reason for a man to wish that he was born a woman as for women to do otherwise—thus struck many responsive chords in his audience.

If Gandhi had had his way, there would be no art or poetry celebrating woman's beauty.

I am told that our literature is full of even an exaggerated apotheosis of women. Let me say that it is an altogether wrong apotheosis. Let me place one simple fact before you. In what light do you think of them when you proceed to write about them? I suggest that before you put your pens to paper think of woman as your own mother, and I assure you the chastest literature will flow from your pens, even like the beautiful rain from heaven which waters the thirsty earth below. Remember that a woman was your mother, before a woman became your wife.[83]

Although Gandhi's wished-for feminization was defensive in origin, we cannot deny the development of its adaptive aspects. Others, most notably Erik Erikson, have commented upon Gandhi's more or less conscious explorations of the maternal stance and feminine perspective in his actions.[84] In spite of a welter of public demands on his time, we know of the motherly care he could extend to the personal lives of his followers, and the anxious concern he displayed about their health and well-being, including solicitous inquiries about the state of their daily bowel movements.[85] We also know of the widening of these maternal–feminine ways—teasing, testing, taking suffering upon oneself, and so on—in the formulation of his political style and as elements of his campaigns of militant nonviolence.

We have seen that for Gandhi, the cherished oneness with the maternal-feminine could not always be maintained and was often threatened by the intrusion of phallic desire. His obsession with food at these times, evident in the letters and writings, not only represented a preparation for erecting physiological barriers against desire, but also the strengthening of his psychological defences, and thus a reinforcement of his spiritual armamentarium. In other words, in his preoccupation with food (and elimination), in his persistent investment of edible physical substances with psychological qualities, Gandhi plays out the 'basic oral fantasy', as described by the psychoanalyst Donald Winnicott—'when hungry I think of food, when I eat I think of taking food in. I think of what I like to keep inside and I think of what I want to be rid of and I think of getting rid of it'—whose underlying theme is of union with the mother. His experiments with various kinds of food and a reduction in its intake—in his later years, he abjured milk completely so as not to eroticize his viscera—appear as part of an involuted and intuitive effort to recover and maintain his merger with his mother.

Gandhi's relationship with women and the passions they aroused are, then, more complex than what he reveals in his own impassioned confession. Nor does recourse to traditional Hindu explanations and prescriptions for their 'diagnosis and cure' reflect adequately the depths of the inner life in which his desires found their wellsprings. Beset by conflicts couched in moral terms familiar to Christian and classical psychoanalyst alike, he struggled with the yearnings aroused by the goddess of longing besides the passions provoked by the god of desire. Or, to use a well-known Indian metaphor in which a woman is said to have two breasts, one for her child, another for her husband, Gandhi's unconscious effort to shift from the one breast to the other—from man to child—was not always successful. He was a man in spite of himself. We know that the sensuality derived from the deeply felt oneness with a maternal world, a sensuality that challenges death, energized Gandhi's person, impelled his transcendent endeavours, and advanced him on the road to a freedom of spirit from which India, as well as the world, has profited. Yet we have seen that throughout his life, there were profound periods of emotional turmoil when this original and ultimately illusory connection broke down, emptying him of all inner 'goodness' and 'power'.

Notes and References

1 For psychoanalytic perspectives on autobiography, see Steele, Robert, 1986, 'Deconstructing Histories: Toward a Systematic Criticism of Psychological Narratives', in T.R. Sarbin (ed.), *Narrative Psychology*, New York: Praeger. See also Erikson, Erik H., Summer 1968, 'In Search of Gandhi: On the Nature of Psychohistorical Evidence', *Daedalus*.

2 For a discussion of Nabokov's *Speak, Memory*, see Kakar, Sudhir and John Ross, 1987, *Tales of Love, Sex, and Danger*, London: Unwin Hyman, ch. 8.

3 Gandhi, M.K., 1927, *Satya no Prayoga athva Atma-Katha* (translated by Mahadev Desai as *The Story of My Experiments with Truth)*, Ahmedabad: Navjivan Prakashan Mandir, p. 10; henceforth referred to as *Autobiography.*

4 Ibid., p. 31.

5 Naipaul, V.S., 1976, *India: A Wounded Civilization*, New York: Knopf, pp. 102–6.

6 Gandhi, *Autobiography*, p. 75.

7 Ibid., p. 69.

8 Ramanujan, A.K., 1982, 'Hanchi: A Kannada Cinderella', in A. Dundes (ed.), *Cinderella: A Folklore Casebook*, New York: Garland Publishing, p. 272.

9 Gandhi, M.K., 1960, *Bibi Amtussalam ke nam patra* [*Letters to Bibi Amtussalam*], Ahmedabad: Navjivan, p. 70.

10 Gandhi, *Autobiography*, p. 91.

11 Ibid, p. 205.

12 Pyarelal, *Mahatma Gandhi: The First Phase*, Bombay: Sevak Prakashan, p. 213.

13 Ibid, p. 207.

14 Gandhi, M.K., 1958, *The Collected Works of Mahatma Gandhi*, Delhi: Publication Division, Government of India, vol. 3, letters of 30 June 1906 to Chaganlal Gandhi and H.V. Vohra, pp. 352–4; henceforth referred to as *Collected Works.*

15 Ibid, pp. 208–9.

16 Gandhi, *Collected Works*, vol. 5, p. 56.

17 Gandhi, M.K., 1943, *To the Women*, Karachi: Hingorani, pp. 49–50, 52.

18 Gandhi, *To the Women*, p. 194.

19 Gandhi, M.K., 1968, 'Yervada Mandir', in *Selected Works*, vol. 4, Ahmedabad: Navjivan, p. 220.

20 Ibid.

21 Gandhi, 'Hind Swaraj,' in *Collected Works.*

22 Polak, Millie G., 1949, *Mr. Gandhi: The Man*, Bombay: Vora & Co., pp. 63–4.

23 Gandhi, 'Yervada Mandir', p. 223.

24 St Augustine, 1949, *The Confessions* (translated by E.R. Pusey), New York: Modern Library, p. 227.

25 Ibid, p. 228.

26 Gandhi, *Autobiography*, p. 324.

27 Ibid, p. 210.

28 Ibdi., p. 501.

29 Ibid., p. 24.

30 St Augustine, *Confessions*, p. 162.

31 'Speech on the Birth Centenary of Tolstoy', 10 September 1928, in Gandhi, *Collected Works*, vol. 37, p. 258.

32 Ibid., p. 265.

33 Gandhi, *Autobiography*, in Gandhi, *Collected Works*, vol. 37, p. 209.

34 Gandhi, *Collected Works*, vol. 37, p. 258.

35 'Letter to Harjivan Kotak', in Gandhi, *Collected Works*, vol. 36, p. 378.

36 Gandhi, 'Ek Tyag', in *Harijanbandhu*, 22.9.35.

37 Gandhi, M.K., 1960, *Kumari Premaben Kantak ke nam patra* [*Letters to Premaben Kantak*], Ahmedabad: Navjivan, pp. 260–2 (my translation).

38 The best eyewitness account of Gandhi's Bengal period is by N.K. Bose, Gandhi's temporary secretary, who was both a respectful follower and a dispassionate observer; see Bose, 1953, *My Days with Gandhi*, Calcutta: Nishana.

39 Ibid., p. 52.

40 Ibid., p. 189.

41 In his *Key to Health*, rewritten in 1942 in the middle of another depressive phase following the widespread violence of the 'Quit India' movement and the death of his wife in prison, Gandhi had hinted at this kind of self-testing: 'Some of my experiments have not reached a stage when they might be placed before the public with advantage. I hope to do so some day if they succeed to my satisfaction. Success might make the attainment of *brahmacharya* comparatively easier.' See *Selected Works*, vol. 4, p. 432. For a compassionate and insightful discussion of these experiments, see also Erikson, Erik H., 1969, *Gandhi's Truth*, New York: Norton, p. 404.

42 Gandhi, *Kumari Premaben Kantak ke nam patra*, p. 16.

43 Ibid., p. 19.

44 Ibid., p. 188.

45 Ibid.

46 Ibid., p. 39.

47 Ibid.

48 Ibid.

49 Ibid.

50 Ibid., p. 190.

51 Ibid., p. 151.

52 Ibid., p. 173.

53 Ibid., p. 369.

54 See Mira Behn (ed.), 1949, *Bapu's Letters to Mira* (1924–48), Ahmedabad: Navjivan and 1960, *The Spirit's Pilgrimage*, London: Longman.

55 Behn (ed.), *Bapu's Letters to Mira*, pp. 27–8.

56 Greenson, R., 1967, *The Technique and Practice of Psychoanalysis*, New York: International University Press, pp. 338–41.

57 See Bergman, Martin S., 1985–6, 'Transference Love and Love in Real Life', *International Journal of Psychoanalytic Psychotherapy* (edited by J.M. Ross), 11, pp. 27–45.

58 Behn (ed.), *Bapu's Letters to Mira*, p. 42.

59 Ibid.

60. Ibid., p. 43.

61 Ibid., p. 71.

62 Ibid., p. 88.

63 Ibid., p. 166.

64 For an elaborate description of some of these popular psychological ideas in English, see Swami Sivananda, 1974, *Mind: Its Mysteries and Control*, Sivanandanagar Divine Life Society, ch. 28, and Swami Narayanananda, 1965, *The Mysteries of Man, Mind, and Mind-Functions*, Rishikesh: Universal Yoga Trust, ch. 19.

65 Gandhi, *To the Women*, p. 71.

66 Bose, G., 1947, 'All or None Attitude in Sex', *Samiksa*, 1, p. 14.

67 O'Flaherty, Wendy, 1980, *Women, Androgynes, and Other Mythical Beasts*, Chicago: University of Chicago Press, p. 45.

68 See O'Flaherty, Wendy, 1973, *Asceticism and Eroticism in the Mythology of Siva*, London: Oxford University Press, p. 55.

69 B*rahmavaivarta Purana*, 4.31, 4.32, 1.20, 4.33, 1.76; English translation abridged from O'Flaherty, *Asceticism and Eroticism*, p. 51.

70 Cited in Dimock, Edward C. Jr., 1966, *The Place of the Hidden Moon*, Chicago: University of Chicago Press, p. 154.

71 Ibid, p. 54.

72 Ibid, p. 156.

73 See Gandhi, Ramchandra, 1981, *Brahmacharya*, Department of Philosophy, Univexsity of Hyderabad, unpublished, p. 26.

74 Mann, Thomas, 1959, *Joseph and his Brothers*, London: Seeker and Warburg, p. 719.

75 Freud, Sigmund, 1908, 'Civilized Sexual Morality and Modern Nervousness', *Standard Edition*, vol. 9, p. 197.

76 St Augustine, *Confessions*, p. 165.

77 Gandhi, *To the Women*, p. 81.

78 Ibid., p. 60.

79 Ibid., p. 57.

80 Polak, *Mr. Gandhi*, p. 34.

81 Gandhi, *To the Women*, pp. 28–9.

82 Behn (ed.), *Bapu's Letters to Mira*, p. 141.

83 Gandhi, *To the Women*, p. 102.

84 Erikson, *Gandhi's Truth.*

85 Mehta, Ved, 1977, *Mahatma Gandhi and his Apostles,* New Delhi: Indian Book Co., p. 13.

86 Winnicott, D.W., 1958, 'Appetite and Emotional Disorder', in *Collected Papers*, London: Tavistock Publications, p. 34.

Lovers in the Dark*

WHEN I WAS GROWING UP in the 1940s, going to the cinema, at least in the Punjab and at least among the middle and upper classes, was regarded as slightly dissolute, if not outright immoral, and the habit was considered especially dangerous to the growing sensibilities of young children. Of course, not all films were equally burdened with disapproval. Like everything else in India—from plants to human beings—there was (and still is) a strict hierarchical classification. In the movie caste system, stunt films, the Indian version of Kung Fu movies, were the low-caste *Shudras* at the lowest rung of the ladder while the *Brahmin* 'mythological' and the *Kshatriya* 'historical' vied for supremacy at the top. The only time I was admitted to the owner's box of Prabhat Talkies—the cinema owned by a grand-uncle in Lahore—was to see an eminently forgettable mythological called *Kadambari.* In childhood, stunt films were my favourite, although my taste was quite catholic, consisting as it did of indiscriminate adoration. With the complicity of a friendly doorman who doubled as an odd job man in my grand-uncle's adjoining house, I was in the fortunate position of being able to indulge my secret passion for films whenever we visited Lahore. I use the word 'passion' literally and not as a metaphor, since my craving for movies was insatiable and my consumption equally remarkable; I saw *Ratan* sixteen times, *Shikari*

*From *Intimate Relations: Exploring Indian Sexuality,* Delhi: Viking-Penguin, 1989; University of Chicago Press, 1990.

fourteen times, and even *Kadambari* three times after that first viewing from the owner's box.

I remember my movie-going with a nostalgia which cloaks childhood events, at least the good ones, in a unique glow of permanence and ephemerality. In the anonymity of a darkness pierced by the flickering light which gave birth to a magical, yet familiar, world on the screen, I was no longer a small boy but a part of the envied world of adulthood, although I sensed its rituals and mysteries but dimly. I always joined in the laughter that followed a risqué comment, even if its exact meaning escaped me. I, too, would hold my breath in the hushed silence that followed a particularly well-enacted love scene and surreptitiously try to whistle with the O of the thumb and the index finger under the tongue, in imitation of the wolf whistles that greeted the obligatory scene in which the heroine fell into the water or was otherwise drenched. Recently, when in *Satyam Shivam Sundaram* Miss Zeenat Aman's considerable charms were revealed through her wet and clinging saree at the receiving end of a waterfall, I felt grateful to the world of Hindi movies for providing continuity in an unstable and changing world. When I was a child, the movies brought the vistas of a desirable adulthood tantalizingly close; as an adult, I find that they help to keep the road to childhood open.

I have described my engagement with the world of Hindi films at some length, not in order to claim any vast personal experience or specialized knowledge but to stress the fact of an enduring empathic connection with the world of Indian popular cinema. Today, this cinema, which draws upon images and symbols from the traditional regional cultures and combines them with more modern western themes, is the major shaper of an emerging, pan-Indian popular culture. Though its fixed repertoire of plots, with which the audience is presumably thoroughly familiar, has striking parallels with traditional folk theatre, the popular culture represented by the cinema goes beyond both classical and folk elements even while it incorporates them.

The appeal of the film is directed to an audience so diverse that it transcends social and spatial categories. Watched by almost 15 million people every day, popular cinema's values and language have long since crossed urban boundaries to enter the folk culture of the rural-based population, where they have begun to influence Indian ideas of the good life and the ideology of social, family, and love relationships. The folk dance of a region or a particular musical form such as the devotional *bhajan*, after it has crossed the portals of a Bombay or Madras studio, is transmuted into a film dance or a film bhajan by the addition of musical and dance motifs from other regions as perhaps also from the West, and is then relayed back in full technicolour and stereophonic sound to decisively alter the original. Similarly, film situations, dialogue, and decor have begun to colonize folk theatre. Even the traditional iconography of statues and pictures for religious worship is paying homage to film representations of gods and goddesses.[1]

My own approach to popular cinema is to think of film as a collective fantasy, a group daydream. By 'collective' and 'group' I do not mean that Hindi film is an expression of a mythic collective unconscious or of something called a group mind. Instead, I see the cinema as the primary vehicle for shared fantasies of a vast number of people living on the Indian subcontinent who are both culturally and psychologically linked. I do not use 'fantasy' in the ordinary sense of the word, with its popular connotations of whimsy, eccentricity, or triviality, but as another name for that world of imagination which is fuelled by desire and which provides us with an alternative world where we can continue our longstanding quarrel with reality. Desire and fantasy are, of course, inexorably linked. Aristotle's dictum that there can be no desire without fantasy contains even more truth in reverse. Fantasy is the *mise-en-scène* of desire, its dramatization in a visual form.

The origins of fantasy lie in the unavoidable conflict between many of our desires, formulated as demands on the environment (especially on people), and the environment's inability or unwillingness to fulfil our desires, where it does not proscribe them altogether. The power of fantasy, then, comes to our rescue by extending or withdrawing the desires beyond what is possible or reasonable, by remarking the past and inventing a future. Fantasy, the 'stuff that dreams are made of,' is the bridge between desire and reality, spanning the chasm between what is asked for and what is granted. It well deserves psychoanalyst Robert Stoller's paean as 'the vehicle of hope, healer of trauma, protector from reality, concealer of truth, fixer of identity, restorer of tranquility, enemy of fear, and sadness, cleanser of the soul.'[2] Hindi films, perhaps more than the cinema of many other countries, are fantasy in this special sense.

The sheer volume of unrelieved fantasy in one film after another is indeed overwhelming, and it is disquieting to reflect that this exclusive preoccupation with magical explanations and fairytale solutions for life's problems could be an expression of a deep-seated need in large sections of Indian society. Some may even consider such a thoroughgoing denial of external reality in Indian cinema to be a sign of morbidity, especially since one cannot make the argument that fantasy in films fulfils the need for escapism of those suffering from grinding poverty. In the first place, it is not the poor who constitute the bulk of the Indian film clientele. In the second, one does not know the cinema of any other country which, even in the worst periods of economic deprivation and political uncertainty, dished out such uniformly fantastic fare. Neither German cinema during the economic crisis of the 1920s nor Japanese cinema in the aftermath of the Second World War elevated fantasy to such an overwhelming principle. And if one considers that neorealism even flourished in Italy during the economic chaos following the Allied victory, then one must acknowledge that economic conditions alone cannot explain the fantasia permeating Indian films.

The reason for the ubiquity of fantasy in the Hindi cinema, I suspect, lies in the realm of cultural psychology rather than in the domain of socioeconomic conditions. Now, as in other cultures, we, too, have our film addicts. These are the unfortunate people who are pressed in childhood to view reality in an adult way and now need the fantasy of the film world to fill up the void left by a premature deprivation of magic in early life. Leaving aside this group, no sane Indian believes that Hindi films depict the world realistically, although I must admit I often feel that our willingness to suspend disbelief is relatively greater than in many other cultures. This is not because the thought processes of Indians are fantasy-ridden. The propensity to state received opinion and belief as observation, to look for confirmation of belief rather than be open to disturbing new knowledge, to generally think in a loose, associative rather than a rigorous and sequential way, is neither Indian, American, Chinese, Japanese, or German, but common to most human beings. However, I would hypothesize, without passing any value judgement, that relatively speaking, in India the child's world of magic is not as far removed from adult consciousness as it may be in some other cultures. Because of a specific thrust of culture and congruent child-rearing practices which I have described in detail elsewhere, the Indian ego is flexible enough to regress temporarily to childhood modes without feeling threatened or engulfed.[3] Hindi films seem to provide this regressive haven for a vast number of our people.

If, as I have indicated above, I regard the Indian cinema audience not only as the reader but also as the real author of the text of Hindi films, what is the role played by their ostensible creators—the producers, directors, scriptwriters, music directors, and so on? In my view, their functions are purely instrumental and akin to that of a publisher who chooses, edits, and publishes a particular text from a number of submitted manuscripts. The quest for the comforting sound of busy cash registers at the box office ensures that the filmmakers select and develop a daydream which is not idiosyncratic. They must intuitively appeal to those concerns of the audience which are shared; if they do not, the film's appeal is bound to be disastrously limited. As with pornography, the filmmakers have to create a work which is singular enough to fascinate and excite, and general enough to excite many. Moreover, in their search for the 'hit', the ten to fifteen films out of the roughly 700 produced every year which evoke the most enthusiastic response, the filmmakers repeat and vary the daydreams as they seek to develop them into more and more nourishing substitutes for reality. Under the general rubric of fantasy, which can range all the way from the most primal images in dreams to the rationalized misinterpretations of reality in everyday life, the Hindi film is perhaps closest to the daydream. Indeed, the visual landscape of these films has a strong daydream quality in that it is not completely situated outside reality but is clearly linked to it. As Arjun Appadurai and Carol Breckenridge point out, while the landscape of the popular film contains places, social types, topological features, and situations which are reminiscent of ordinary experience, these elements are transformed or transposed so as to create a subtly fantastic milieu.[4] Even film speech is reminiscent of real speech. Thus, the frequently heard admonition in 'Indinglish,' 'Don't *maro filmi dialogues, yaar* (Don't spout dialogues from films at me, friend)', is often addressed to someone expressing highly inflated sentiments of friendship, love, or hostility which typify exchanges between the characters of Indian cinema.

Like the adult daydream, the Hindi film emphasizes the central features of fantasy—the fulfilment of wishes, the humbling of competitors, and the destruction of enemies. The stereotyped twists and turns of the film plot ensure the repetition of the very message that makes, for instance, the fairytale so deeply satisfying to children—namely, that the struggle against difficulties in life is unavoidable, but if one faces life's hardships and its many, often unjust impositions with courage and steadfastness, one will eventually emerge victorious.[5] At the conclusion of both films and fairytales, parents are generally happy and proud, the princess is won, and either the villains are ruefully contrite or their battered bodies satisfactorily litter the landscape. Evil in film, too, follows the same course it does in fairytales; it may be temporarily in ascendance or usurp the hero's legitimate rights, but its failure and defeat are inevitable. Like the temptations of badness for a child who is constantly forced to be good, evil in Hindi cinema is not quite without its attractions of sensual licence and narcissistic pleasure in the unheeding pursuit of the appetites. It is usually the unregenerate villain who gets to savour the pleasures of drinking wine and the companionship, willing or otherwise, of sexy and attractive women.

Another feature common to both Hindi films and fairytales is the oversimplification of situations and the elimination of detail, unless the detail is absolutely essential. The characters of the film are always typical, never unique, and without the unnerving complexity of real people. The Hero and the Villain, the Heroine and Her Best Friend, the Loving Father and the Cruel Stepmother, are never ambivalent, never the mixed ticket we all are in real life. However, unlike in novels, the portrayal of characters in film is neither intended to enhance our understanding of the individual complexities of men and women nor to assist our contemplation of the human condition. Their intention is to appeal to the child within us, to arouse quick sympathies and antipathies, and thus encourage the identifications that help us to savour our fantasies more keenly.

When dogmatic rationalists dismiss Hindi films as unrealistic and complain that their plots strain credibility and their characters stretch the limits of the believable, this condescending judgement is usually based on a restricted vision of reality. To limit and reduce the real to that which can be demonstrated as factual is to exclude the domain of the psychologically real—all that is felt to be, enduringly, the actuality of one's inner life. Or, to adapt Bruno Bettelheim's observation on fairytales, Hindi films may be unreal in a rational sense but they are certainly not untrue. Their depiction of the external world may be flawed and their relevance to the external life of the viewer remote; yet, as we shall see, in their focus on the unconsciously perceived fantasy rather than the consciously perceived story, the Hindi film demonstrates a confident and sure-footed grasp of the topography of desire. The stories they tell may be trite and limited in number, with simple, recognizable meanings which on the surface reinforce rather than challenge cultural convention, yet beneath the surface, the fantasies they purvey, though equally repetitious, are not so trite and add surprising twists to the conscious social understanding of various human relationships in the culture.

Having described the relationship between Indian cinema, culture, and psyche is some detail, let me now turn to the cinema audience's internal theatre of love as they watch the images flicker by on the screen. The composite love story I seek to present here is culled largely from a score of the biggest box-office hits of the last twenty years. Since it would be impossible as well as tedious to narrate the plots of all these films, I will take as my illustrative text only one film, Raj Kapoor's *Ram*

Teri Ganga Maili (*Rama, Your Ganga Is Polluted*), the top box-office hit for the year 1986. I shall then use examples from other films to amplify and otherwise complete the prototypical love story of Hindi cinema.

Narendra, the hero of the film, is a student of a Calcutta college and the son of a rich, thoroughly corrupt businessman. His father is a close associate of Bhag Choudhary, a villainous politician, whose only daughter, Radha, is romantically interested in our young hero. Narendra, however, is unaware of Radha's feelings for him. He ignores her not-so-subtle advances and generally treats her in a friendly asexual fashion.

Narendra goes on a college trip to Gangotri, the source of the sacred river Ganges, in the Himalayan hills. He has promised to bring his doting grandmother pure Ganges water from the river's very source, since the water is polluted by the time it reaches the sea at Calcutta. He clambers down a mountainside to reach the stream, but the pitcher he has brought with him slips from his hand and rolls down the slope. As Narendra seeks to retrieve the pitcher, he is saved from falling over a cliff by a shouted warning from the heroine of the movie, Ganga. Ganga is a pretty, young girl of the hills, unspoilt and innocent, and frankly expresses her liking for the city boy. Often enough, she takes the initiative in their budding relationship. She leads him by the hand on their excursions through the mountains, barefooted and impervious to the cold, while he both stumbles and shivers. During their courtship, they sing duets in meadows full of wild flowers and frolic through streams which, of course, make Ganga's thin white sari wet and cling revealingly to her well-formed breasts. Narendra saves Ganga from being raped by one of his college friends, which deepens the girl's feelings for the boy and increases their mutual attachment.

Although Ganga has been promised in marriage to one of her own people, she decides to break the engagement and marry Narendra. The marriage ceremony is preceded by a rousing (and arousing) folk dance and is succeeded by the wedding night. While inside the room, Narendra undresses Ganga with the gravity and devotion of a priest preparing the idol of the goddess for the morning worship, Ganga's brother and her enraged ex-fiancé are engaged outside in a murderous fight which will end in both their deaths.

Narendra goes back to Calcutta, promising to send for Ganga as soon as he has informed the family of his marriage. There he discovers that his grandmother has betrothed him in his absence to Radha, the politician's daughter, a match welcomed by both the families. After many emotional scenes involving the boy and his parents, in the course of which his grandmother suffers a heart attack and eventually dies, Narendra, defying his parent's wishes, sets out for the hills to fetch Ganga. By virtue of the political influence exercised by Choudhary, he is forcibly taken off the bus by the police before he can reach her village in the hills and is brought back to Calcutta.

In the meanwhile, a letter by Narendra's grandmother to her grandson reaches Ganga, from which she learns of the family's plans for Narendra's betrothal; Ganga believes her husband now to be married to another woman. Their wedding night, however, has had consequences and Ganga gives birth to a child. Since in Hindu tradition children belong to the father, Ganga nobly decides to take the infant son to far off Calcutta and hand him over to Narendra. It is now that the perils of Ganga begin. Alighting from the bus at the foot of the hills and looking for the train station from where she can take the train to Calcutta, Ganga is instead guided to a cheap whorehouse. There she is sold to a customer who would rape her but Ganga manages to escape with the baby clutched to her breast. She then approaches an old priest for directions to the station. He, too, turns out to be lecherous. Ganga is saved from his attentions by the timely arrival of the police. Finally put on the train to Calcutta by a kindly police officer—who for a change does not try to rape her—Ganga is kidnapped on the way by a pimp who brings her to a *kotha* in Benares, a brothel whose customers are first entertained by song and dance in the traditional style of the Indian courtesan. Ganga becomes a well-known dancing girl though all the while retaining her mysterious purity, that 'purity of the Ganges which lies in a woman's heart and which makes a man attracted to her, merge into her'.

Ganga is now sold by the owner of the kotha to Choudhary who has come to Benares to find a girl to keep him company in his declining years. Choudhary, her husband's future father-in-law, installs the girl in a house in Calcutta and one day brings Narendra's father along with him to show off the girl's charms. He promises to share Ganga with him once the marriage of their children has been solemnized. On the day of the marriage, Ganga is called upon by Choudhary to entertain the wedding guests. As she sings and dances, Narendra recognizes her and without completing the marriage rites, rushes to her side. His father and especially Choudhary and his goons try to stop him but Narendra and Ganga are finally united. Together with their infant son, they go away from the corruption of a degraded older generation towards a hopeful new future.

Superficially, *Ram Teri Ganga Maili* is a syrupy tale of the eternally pure woman whose devotion and innocence triumph over the worst efforts of lustful (mostly older) males to enslave and exploit her. As the third ear is deemed essential for listening in the analytic hour, similarly the analyst may need a third eye to break up the cloying surface of the film into less obvious patterns. Unlike Shiva's third eye which destroys all reality, the Freudian one merely cracks reality's stony surface to release its inner shape of fantasy. Like the dreamer who is not only the author, producer, and director of his dream but often plays all the important leads himself, the creator–audience of the film, too, is not limited to existing within the skin of the hero or the heroine but spreads out to cover other characters. The analyst may then reassign different values to the characters of the story than what has been the dreamer's manifest intent. He will, for instance, be mindful that besides experiencing the overt pity aroused by the hapless Ganga, the audience may well be deriving secret pleasure in the sexual villainy as well as surreptitiously partaking of the masochistic delight of her ordeals. Moreover, the third eye also destroys the very identities of the film's characters, replacing them with those of a child's internal family drama. Thus Ganga's screen image, with the infant clutched perpetually to her breast, becomes the fantasized persona of the mother from a particular stage of childhood. The faces of the various villains, on the other hand, coalesce into the visage of the 'bad' aggressive father, forcing the poor mother to submit to his unspeakable desire. It is then with the third eye that we look at Indian men and women as lovers and at some of the situations and spaces of love they project on the screen.

Bearing a strong resemblance to another girl from the hills, Reshma, played by Nargis in Raj Kapoor's first film *Barsaat* four decades ago, Ganga is the latest reincarnation of the heroine who is totally steadfast in her devotion to a hero who is passive, absent, or both. Independent and carefree before being struck by the love-god Kama's flowery arrows, all that love brings her is suffering and humiliation, particularly of the sexual kind. Indeed, her suffering, like that of such legendary heroines as Laila and Sohni, seems almost a punishment for breaking social convention in daring to love freely. Rape, actual or attempted, is of course the strongest expression, the darkest image of the degradation she must undergo for her transgression.

The question of why rape is a staple feature of Indian cinema where otherwise even the kiss is taboo, why the sexual humiliation of the woman plays such a significant role in the fantasy of love, is important. That this rape is invariably a fantasy rape, without the violence and trauma of its real life counterpart, is evident in the manner of its visual representation. Villains, moustachioed or stubble-chinned, roll their eyes and stalk their female prey around locked rooms. With deep-throated growls of gloating, lasciviously muttering a variant of 'Ha! You cannot escape now', they make sharp lunges to tear off the heroine's clothes and each time come away with one more piece of her apparel. The heroine, on the other hand, retreats in pretty terror, her arms folded across her breasts to protect her disheveled modesty, pleading all the while to be spared from the fate worse than death. As in the folk theatre presentations of the scene from the Mahabharata where Dushasana is trying to undrape Draupadi, what is being enjoyed by the audience is the sadomasochistic fantasy incorporated in the defencelessness and pain of a fear-stricken woman.

Now masochism is usually defined as the seeking of pain for the sake of sexual pleasure, with the qualification that either the seeking or the pleasure, or both, are unconscious rather than conscious. The specific locus of the rape fantasy for men is the later period of childhood which I have elsewhere called the 'second birth', when the boy's earlier vision of the mother as an overwhelming feminine presence is replaced by her image, and that of the woman generally, as a weak, castrated, suffering, and humiliated being. This is less a consequence of the boy's confrontation with female reality in the Indian family setting and more a projection of what would happen to him if he sexually submitted to the father and other elder males. As the boy grows up into a man, this fantasy needs to be repressed more and more, banished into farther and farther reaches of awareness. In the cavernous darkness of the cinema hall, the fantasy may at last surface gingerly and the associated masochistic pleasure be enjoyed vicariously in the pain and subjugation of the woman with whom one secretly identifies.

The effect of the rape scene on the female part of the audience, even if the movie rape is highly stylized and eschews any pretence to reality, is more complex. On the one hand, the sexual coercion touches some of her deepest fears as a woman. On the other hand, we must note the less conscious presence of a sexual fantasy due to the fact that the raping 'baddies' of Indian cinema are very often older men on whom the woman is dependent in some critical way: employers, zamindars (landlords), and so on. The would-be rapists in *Ram Teri Ganga Maili*, apart from the anonymous brothel customer, are the priest and the powerful Choudhary, the future father-in-law of Ganga's husband. In many other movies, the face of the father behind the rapist's mask is more clearly visible. Thus in *Karz*, a box-office hit of 1979, the heroine's stepfather stages a mock rape of his stepdaughter to test the suitability of the hero as her future spouse. Wendy O'Flaherty has linked the power of this particular scene to the ancient myth in which the father–god (Brahma, Prajapati, or Daksha) attempts to rape his own daughter until she is rescued by the hero, Shiva.[7] She points out that this well-known myth is tolerated and viewed positively in Hindu texts which tell of the birth of all animal life from the incestuous union of father and daughter. I would, on the other hand—a case of cultural psychology complementing mythology—trace the woman's allurement in the fantasy of rape by the villainous father figure to many an Indian woman's adolescence. This is perhaps the most painful period of a girl's life, in which many renunciations are expected of her and where her training as an imminent daughter-in-law who must bring credit to her natal family is painfully stepped up. Psychoanalysis regularly brings up the powerful wish from this period for an intimacy with the father in which the daughter is simultaneously indulged as a little girl and treated as a young woman whose emerging womanhood is both appreciatively recognized and appropriately reacted to. In part, this is a universal fantasy among women, arising from the fact that a father often tends to withdraw from his daughter at the onset of puberty, feeling that he should no longer exhibit physical closeness, doubtless also because of the sexual feelings the daughter arouses in him. The daughter, however, learning to be at home in a woman's body and as yet insecure in her womanly role, may interpret the father's withdrawal as a proof of her feminine unattractiveness. The wished for father–daughter intimacy becomes a major fantasy in India because of the fact that in the Indian family, the father's withdrawal from his daughter is quite precipitate once she attains puberty. The daughter is completely given over to the woman's world which chooses precisely this period of inner turmoil to become increasingly harsh. The rape by the father is then the forbidden, sexual aspect of her more encompassing longing for intimacy. The fearful mask worn by the father is a projection of the daughter's own villainous desire which frees her from the guilt for entertaining it.

Narendra, the hero of the movie, is a passive, childlike character, easily daunted by his elders who put obstacles in the path of the lovers' union. He is a pale shadow of the more ubiquitous romantic hero who suffers the despair of separation or disappointment in love with a suprahuman intensity (by which I mean less that of an inconstant god than of the faithful child lover). Such a hero used to be very popular in Indian films until about twenty years ago. Since in India nothing ever disappears, whether religious cults, political parties, or mythological motifs, the romantic lover too lives on, though at present he is perhaps in the trough rather than at the crest of the wave. For my generation, however, the images of this lover, as played for example by Dilip Kumar in *Devdas* or Guru Dutt in *Pyasa*, remain unforgettable.

The Majnun–lover, as I would like to label this type after the hero of the well-known Islamic romance, has his cultural origins in a confluence of Islamic and Hindu streams. His home is as much in the Indo-Persian *ghazal* (those elegies of unhappy love where the lover bemoans the loss, the inaccessibility, or the turning away of the beloved) as in the lover's laments of separation in Sanskrit and Tamil *viraha* poetry—of which Kalidasa's *Meghaduta* (*The Cloud Messenger*) is perhaps the best known example.

Elsewhere, I have discussed the psychological origins of the Majnun-lover as part of the imperious yet vulnerable erotic wishes of infancy.[8] His is the wish for a total merger with the woman; his suffering, the wrenching wail of the infant who finds his budding self disintegrating in the mother's absence. What he seeks to rediscover and reclaim in love is what is retrospectively felt to be paradise lost—the postpartum womb of life before 'psychological birth', before the separation from the mother's anima took place. These wishes are of course part of every man's erotic being and it is only the phallic illusion of modern western man which has tended to deny them legitimacy and reality.

All soul, an inveterate coiner of poetic phrases on the sorrows and sublimity of love, the romantic lover must split off his corporeality and find it a home or, rather, an orphanage. The kotha, the traditional-style brothel, is Hindi cinema's favourite abode for the denied and discarded sexual impulses, a home for vile bodies. Sometimes replaced by the shady night club, a more directly licentious import from the West, the kotha provides the alcohol as well as the rhythmic music and dance associated with these degraded impulses. Enjoyed mostly by others, by the villain or the hero's friends, for the romantic lover the sexual pleasures of the kotha are generally cloaked in a pall of guilt, to be savoured morosely in an alcoholic haze and to the nagging beat of self-recrimination.

The Krishna-lover is the second important hero of Indian films. Distinct from Majnun, the two may, in a particular film, be sequential rather than separate. The Krishna-lover is physically importunate, what Indian–English will perhaps call the 'eve-teasing' hero, whose initial contact with women verges on that of sexual harassment. His cultural lineage goes back to the episode of the mischievous Krishna hiding the clothes of the *gopis* (cowherdesses) while they bathe in the pond and his refusal to give them back in spite of the girls' repeated entreaties. From the Dev Anand movies of the 1950s to those (and especially) of Shammi Kapoor in the 1960s and of Jeetendra today, the Krishna-lover is all over and all around the heroine who is initially annoyed, recalcitrant, and quite unaware of the impact the hero's phallic intrusiveness has on her. The Krishna-lover has the endearing narcissism of the boy on the eve of the Oedipus stage, when the world is felt to be his 'oyster.' He tries to draw the heroine's attention by all possible means—aggressive innuendoes and double entendres, suggestive song and dance routines, bobbing up in the most unexpected places to startle and tease her as she goes about her daily life (Jeetendra is affectionately known as 'jack-in-the-box'). The more the heroine dislikes the lover's incursions, the greater is his excitement. As the hero of the film *Aradhana* remarks, 'Love is fun only when the woman is angry'.

For the Krishna-lover, it is vital that the woman be a sexual innocent and that in his forcing her to become aware of his desire she get in touch with her own. He is phallus incarnate, with distinct elements of the 'flasher' who needs constant reassurance by the woman of his power, intactness, and especially his magical qualities that can transform a cool Amazon into a hot, lusting female. The fantasy is of the phallus—Shammi Kapoor in his films used his whole body as one—humbling the pride of the unapproachable woman, melting her indifference and unconcern into submission and longing. The fantasy is of the spirited androgynous virgin awakened to her sexuality and thereafter reduced to a grovelling being, full of a moral masochism wherein she revels in her 'stickiness' to the hero. Before she does so, however, she may go through a stage of playfulness where she presents the lover a mocking version of himself. Thus in *Junglee*, it is the girl from the hills—the magical fantasy land of Indian cinema where the normal order of things is reversed—who throws snowballs at the hero, teases him, and sings to him in a good-natured reversal of the man's phallicism, while it is now the hero's turn to be provoked and play the reluctant beloved.

The last fifteen years of Indian cinema have been dominated, indeed overwhelmed, by Amitabh Bachchan who has personified a new kind of hero and lover. His phenomenally successful films have spawned a brand new genre which, though strongly influenced by Hollywood action movies such as those of Clint Eastwood, is neither typically western nor traditionally Indian.

The Bachchan hero is the good–bad hero who lives on the margins of his society. His attachments are few but they are strong and silent. Prone to quick violence and to brooding periods of withdrawal, the good–bad hero is a natural law-breaker, yet will not deviate from a strict private code of his own. He is often a part of the underworld but shares neither its sadistic nor its sensual excesses. If cast in the role of a policeman, he often bypasses cumbersome bureaucratic procedures to take the law into his own hands, dealing with criminals by adopting their own ruthless methods. His badness is not shown as intrinsic or immutable but as a reaction to a development deprivation of early childhood, often a mother's loss, absence, or ambivalence towards the hero.

The cultural parallel of the good–bad hero is the myth of Karna in the Mahabharata. Kunti, the future mother of the five Pandava brothers, had summoned the Sun when she was a young princess. Though her calling the Sun was a playful whim—she was just trying out a *mantra*—the god insisted on making something more of the invitation. The offspring of the resulting union was Karna. To hide her shame at Karna's illegitimate birth, Kunti abandoned her infant son and cast him adrift on a raft. Karna was saved by a poor charioteer and grew up into a formidable warrior and the supporter of the evil Duryodhana. On the eve of the great battle, Kunti approaches Karna and reveals to him that fighting on Duryodhana's side would cause him to commit the sin of fratricide. Karna answered:

> It is not that I do not believe the words you have spoken, *Kshatriya* (warrior caste) lady, or deny that for me the gateway to the Law is to carry out your behest. But the irreparable wrong you have done me by casting me out has destroyed the name and fame I could have had. Born a *Kshatriya*, I have yet not received the respect due to a baron. What enemy could have done me greater harm than you have? When there was time to act you did not show your present compassion. And now you have laid orders on me, the son to whom you denied the sacraments. You have never acted in my interest like a mother, and now, here you are, enlightening me solely in your own interest.[9]

Karna, though, finally promises his mother that on the battlefield he will spare all her sons except Arjuna—the mother's favourite.

The good–bad Bachchan hero is both a product of and a response to the pressures and forces of development and modernization taking place in Indian society today and which have accelerated during the last two decades. He thus reflects the psychological changes in a vast number of people who are located in a halfway house—in the transitional sector—which lies between a minuscule (yet economically and politically powerful) modern and the numerically preponderant traditional sectors of Indian society. Indeed, it is this transitional sector from which the Bachchan movies draw the bulk of their viewers.

The individual features of the good–bad hero which I have sketched above can be directly correlated with the major psychological difficulties experienced by the transitional sector during the course of modernization. Take, for instance, the effects of overcrowding and the high population density in urban conglomerations, especially in slum and shanty towns. Here, the lack of established cultural norms and the need to deal with relative strangers whose behavioural cues cannot be easily assessed compel the individual to be on constant guard and in a state of permanent psychic mobilization. A heightened nervous arousal, making for a reduced control over one's aggression, in order to ward off potential encroachments, is one consequence *and* a characteristic of the good–bad hero.

Then there is bureaucratic complexity with its dehumanization which seems to be an inevitable corollary of economic development. The cumulative effect of the daily blows to feelings of self-worth, received in a succession of cold and impersonal bureaucratic encounters, so far removed from the familiarity and predictability of relationships in the rural society, gives rise to fantasies of either complete withdrawal or of avenging slights and following the dictates of one's personal interests, even if this involves the taking of the law into one's own hands. These, too, form a part of our hero's persona.

Furthermore, the erosion of traditional roles and skills in the transitional sector can destroy the self-respect of those who are now suddenly confronted with a loss of earning power and social status. For the families of the affected, especially the children, there may be a collapse of confidence in the stability of the established world. Doubts surface whether hard work and careful planning can guarantee future rewards of security. The future itself begins to be discounted to the present.[10] The Bachchan hero, neither a settled family man nor belonging to any recognized community of craftsmen, farmers, et cetera, incorporates the transitional man's collective dream of success without hard work and of life lived primarily, and precariously, in the here-and-now.

The last feature of the portrait is the core sadness of the good–bad hero. On the macro level, this may be traced back to the effects of the population movements that take place during the process of economic development. The separation of families, the loss of familiar village neighbourhoods and ecological niches, can overwhelm many with feelings of bereavement. Sometimes concretized in the theme of separation from the mother, these feelings of loss and mourning are mirrored in the Bachchan hero and are a cause of his characteristic depressive detachment, in which the viewers, too, can recognize a part of themselves.

As a lover, the good–bad hero is predictably neither overly emotional like Majnun nor boyishly phallic like the Krishna lover. A man of controlled passion, somewhat withdrawn, he subscribes to the well-known lines of the Urdu poet Faiz that 'Our world knows other torments than of love and other happinesses than a fond embrace.' The initial meeting of the hero and heroine in *Deewar*, Bachchan's first big hit and widely imitated thereafter, conveys the essential flavour of this hero as a lover. The setting is a restaurant–night club and Bachchan is sitting broodingly at the bar. Anita, played by Parveen Babi, is a dancer—the whore with a golden heart—who comes and sits next to him. She offers him a light for his cigarette and tells him that he is the most handsome man in the bar. Bachchan, who must shortly set out for a fateful meeting with the villain, indifferently accepts her proffered homage as his due while he ignores her sexually provocative approach altogether. Indeed, this narcissistically withdrawn lover's relationships with his family members and even his best friend are more emotionally charged than with any woman who is his potential erotic partner. Little wonder that Shashi Kapoor, who played the hero's brother or best friend in many movies, came to be popularly known as Amitabh Bachchan's favourite heroine!

Afraid of the responsibility and effort involved in active wooing, of passivity, and dependency upon a woman—urges from the earliest period of life which love brings to the fore and intensifies—the withdrawn hero would rather be admired than loved. It is enough for him to know that the woman is solely devoted to him while he can enjoy the position of deciding whether to take her or leave her. The fantasy here seems of revenge on the woman for a mother who either preferred someone else—in *Deewar*, it is the brother—or only gave the child conditional love and less than constant admiration.

The new genre of films, coexisting with the older ones, has also given birth to a new kind of heroine, similar in some respects to what Wolfenstein and Leites described as the masculine–feminine girl of the American movies of the 1940s and 1950s.[11] Lacking the innocent androgyny of Krishna's playmate, she does not have the sari-wrapped femininity (much of the time she is clad in jeans anyway!) of Majnun's beloved either. Like the many interchangeable heroines of Bachchan movies, she is more a junior comrade to the hero than his romantic and erotic counterpart.

Speaking a man's language, not easily shocked, she is the kind of woman with whom the new hero can feel at ease. She is not an alien creature of feminine whims, sensitivities, and susceptibilities, with which a man feels uncomfortable and which he feels forced to understand. Casual and knowing, the dull wholesomeness of the sister spiced a little with the provocative coquetry of the vamp, she makes few demands on the hero and can blend into the background whenever he has more important matters to attend to. Yet, she is not completely unfeminine, not a mere mask for the homosexual temptation to which many men living in the crowded slums of big cities and away from their womenfolk, are undoubtedly subject. She exemplifies the low place of heterosexual love in the life of the transitional man, whose fantasies are absorbed more by visions of violence than of love, more with the redressal of narcissistic injury and rage than with the romantic longing for completion—a gift solely in the power of a woman to bestow.

Having viewed some dreams in Indian popular cinema with the enthusiast's happy eye but with the analyst's sober perspective, let me reiterate in conclusion that *oneiros*—dream, fantasy—between the sexes and within the family, does not coincide with the cultural propositions on these relationships. In essence, oneiros consists of what seeps out of the crevices in the cultural floor. Given secret shape in narrative, oneiros conveys to us a particular culture's versions of what Joyce McDougall calls the Impossible and the Forbidden,[12] the unlit stages of desire where so much of our inner theatre takes place.

Notes and References

1 On the influence of film values on Indian culture, see Bahadur, Satish, n.d., *The Context of Indian Film Culture*, Poona: National Film Archives of India. See also the various contributions in *Indian Popular Cinema: Myth, Meaning, and Metaphor*, special issue of the *India International Quarterly*, 8 (1), 1980.

2 Stoller, Robert J., 1975, *Perversion*, New York: Pantheon Books, p.55.

3 Kakar, Sudhir, 1978, *The Inner World: A Psychoanalytic Study of Childhood and Society in India*, Delhi: Oxford University Press, ch. 3.

4 Appadurai, Arjun and Carol Breckenridge, July 1986, 'Public Culture in Late Twentieth Century India', Department of Anthropology, Pittsburgh: University of Pennsylvania, unpublished.

5 See Bettleheim, Bruno, 1976, *The Uses of Enchantment*, New York: Knopf.

6 Some of these films are *Junglee, Bees Saal Baad, Sangam, Dosti, Upkaar, Pakeeza, Bobby, Aradhana, Johnny Mera Nam, Roti, Kapda aur Makan, Deewar, Zanjeer, Sholay, Karz, Muqaddar ka Sikandar,* and *Ram Teri Ganga Maili.*

7 O'Flaherty, Wendy, 'The Mythological in Disguise: An Analysis of *Karz*', in *Indian Popular Cinema*, note 1 above, pp. 23–30.

8 Kakar, Sudhir and John M. Ross, 1987, *Tales of Love, Sex, and Danger*, London: Unwin Hyman, ch. 3.

9 *Mahabharata*, 5. 144. pp. 5–10. The English translation is taken from *The Mahabharata* (edited and translated by J.A.B. von Buitenen), Chicago: University of Chicago Press 1978, p. 453.

10 The psychological effects of modernization have been discussed in E. James Anthony and C. Chiland (eds), *The Child in His Family: Children and Their Parents in a Changing World*, New York: John Wiley, 1978.

11 Wolfenstein, Martha and Nathan Leites, 1950, *Movies: A Psychological Study*, Glencoe, Ill.: Free Press.

12 McDougall, Joyce, 1986, *Theatres of the Mind*, New York: Basic Books.

Indian Sexuality*

THERE ARE VERY FEW ASPECTS of Indic civilization where the disjunction between its 'classical' and modern ages is as striking as in the area of sexuality. Compared to contemporary conservative sexual attitudes and oppressive mores, the stance of ancient Hindus towards erotic and sensual life, at least as it comes through to us in literary and scholarly texts, as also in temple sculptures, seems to belong to a culture long ago and a galaxy far away. Often repressed or denied, the terrain of ancient Indian sexuality is home to a siren's song to which most contemporary Indians continue to shut their ears.

Sex in Ancient India

No discussion of Indian sexuality, ancient or modern, can begin without a respectful nod, or rather a bow towards the *Kamasutra* which has been pivotal in forming the rest of the world's ideas on Indian sexuality. People who find it difficult to name one Sanskrit book or are not even aware of the existence of Sanskrit as the classical language of ancient India, have no trouble in identifying the *Kamasutra*. The name alone conjures up titillating visions of erotic frescos in which 'regal maharajas with outsized genitals cavort with naked bejeweled nymphs in positions exotic enough to slip the discs of a yoga master.'[1]

* From *The Indians: Portrait of a People*, Delhi: Viking–Penguin, 2007.

Few, of course, have read this third century treatise on erotic love, even the 'good' parts about positions in sexual intercourse that have given it the reputation of 'that racy sex manual from India'. What the *Kamasutra* is *really* about is the art of living—about finding a partner, maintaining power in marriage, committing adultery, living as or with a courtesan, using drugs—and also about positions in sexual intercourse. It has attained its classical status as the world's first comprehensive guide to erotic love because it is, at the bottom, about essential, unchangeable human attributes—lust, love, shyness, rejection, seduction, manipulation—that are also a part of human sexuality.

The *Kamasutra* can be viewed as an account of a 'psychological war' of independence that took place in India some two thousand years ago. The first aim of this struggle, the rescue of erotic pleasure from the crude purposefulness of sexual desire, from its biological function of reproduction alone, has been shared by many societies at different periods of history. Today, the social forces and the moral orders that would keep sexuality tied to reproduction and fertility are no longer of such fateful import, at least in what is known as the 'modern West' (and its enclaves in the more traditional societies around the world), although this was not the case even a hundred years ago.

The first European translators of the *Kamasutra* in the late nineteenth century, clearly on the side of sexual pleasure in a society where the reigning Christian morality sought to subordinate, if not altogether eradicate it in service of a divinely ordained reproductive goal, regarded the ancient Sanskrit text devoted to the god of love without even a nod to the divinities who preside over fertility and birth, as a welcome ally. To them, the *Kamasutra* was the product of a place and people who had raised the search for sexual pleasure to the status of a religious quest. Lamairesse, the French translator, even called it 'Theologie Hindoue' that revealed vital truths regarding man's fundamental, sexual nature while Richard Schmidt, the German translator, would wax lyrical:

> The burning heat of the Indian sun, the fabulous luxuriance of the vegetation, the enchanted poetry of moonlit nights permeated by the perfume of lotus flowers and, not in the least, the distinctive role the Indian people have always played, the role of unworldly dreamers, philosophers, impractical *Schwärmer*—all combine to make the Indian a real virtuoso in love.[2]

Vatsyayana and other ancient Indian sexologists can certainly be viewed as flag bearers for sexual pleasure in an era where the sombre Buddhist view of life, which equated the god of love with *Mara* ('death', 'destruction'), was still influential. However, they were also inheritors of another worldview, that of the epics of the Mahabharata and the *Ramayana*, where sexual love is usually a straightforward matter of desire and its gratification. This was especially so for the man for whom a woman was an instrument of pleasure and an object of the senses—one physical need among many others. There is an idealization of marriage in the epics, yes, but chiefly as a social and religious act. The obligation of conjugal love and the virtue of chastity within marriage were primarily demanded of the wife, while few limits were set on a husband who lived under and looked up at a licentious heaven teeming with lusty gods and heavenly whores, otherworldly and utterly desirable at once, and most eager to give and take pleasure. The Hindu pantheon of the epics was not unlike the Greek Olympus where gods and goddesses sported and politicked with a welcome absence of moralistic subterfuge.

Vatsyayana and the early sexologists were thus also heirs to a patrimony where sexual desire ran rampant, unchecked by moral constraints. Indeed, Shvetaketu Auddalaki, the legendary composer of the first textbook on sex, was credited with trying to put an end to unbridled sexual coupling and a certain profligacy in relation to intercourse with married women, which is so prominent in the Mahabharata. Prior to Shvetaketu's treatise, both married and unmarried women were viewed as items for indiscriminate consumption, 'like cooked rice'. Shvetaketu was the first to make the novel suggestion that men should not generally sleep with the wives of others.

Besides the rescue of erotic pleasure from the confining morality of fertility and reproduction, the *Kamasutra*'s 'freedom struggle', thus, also had a second aim. This was to find a haven for the erotic from the ferocity of unchecked sexual desire. For desire has an open, lustful intent, imperiously and precipitously seeking satisfaction for its own sake, a tidal rush of gut instinct. Human beings have always sensed that sexual desire may also have other aims besides the keen pleasure of genital intercourse and orgasm. For instance, the sexual fantasies of men and women are often coloured with the darker purposes of destructive aggression. Without an imagined violence, however minimal, attenuated and distant from awareness, many men fail to be gripped by powerful sexual excitement. Aggressiveness towards the woman is as much a factor in their potency as their loving feelings. One of their major fantasies is of taking by force that which is not easily given. Some imagine the woman not wishing to participate in the sexual experience but then being carried away by the man's forcefulness despite herself. We find a variant of the 'possession fantasy' in classical Sanskrit love poetry, with its predilection for love scenes where the woman trembles in a state of diffuse bodily excitement as if timorously anticipating a sadistic attack, her terror a source of excitement for both herself and her would-be assailant. In Kalidasa's *Kumara Sambhava*, a fifth-century(?) masterpiece of erotic poetry, Siva's excitement reaches a crescendo when Parvati 'in the beginning felt both fear and love.'[3]

Sexual desire, then, in which the body's wanting and violence, the excitement of orgasm and the exultation of possession, all flow together, can easily overwhelm erotic pleasure. Today, when what were once called 'perversions' are normal fare of television channels, video films, and internet sites, where small but specialized professions exist for the satisfaction of every sexual excess, the *Kamasutra*'s second project of rescuing the erotic from the rawly sexual would find many supporters. In today's post-moral world, the danger to erotic pleasure is less from the icy frost of morality than from the fierce heat of instinctual desire. *Kamasutra*'s most valuable insight, then, is that pleasure needs to be cultivated, that in the realm of sex, nature requires culture.

Culture, in *Kamasutra*'s sense, the sixty-four arts that need to be learnt and so on, needs leisure and means, time and money. These were not in short supply for the text's intended audience, an urban (and urbane) elite consisting of princes and barons, high state officials, and wealthy merchants who had the leisure time to seduce virgins and other men's wives and a considerable amount of money to buy the gifts needed for the purpose.

Despite the role of violence in sexuality, the feeling-tone of *Kamasutra*'s eroticism is primarily of lightness. In its pages, we meet leisured gallants who spend hours in personal grooming and teaching their mynah birds and parrots to speak. Their evenings are devoted to drinking, music, and dance; that is, when they are not busy talking poetry and engaging in light-hearted sexual banter with artful courtesans. In its light-hearted eroticism, the *Kamasutra* is part of a literary climate during the first six centuries of the Christian calendar where the erotic was associated with all that was bright, shining, and beautiful in the ordinary world. The Sanskrit poems and dramas of this period are also characterized by this quality, an eroticism more hedonist than impassioned. The mood is of a playful enjoyment of love's ambiguities, a delighted savoring of its pleasures, and a consummately refined suffering of its sorrows. The poems are cameos yielding glimpses into arresting erotic moments, their intensity enhanced by the accumulation of sensuous detail. The aesthetic of this period could confidently proclaim that certain emotions such as laziness, violence, and disgust do not belong to a depiction of the erotic. Today, the 'flavour' or 'essence'—*rasa*—of sexual love knows no such limits.

Women in the *Kamasutra*

Another aspect of the *Kamasutra* is the discovery of the woman as a subject and full participant in sexual life. The text both reflects and fosters the woman's enjoyment of her sexuality. Vatsyayana expressly recommends the study of *Kamasutra* to women, even before they reach puberty. Two of the book's seven parts are addressed to women, the fourth to wives, and sixth to courtesans. The woman is very much a subject in the erotic realm, not a passive recipient of the man's lust. Of the four embraces in preliminary love play, the woman takes the active part in two. In one, she encircles her lover like a vine does a tree, offering and withdrawing her lips for a kiss, driving the man wild with excitement. In the other—familiar from its sculpted representation in the temple friezes of Khajuraho—she rests one of her feet on the man's and the other against his thigh. One arm is across his back and with the other clinging to his shoulder and neck she makes the motion of climbing him as if he was a tree. In the final analysis, though, given the fact that the text was composed by a man, primarily for the education of other men, the fostering of a woman's sexual subjectivity is ultimately in the service of an increase in the man's pleasure. The *Kamasutra* recognizes that a woman who actively enjoys sex will make it much more enjoyable for him.

Women in the *Kamasutra* are thus not only presented as erotic subjects but as sexual beings with feelings and emotions which a man needs to understand for the full enjoyment of erotic pleasure. The third part of the text instructs the man on a young girl's need for gentleness in removing her virginal fears and inhibitions. Erotic pleasure demands that the man be pleasing to his partner. In recommending that the man not sexually approach the woman for the first three nights after marriage, using this time to understand her feelings, win her trust and arouse her love, Vatsyayana takes a momentous step in the history of Indian sexuality by introducing the notion of love in sex. He even goes so far as to advance the radical notion that the ultimate goal of marriage is to develop love between the couple and thus considers the love-marriage (still a rarity in contemporary Indian society), ritually considered as 'low' and disapproved of in the religious texts, as the pre-eminent form of marriage.

The *Kamasutra* is a radical advocate of women's empowerment in a conservative, patriarchal society in other ways, too. The law books of the time come down hard on women contemplating divorce: 'A virtuous wife should constantly serve her husband like a god, even if he behaves badly, freely indulges his lust, and is devoid of any good qualities.'[4] Vatsyayana, on the other hand, views the prospect of wives leaving their husbands with equanimity; he tells us that a woman who does not experience the pleasures of love may hate her man and leave him for another. He is equally subversive of the prevailing moral order between the sexes when he advises courtesans (and by extension, other women readers of the text) on how to get rid of a man she no longer wants:

She does for him what he does not want, and she does repeatedly what he has criticized … She talks about things he does not know about … She shows no amazement, but only contempt, for the things he does know about. She punctures his pride. She has affairs with men who are superior to him. She ignores him. She criticizes men who have the same faults. And she stalls when they are alone together. She is upset by the things he does for her when they are making love. She does not offer him her mouth. She keeps him away from between her legs. She is disgusted by wounds made by nails or teeth when he tries to hug her, she repels him by making a 'needle' with her arms. Her limbs remain motionless. She crosses her thighs. She wants only to sleep. When she sees that he is exhausted, she urges him on. She laughs at him when he cannot do it, and she shows no pleasure when he can. When she notices that he is aroused, even in the daytime, she goes out to be with a crowd.

She intentionally distorts the meaning of what he says. She laughs when he has not made a joke, and when he has made a joke, she laughs about something else …[5]

Yes! That would get rid of him!

It is not that Vatsyayana idealizes women; only that he is equally cynical about men and women as far as sex is concerned. The Hindu law books are traditionally patriarchal in discussing why women commit adultery: 'Good looks do not matter to women, nor do they care about youth; "A man!" they say, and enjoy sex with him, whether he is good looking or ugly.'[6] The *Kamasutra*, on the other hand, is more egalitarian: 'A woman desires any attractive man she sees, and, in the same way, a man desires a woman. But, after some consideration, the matter goes no further.'[7]

Love in the Age of the *Kamasutra*

The erotic love of the *Kamasutra* is not of the romantic variety as we know it today. Its tenderness and affection for the partner is still, largely, in the service of sexual desire. Thus, Vatsyayana's detailed instructions to the man on the tender gestures required of him at the end of sex, 'when their passion has ebbed', end with the words, 'Through these and other feelings, the young couple's passion grows again.'[8] The literary birth of romantic love in the twelfth century, Bedier's *The Romance of Tristan and Iseult* in Europe and Nizami's *The Story of Layla and Majnun* in the Islamic world, still lay far into the future.

What distinguishes romantic love from the erotic love of the *Kamasutra* is the pervasive presence in the former of what may be called 'longing.' In its quest for oneness with the beloved, longing emphasizes a willing surrender, adoration and cherishing of the person for whom one lusts. Longing presupposes, first, a special kind of identification that makes the person of the beloved attain for the lover a centrality at least equal to his own. It also requires an idealization which makes him experience the loved one as an infinitely superior being to whom he willingly subordinates his desire. Romantic love finds fulfillment only when the lover becomes metaphorically porous to the beloved. Possessive desire aspires to overpower its object while tender longing would have her or him indestructible; longing lends desire permanence and stability.

The porosity, the surrender, the identification, and the idealization, are not a part of the erotic love we find in the *Kamasutra* or, for that matter, in the classical literature of that period. In the Sanskrit and Tamil love poems, as in the textbooks of erotics, the beloved is a partner who is a source of excitement and delight, enlivening the senses but not a beacon for the soul. She is to be explored thoroughly, in enormous detail, and therefore, she is not quickly abandoned. Yet, her inner life or her past and future are not subjects of entrancement; the impulse is not of fierce monogamy.

For most modern readers who have an affinity for the personal and the subjective, this emphasis on love as a depersonalized voluptuous state, while delighting the senses, does not touch the heart. For those whose sensibility has been moulded by romanticism and individualism, it is difficult to identify with the impersonal protagonists of the poems. These are not a particular man or woman but man and woman as such, provided he is handsome, she beautiful, and both young. The face of the heroine, for instance, is always like a moon or lotus flower, eyes like water lilies or those of a fawn. She always stoops slightly from the weight of her full breasts, improbable fleshy flowers of rounded perfection that do not even admit a blade of grass between them. The waist is slim, with three folds, the thighs round and plump, like the trunk of an elephant or a banyan tree. The navel is deep, the hips heavy. These lyrical yet conventional descriptions of body parts seem to operate like collective fetishes, culturally approved cues for the individual to allow himself to indulge in erotic excitement without the risk of surrender so longed for in romantic love.

Whereas the erotic love of the Kamasutra and the classical Sanskrit literature of the period is bright and shiny, romantic love, in spite of its exquisite transports of feeling, is often experienced by the lovers as dark and heavy. In its full flowering, sexual desire loses its primacy as the lover strives to disappear in the contours of another, a person whose gender fits the mould but whose flesh is almost incidental to the quest for wholeness.[9] Sexual desire becomes a mere vehicle for a yearned for merger of souls, a consummation that is impossible as long as lovers have bodies. The impossibility of merger, making the lovers aware of their elemental separation, is the potential tragedy of romantic love, its anguish and torment. This is its inherent heaviness wherein lovers through the ages, and not only fictional ones, have cursed it as a plague and affliction.

The suffering of erotic love, on the other hand, the dark spot on its brightness, has less to do with the soul's elemental longing to end separation than with the bodily nature of sexual desire. Sexual desire does not subside with seeming satiation. Memory as well as the deliciousness of pleasure's ache gnaw further, making for the distress that marks the separation of lovers in erotic love. This sentiment casts only a small shadow on the *Kamasutra*, where it takes the rather different form of the sufferings of the rejected wife and the anxiety of the not-yet-successful suitor. The erotic love of *Kamasutra* is then a precarious balancing act between the possessiveness of sexual desire and the tenderness of romantic longing, between the disorder of instinctuality and the moral forces of order, between the imperatives of nature and the civilizing attempts of culture. It is a search for harmony in all the opposing forces that constitute human sexuality, a quest often destined to be futile by the very nature of the undertaking. As Vatsyayana remarks, 'When the wheel of sexual ecstasy is in full motion, there is no textbook at all, and no order.'[10]

Sexuality in Temples and Literature of Medieval India

From all available evidence (and the *Kamasutra* provides the bulk of it), there was little sexual repression in ancient India, at least among the upper classes, the *Kamasutra*'s primary audience. The demands of sexuality had to be reconciled with those of religion, yes, but it was a reconciliation rather than suppression when the two were in conflict.

The uninhibited sexuality of the *Kamasutra,* where nothing is taboo in imagination and very little in reality, which combines tenderness with playful aggressiveness in lovemaking, where gender roles in the sexual act are neither rigid nor fixed, is brought to its visual culmination in the temples of Khajuraho.

This group of originally over eighty temples of which twenty-nine still stand, was rediscovered in a village in central India in the middle of the nineteenth century. The sculptures and friezes of the temples, built between the tenth and eleventh centuries are generally regarded as being among the masterpieces of Indian art and architecture. Besides the religious motifs, the temple walls also represent the world of the worshippers and portray life in all its fullness. Temples of this time were not only places of worship. They were centres of social, cultural, and political life where musical and dance performances were held, literary and religious discussions took place, and people met to discuss community issues.

Khajuraho's contemporary fame, even notoriety, however, is chiefly due to its profusion of erotic carvings. Among the most beautiful are the *apsaras*, the heavenly whores, in a variety of moods and in various states of undress, exposing themselves with erotic suggestiveness. Then there are graphic depictions of sexual intercourse, group orgies, and sex with animals. If there is one clear and unambiguous message in the sensuality of the sculpted representations of Khajuraho and Konarak, it is that the human soul is pre-eminently amorous, and nothing if not amorous.

The loving couple (the so-called *mithuna* motif) occurs in Indian temples from very early times, at least from third century BC. The couple may well represent the union of the individual soul with the Supreme soul—the highest goal of Hindu religiosity. A necessary auspicious element in Indian temples, the loving couple becomes elaborated through the centuries. By the time of Khajuraho, the artistic imagination of the temple sculptors had begun to depict the couple as one engaged in sexual intercourse. The progress from the more abstractly loving couple to the one engaged in intercourse is possible because the sexual act in Hindu tradition does not lie outside but within the holiness of life. An authoritative religious text asserts that: 'The whole universe, from Brahman to the smallest worm, is based on the union of the male and female. Why then should we feel ashamed of it, when even Lord Shiva was forced to take four faces on account of his greed to have a look at a maiden?'[11]

Here, we must remember that the Indian combination of religiosity and eroticism is not unique to Khajuraho. From the ninth to the thirteenth centuries, when there was a remarkable temple building activity all over India, erotic sculptures were common. The infusion of religion with sexuality is not limited to sculpture but also extends to literature, preeminently the poetry and songs of *bhakti*, the devotional religiosity that first emerged in the sixth century in the south and then went from strength to strength to become the dominant form of Hindu religious expression all over the country. Bhakti's principal mood has always been erotic, extolling possessing and being possessed by the god as its ideal state. Here, religion is not an enemy of erotic sentiment but its ally. Even the highest of gods delights in the many hues of sexuality as much as mortals. In Jayadeva's *Gita Govinda*, perhaps the swan song of this era which was coming to an end by the twelfth century, after their ecstatic lovemaking has subsided in orgasmic release, a playful Radha (the emblem of the human soul) asks Krishna (an incarnation of the Divine) to rearrange her clothes and tousled hair:

Paint a leaf on my breasts,
lay a girdle on my hips,
twine my heavy braid with flowers,
fix rows of bangles on my hands
and jeweled anklets on my feet.
Her yellow-robed lover
did what Radha said. [12]

Jayadeva, legend has it, hesitant to commit sacrilege by having God touch Radha's feet, a sign of abnegation, was unable to pen the last lines and went out to bathe; when he returned, he found Krishna himself had completed the verse in his absence ... Bhakti poetry's erotic love for Krishna (or Shiva in Tamil or Kannada poetry), similar to the sentiments expressed towards Jesus by such female medieval mystics as Teresa of Avilla, is not an allegory for religious passion but *is* religious passion; the Indian poets refuse to make a distinction between the religious and the erotic.

The sculptures of Khajuraho, Konark and other medieval Indian temples as also the erotic transports of bhakti poetry, then, do not need fanciful explanations. They are the art of and for an energetic and erotic people. As we look back over the centuries, the Indians of a bygone era are involved in the metaphysical questions raised by death, certainly.

Yet they do not let the search for answers dominate the living of their lives; nor do they withdraw from life's possible joys because of the probable sorrows. Khajuraho represents the attitude of a people who, as Vatsyayana remarked centuries earlier, have doubts about the rewards of austerities and an ascetic way of life and believe that 'better a dove today than a peacock tomorrow.'

Contemporary Sexuality

Modern, urban Indians, feasting their eyes on the erotic gyrations of scantily clad nymphs in gorgeously mounted Bollywood movies and fed on a steady diet of stories and surveys in the English language media that proclaim a sexually rising India, may find it hard to believe that vast stretches of contemporary India remain covered in sexual darkness. In spite of somewhat more relaxed sexual attitudes in the upper and upper-middle classes, Indian sexuality remains deeply conservative if not puritanical, lacking that erotic grace which frees sexual activity from imperatives of biology, uniting the partners in sensual delight and metaphysical openness.

Between the land of the *Kamasutra* and contemporary India lie many centuries during which Indian society has successfully managed to enter the sexual dark ages. Many observers wonder as to what could have happened to the same people to turn contemporary Indian eroticism into a sexual wasteland, a country where till recently kissing was banned in films, yet where temple panels of Khajuraho and Konarak blithely show the pleasures of oral sex. Some blame the Muslim invasions and the medieval Muslim rule, although there is little evidence that Islam is a sexually repressive creed. At least in the upper classes, sexual love in most Islamic societies has been marked by a cheerful sensuality.[13] Indeed, a number of *hadith*s, the commentaries on the Koran, strongly favour the satisfaction of the sexual instinct. At least, that is, for the privileged male.

Others blame the Victorian morality of British colonial rule, itself the consequence of Christianity's uneasy relationship with the body, for a state of affairs where modern Indians are embarrassed by Khajuraho's sculptures and feel the need to explain them away in convoluted religious metaphors and symbols or to dismiss them as a product of a 'degenerate' era.

For the 'fault', if it can be called one, one must look within Hindu culture itself, to its holding fast to the ascetic ideal and the virtues of celibacy. At the same time the *Kamasutra* came into existence, there were other texts painting scary pictures of what the loss of semen could entail for the man and elaborating a whole mythology of the woman 'draining' the man in the sexual act. This ascetic ideal, intimately linked with the Hindu concept of purity and impurity, proposes that what is most pure needs the greatest protection. Semen, the purest bodily product of a man and the source of his power, needs to be protected from the woman's ferocious and insatiable desire. Innumerable myths equate bodily weakness or loss of spiritual power in a man or a god with a loss of semen. These myths and legends vividly demonstrate why the ideals of sexual restraint and celibacy enjoy such a high status in Indian culture. In the ascetic imagination, women and their power to attract men is a temptation that is feared the most. This is an imagination scarred by the threat posed by women who are regarded as lustful and sexually rapacious by nature; that is, as long as they have not become mothers.

The ascetic ideal, too, is then quintessentially Indian, perennially in competition with the erotic one for possession of the Indian soul. It is very unlikely that ancient Indians could be or were ever as unswerving in their pursuit of pleasure as, for instance, the ancient Romans. Although today there are again signs of a change, a tentative re-emergence of the erotic in the upper class urban elite, the strain of asceticism, the road to spirituality through celibacy, held aloft through centuries by the Hindu version of William Blake's 'priests in black gowns … binding with briars my joys and desires', has dominated Indian sexual discourse for the last few centuries.

Sexuality and Health

One of the ways the ascetic discourse has sought to assert its pre-eminence over the erotic one is by associating sexuality with fears relating to health. By this, we do not only mean diseases that the Hindu medical tradition explicitly relates to sexuality. For instance, 'overheating' due to too much sex is said to lead to venereal disease; sexual intercourse with a menstruating woman and adultery are held to cause other physical and mental diseases.

The relation between sexuality and ill health in the ascetic discourse is more complex than a simple matter of the sexual origin of diseases. Indeed, the ascetic imagination often seems to be obsessed with sex, for instance in the frequent and long descriptions of the dramatic combat of celibate Yogis with the god of desire—assisted by his host of beautiful apsaras—while they seek to conquer and transform their sexuality into spiritual power.

In traditional ascetic discourse, spirituality is intended to be an intensely practical affair, concerned with the 'alchemy' of the libido that would transform it into spiritual power. It is the sexual fire that stokes the alchemical transformation, wherein the cooking pot is the body and the cooking oil is a distillation from sexual fluids.

In its popular form, the theory of sexual sublimation goes something like this ... Physical strength and mental power have their source in *virya*, a word that stands for both sexual energy and semen. Either virya can move downward in sexual intercourse, where it is emitted in its gross physical form as semen, or it can move upward through the spinal chord and into the brain in its subtle form known as *ojas*. Semen, we should note here, is the meeting point of medicine and spirituality. Indeed, for Sushruta, the author of one of the two foundational texts of traditional Indian medicine, Ayurveda, semen is the material form of the individual soul.

Ascetic discourse regards the downward movement of sexual energy and its emission as semen as enervating, a waste of vitality and essential energy. Of all the emotions, it is said, lust throws the physical system into the greatest chaos, with every passionate embrace destroying millions of red blood cells.

On the other hand, if semen is retained, converted into ojas, and moved upward by observing celibacy, it becomes a source of spiritual life rather than a cause of physical decay. The belief in the possibility of sublimating sexuality into spirituality is shared by most Hindus—Mahatma Gandhi was only one of its best-known advocates and practitioners.

Virgins and Othershead

Sexuality is notorious for not conforming to commands of the culture's moral guardians. Especially in the young, its unruliness has a tendency to seep through the crevices in the cultural floor. Although Indian mores taboo any expression of adolescent sexual behaviour before marriage, various studies from different parts of India suggest that the injunction is flouted by 20 to 30 per cent of the young men.[15] It is more successful in the case of young women, urban or rural, affluent or poor, where these studies report premarital sexual activity in less than 10 per cent of young women. The greater incidence of sexual activity reported by young men is due to the fact that their sexual partners not only include girls of their own age—both 'time pass' and 'true love' affairs—but also commercial sex workers and older married women in the neighborhood they call 'aunties'.

A part of the gender difference in sexual behaviour during youth may also be the result of (boastful) over-reporting by men and (inhibited) under-reporting by women. Girls tend to be secretive of their sexual relationships since even the hint of a friendship with a boy can ruin her reputation, her marriage prospects, and the social status of her entire family. If asceticism is a way of controlling male sexuality, then chastity before (and faithfulness in) marriage are the indispensable checks on female sexuality.

Leaving aside a small upper-class crust in the metropolitan centres, chastity remains the highest commandment for young unmarried women. Whether she belongs to a protective, upwardly mobile middle-class family or lives in the slum of a large city, an Indian girl learns early in life that she must move and behave with utmost modesty in public spaces. In contrast to boys, girls who make even the slightest public show of sexual interest are not only risking their reputation but are also setting themselves up as prey for sexual harassment. Families, too, severely limit a girl's interaction with boys who are not part of the family, so as not to jeopardize her 'value' in the marriage market. An eighteen year old college student from Delhi says, 'If someone finds out that a girl has boyfriends, then—oh God!—no one will marry her because she may have gone to bed with them. A woman should only have sex after marriage.'[16]

'There is no problem if my brother had a girlfriend,' says another college student, 'but in my case it would be a scandal. If I got married tomorrow, the neighbours would say, "That girl is a slut. She had boyfriends before marriage." My brother has no such problems. No one will come and say he has had girlfriends. If one of us has a boyfriend, she would keep it a secret. Otherwise she won't be allowed to go to the telephone at home, not allowed to go out … nothing.'[17]

Little wonder that a number of women in psychotherapy report their first sexual contact with a male member of the extended family—uncle, cousin, even an older brother and, in the case of middle- and upper-class women, also with male servants. The contacts rarely extend to penetrative sex but are nevertheless carriers of considerable guilt as the women struggle to repress memories of their own excitement and curiosity-driven participation in episodes of obvious sexual abuse.

In the identity formation of most young women in India, the conflict between individual needs and social norms leads to persistent feelings of guilt around premarital sexual contact. Young girls develop strongly ambivalent feelings around their sexual identity and its bodily expression. Besides guilt, the (hidden) interest in sexuality can also lead to overpowering feelings of shame. These are expressed, for instance, in a marked embarrassment to talk of sexual matters. After a certain age, most girls have never been naked in front of their parents (nor will be with their husbands); nor would they watch sexually explicit scenes on television together with other, especially male family members.

There *are* changes taking place in urban India. Young girls are developing a greater acceptance of their bodies. They have begun to place importance on clothes that accentuate body contours and are eager to inform themselves on the care and ornamentation of the body through television programmes and women's magazines. Yet, this increasing body consciousness stops with deeply internalized feelings of shame around the genitals—one's own and those of the male. Many girls and young women from higher castes do not even have a name for their genitals. At the most, genitals are referred to obliquely—for instance as 'the place of peeing', though even this euphemism carries a strong emotional charge. A twenty-three year old Sikh patient, educated in England, did not have any trouble mentioning her sexual parts as long as she could do so in English. If asked to translate the words into her mother tongue, the language nearer her early bodily experience, she would either 'forget' the appropriate words or freeze into a long silence.[18] Sexual ignorance, of course, thrives in the socially mandated pall of silence. A college-educated patient believed well into her late teens that menstrual blood, urine, and babies all came through the urethra. Another woman, brought up in a village and presumably more familiar with the 'barnyard' facts of life, realized with consternation, only when giving birth to her first child, that babies were not born through the anus as she had believed.

It is undeniable that in urban India, young girls move more freely in public spaces than was the case with the generation of their mothers. However, it is also indisputable that public space remains a domain of men and there are few signs that this will change in the near future. The writer, V. Geetha, eloquently describes what other women can only confirm from their experience:

> For many of us, nothing captures men's relationship to space as much as the image of the man urinating unconcernedly on a busy thoroughfare, next to

a girl's school building, at a street corner where buses turn, in a public park. Consider flashers: what is it that makes them flash their organs at women, at girls? What notions of intimacy drive men to whisper obscenities into the ears of girls and women on a crowded bus and train? Or pinch their breasts and behinds? Why do men's hands stray, almost unconsciously, as it were, to their crotches, even if they are at a public meeting and on stage? (Women, on the contrary would pull their saris tighter over their breasts) It is as if the public space they claim so effortlessly as their own was defined by their penis and its vagaries.[19]

Sexuality in Marriage

With so many traditional women carrying the baggage of shame and guilt in relation to their (sexual) bodies, and images of insatiable women and notions of sex being an act that drains a man of power and vigour running riot in male cultural imagination, the omens for a joyful sexual life in many marriages are not promising. It is difficult for a man to abandon himself fully to erotic transports if his wife's potential infidelity is a major theme in proverbs of all major Indian languages.[20] 'Only when fire will cool, the moon burn or the ocean fill with tasty water will a woman be pure,' is one of the many pronouncements on the subject. 'A woman if she remains within bounds; she becomes a donkey out of them,' say the Tamils. The exceptional proverbs in praise of wives, for instance in Assamese and Bengali, invariably and predictably address their maternal aspect—'Who could belittle women? Women who bear children!' A Punjabi proverb puts the husband's quandary and its solution in a nutshell: 'A woman who shows more love for you than your mother is a slut.'

Studies show that many Indian men have internalized such proverbs to a considerable extent. Sentiments such as, 'She shouldn't talk to men other than me; even to my brothers and relatives, only in my presence,'[21] are commonly shared, leading to widespread sexual jealousy that can, on occasion, verge on paranoia. Many women cannot even talk to their husbands about taking precautions against unwanted pregnancy without being accused of contemplating adultery.[22] It may well be that some men need this jealousy to stoke their possessive desire and thus heighten their pleasure in sex. The violent promptings of jealousy, though, tend to undermine eroticism, reducing sex to a need of the body alone and removing all controls on the husband's abusive behaviour.

Weighed down by a cultural burden of fear, shame, and guilt, physical love in many traditional Indian marriages often tends to be a sharp stabbing of lust without the full force of energizing erotic passion. Interviews with low-caste poor women in Delhi reveal a sexuality pervaded by hostility and indifference rather than affection and tenderness.[23] Most women portrayed sexual intercourse as a furtive act in a cramped and crowded room, lasting barely a few minutes and with a marked absence of physical or emotional caressing. Most women found it painful or distasteful or both. It was a situation to be submitted to, often from a fear of beating. None of the women removed their clothes for the act since it is considered shameful to do so. Though some of the less embittered women still yearned for physical tenderness from the husband, the act itself was seen as a prerogative and need of the male—'*Aadmi bolna chahta hai* (Man wants to speak).' Another metaphor for what in English is called 'lovemaking' is '*Hafte mein ek baar lagwa lete hain* (I get it done to me once a week)'. In its original Hindustani, the phrase has echoes of a weekly injection, painful perhaps, but necessary for health. The most common expressions for intercourse are *kaam* and *dhandha*, work and business. Sexual intercourse for these women (and men) seems to be structured in terms of contractual and impersonal exchange relations, with the ever-present possibility of one party exploiting or cheating the other.

Studies from other parts of India confirm these observations. For young women of the poorer sections of society, the vast majority, the expectations from their sexual life and of a potential husband are minimal: '... he should not drink, not beat me, and support me and the family.'[24] Most women report that they were unprepared for and ignorant about sexual intercourse until the first night with their husbands. Many experienced some form of sexual coercion and described their first sexual experience as traumatic, distasteful, and painful and involving the use of physical force: 'It was a terrifying experience; when I tried to resist, he pinned my arms above my head. It must have been so painful and suffocating that I fainted.'[24] This India is indeed far removed from the country where, once, the *Kamasutra* guided the newly married man thus:

'For the first three nights after they have been joined together, the couple sleep on the ground, remain sexually continent, and eat food that has no salt or spices. Then, for seven days they bathe ceremoniously to the sound of musical instruments, dress well, dine together, attend performances, and pay their respects to their relatives. All of this applies to all the classes. During this ten-night period, he begins to entice her with gentle courtesies when they are alone together at night.'

The followers of Babhravya say, 'If the girl sees that the man has not made conversation (i.e. sex) for three nights, like a pillar, she will be discouraged and will despise him, as if he were someone of the third nature (i.e., a homosexual).' Vatsyayana says:

> He begins to entice her and win her trust, but he still remains sexually continent. When he entices her he does not force her in any way, for women are like flowers, and need to be enticed very tenderly. If they are taken by force by men who have not yet won their trust they become women who hate sex.[25]

In contrast to much popular Western fiction for women, the Indian 'romantic' yearning is not for an exploring of the depths of erotic passion, or for being swept off the feet by a masterful man. It is a much quieter affair and, when unsatisfied, this longing shrivels the emotional life of many women, making some go through life as mere maternal automatons. Others, though, react with an inner desperation where, as one woman put it, 'even the smell of the husband is a daily torture that must be borne in a silent scream.' The desired intimacy, forever subduing an antagonism between husband and wife, inherent in the division of sexes, is the real *sasural*—the husband's home—to which a girl looks forward after marriage and which a married woman keeps on visiting and revisiting in the hidden vaults of her imagination.

Alternate Sexualities

Except for a few persons belonging to the English-speaking elite in the metropolitan centres, most of them in the higher echelons of advertising, fashion, design, fine and performing arts, men (and women) with same-sex partners neither identify themselves as homosexuals nor admit their sexual preference, often even to themselves. In other words, there are large numbers of men—some married—who have had or continue to have sex with other men; but only a miniscule minority are willing to recognize themselves as 'homosexual'.

The statement that there are hardly any homosexuals in India and yet there is considerable same-sex involvement seems contradictory but simple to reconcile. Sex between men, especially among friends or within the family during adolescence and youth, is not regarded as sex but *masti*, an exciting, erotic playfulness, with overtones of the *mast* elephant in heat. Outside male friendship, it is a way to satisfy an urgent bodily need or, for some, to make money. Sex, on the other hand, is the serious business of procreation within marriage. Almost all men who have sex with other men will get married even if many continue to have sex with men after marriage. Sexual relations with men are not a source of conflict as long as the person believes he is not a homosexual in the sense of having an exclusive preference for men and does not compromise his masculine identity by not marrying and refusing to produce children. As a recent study tells us, 'Even effeminate men who have a strong desire for receiving penetrative sex are likely to consider their role as husbands and fathers to be more important in their self-identification than their homosexual behavior.'[30] Ashok Row Kavi, a well-known gay activist, relates that when he was young and being pressured to marry by his family, especially by the elder sister of his father, he finally burst out that he liked to fuck men. 'I don't care whether you fuck crocodiles or elephants,' the aunt snapped back. 'Why can't you *marry*?'[31]

The cultural ideology that strongly links sexual identity with the ability to marry and procreate does indeed lessen the conflict around homosexual behaviour. Yet, for many, it also serves the function of masking their sexual orientation, of denying them the possibility of an essential aspect of self-knowledge. Those with a genuine homosexual orientation subconsciously feel compelled to maintain an emotional distance in their homosexual encounters and thus struggle against the search for love and intimacy which, besides the press of sexual desire, motivated these encounters in the first place.

The 'homosexual denial', as we would like to call it, is facilitated by Indian culture in many ways. A man's behaviour has to be really flagrant, such as that of the cross-dressing *hijras*, the community of transvestites, to excite interest or warrant comment. For some, the mythology around semen can serve as a cultural defense in denying their homosexual orientation. Kavi tells us about the *dhurrati panthis*, men who love to be penetrated by other men because the semen inside them makes them twice as manly and capable of *really* satisfying their wives. Then there are the *komat panthis* who like to give blow jobs but will not let themselves be touched. Some of these men are revered teachers, 'gurus', in body building gymnasiums who think they will become exceptionally powerful by performing oral sex on younger men. Both will be horrified if one called them homosexual.

Much of the contemporary attitude towards homosexuality goes back in time to ancient India where it was the homosexual (but not homosexual activity) who evoked society's scorn. Actually, in classical India, the disparagement for the homosexual was not devoid of compassion. The homosexual belonged to a deficient class of men called *kliba* in Sanskrit, deficient because he is unable to produce male offspring. Kliba was a catch-all term to include someone who was sterile, impotent, castrated, a transvestite, a man who had oral sex with other men, who had anal sex as a recipient, a man with mutilated or deficient sexual organs, a man who produced only female children, or, finally, a hermaphrodite. Kliba is not a term that exists any longer but some of its remnants—the perception of a deficiency and the combination of pity, dismay, and revulsion towards a man who is unable to marry and produce children—continue to cling to the Indian homosexual.

In *Same Sex Love in India*, Ruth Vanita argues that the relative tolerance, the gray area between simple acceptance and outright rejection of homosexual attraction, can be primarily attributed to the Hindu concept of rebirth.[32] Instead of condemning the couple, others can explain their mutual attraction as involuntary because it is caused by attachment in a previous birth. This attachment is presumed to have the character of 'unfinished business' which needed to be brought to a resolution in the present birth. In ancient texts, folk tales, and in daily conversations, mismatched lovers, generally those with vast differences in status ('a fisherman or an "untouchable" falling in love with a princess'), are reluctantly absolved of blame and the union gradually accommodated because it is viewed as destined from a former birth. When a brave homosexual couple defies all convention by openly living together, its tolerance by the two families and the social surround generally takes place in the framework of the rebirth theory. In 1987, when two policewomen in the state of Madhya Pradesh in central India got 'married', a *cause celebre* in the Indian media, the explanation often heard from those who could no longer regard them as 'just good friends sharing living accommodation' was that one of them must have been a man in a previous birth and the couple prematurely separated by a cruel fate.

In ancient India, homosexual activity itself was ignored or stigmatized as inferior but never actively persecuted. In the dharma (moral law) textbooks, male homoerotic activity is punished, albeit mildly: a ritual bath or the payment of a small fine was often sufficient atonement. This did not change materially in spite of the advent of Islam which unequivocally condemns homosexuality as a serious crime. Muslim theologians in India held that the Prophet advocated severest punishment for sodomy.[33] Islamic culture in India, though, also had a Persian cast wherein homoeroticism is celebrated in literature. In Sufi mystical poetry, both in Persian and later in Urdu, the relationship between divine and human was expressed in homoerotic metaphors. Inevitably, the mystical was also enacted at the human level. At least among the upper classes of Muslims, in the 'men of refinement,' pederasty became an accepted outlet for a man's erotic promptings, as long as he continued to fulfil his duties as a married man.[34]

It seems that the contemporary perception of homosexual activity primarily in images of sodomy can be traced back to the Muslim period of Indian history. In ancient India, in the *Kamasutra* for instance, it is fellatio that is regarded as the defining male homosexual act. The fellatio technique of the closeted man of 'third nature' (the counterpart of the kliba in other Sanskrit texts) is discussed in considerable sensual detail whereas sodomy is mentioned in only one passage and that, too, in the context of heterosexual and *not* homosexual sex. It is the sodomy aspect of male homosexuality which the British colonial authorities, encased in a virulent, homophobic Victorian morality, latched on to in their draconian legislation of 1861. This law, the Section 377 of the Indian Penal Code, states: 'Whoever voluntarily has carnal intercourse against the order of nature with any man, woman or animal shall be punished with imprisonment for life, or with imprisonment of either description for a term which may extend to ten years, and shall be liable to fine.' The law, challenged in the courts by a gay organization and currently awaiting judgement in the Delhi High Court, is still on the statute books. Although the law is rarely used to bring transgressors to court, it is regularly availed of by corrupt policemen to harass and blackmail homosexuals in public places.

If male homosexuals make themselves invisible, then lesbians simply do not exist in Indian society—or so it seems. Again, it is not as if Indians are unaware of lesbian activity. Yet this activity is never seen as a matter of personal choice, a possibility that is theoretically, if reluctantly, granted to 'deficient' men, the men of 'third nature' in ancient India. Lesbian activity, on the other hand, is invariably seen as an outcome of the lack of sexual satisfaction in unmarried women, widows or, women stuck in unhappy, sex-less marriages. This is true even in creative depiction of lesbian activity in fiction or movies. In Deepa Mehta's 1998 movie *Fire*, which caused a huge controversy, with Hindu activists setting fire to cinema halls because the movie showed two women having an affair, both women turn to each other only because they are deeply unhappy in their marriages.

In ancient India, lesbian activity is described in the *Kamasutra* at the beginning of the chapter on harems where many women live together in the absence of men. What the queens have is just one king (preoccupied with affairs of state) to go around. Since none of the kings can be the god Krishna who is reputed to have satisfied each one of his sixteen thousand wives every night, the women use dildos, as well as bulbs, roots, or fruits that have the form of the male organ. The implication is that lesbian activity takes place only in the absence of the 'real thing'. There are hints of other kinds of lesbian activity in the ancient law books: a woman who corrupts a virgin is to be punished by having two of her fingers cut off—a pointer to what the male author thinks two women do in bed. The harsh punishment is not for the activity itself but for the 'deflowering', the heinous crime of robbing a young girl of her chastity. It seems (and this is not surprising) that female homosexuality was punished more severely than homosexuality among men: out of concern for the protection of women's virginity and sexual purity, the traditionalists would say; to exercise control over women's sexual choice and activity, modern feminists would counter.

From medieval India we have the word *chapati* (sticking or clinging together) in Urdu, which is still used today to describe lesbian activity. A modern Hindi commentator on the *Kamasutra* captures the traditional liberal view (all traditionalists are not conservative!) of lesbianism in India when he writes:

> These days, the act of women rubbing their vulvas together is called *chapati*. Vatsyayana has discussed all natural and unnatural means for the satisfaction of unslaked sexual desires. But it is surprising he does not talk of *chapati* intercourse among unsatisfied queens. Perhaps *chapati* intercourse had not yet appeared at Vatsyayana's time; otherwise, it could not have remained hidden from his penetrating gaze. Today, when the emphasis on virginity has increased, the playing of *chapati* and the employment of artificial means for sexual satisfaction among girls is also increasing.[35]

These, then, are some Indian variations on the universal theme of sexuality, that (to borrow from Herman Melville) 'endless ... flowing river in the cave of man.' For sexuality is a country bounded by biological instinct on one side and the imaginative impulse on the other. Erotic spontaneity does not run wild in this terrain but is tamed by an imagination, pre-eminently cultural in origin, introducing fascinating paradoxes in the soul while the body seeks orgasmic release.

Notes and References

1 Castleman, M., 2002, 'Review of Wendy Doniger & Sudhir Kakar's *Kamasutra: A New Translation* (London & New York: Oxford University Press, 2002)', in *Salon.com*, 29 May. Much of the following is from the 'Introduction' in the Doniger and Kakar book in which Doniger was very much the senior author. The quotes from the *Kamasutra*, in Doniger's translation, are from the same book.

2 Schmidt, R., 1911, *Beitraege zur Indischen Erotik. Das Liebesleben der Sanskritvoelker*, Berlin: Verlag Barsdorf, p. 1.

3 Kalidasa, *Kumara Sambhava*, in V.P. Joshi (ed.), 1976, *The Complete Works of Kalidasa*, Leiden: E.J. Brill, 8.1.

4 *Manu*, 5.154.

5 *Kamasutra*, 6.3.41–3.

6 *Manu*, 9.15.

7 *Kamasutra*, 5.1.8.

8 *Ibid.*, 2.10.6–13.

9 Kakar and Ross, *Tales of Love, Sex, and Danger*, p. 202.

10 *Kamasutra*, 2.2.31.

11 Varahamira, *Brihatsamhita*, vol. 2, translated by M.R. Bhat, Delhi: Motilal Banarsidass, 74.20.

12 Jayadeva, 1977, *Gitagovinda*, translated by Barbara Stoler Miller, New York: Columbia University Press, p. 89.

13 Bouhdiba, A., 1975, *La Sexualite en Islam*, Paris: Presses Universitaires de France.

14 O'Flaherty, Wendy, 1971, *Asceticism and Eroticism in the Mythology of Siva*, London: Oxford University Press, p. 51.

15 See Bott, S. and S. Jejeebhoy, 'Adolescent Sexual and Reproductive Behavior: A Review of Evidence from India', in R. Ramasubban and S. Jejeebhoy (eds), 2000, *Women's Reproductive Health in India*, Jaipur: Rawat Publications, pp. 40–101.

16 Poggendorf-Kakar, K., 2002, *Hindu Frauen zwischen Tradition und Moderne*, Stuttgart: Metzler Verlag, pp. 54 and 81.

17 Ibid., p. 82.

18 Kakar, *Intimate Relations*, p. 20.

19 Geetha, V., 'On Bodily Love and Hurt', in M. John and J. Nair (eds), 1998, *A Question of Silence: The Sexual Economies of Modern India*, Delhi: Kali for Women, pp. 304–31.

20 Kakar, *Intimate Relations*, p. 19.

21 Sundari Ravindran, WS–42.

22 Pande, M., 2003, *Stepping Out: Life and Sexuality in Rural India*, Delhi: Ink India.

23 Kakar, *Intimate Relations*, ch. V.

24 Khan, M.E., *et al.*, 1996, 'Sexual Violence within Marriage', *Seminar*, 447: 32–5, cited in S. Jejeebhoy and S. Bott, 2003, *Non-consensual Sexual Experiences of Young People: A Review of Evidence from Developing Countries*, Delhi: Population Council, p. 9. See also, George, A., 'Newly Married Adolescent Women: Experiences

from Case Studies in Urban India', in S. Bott, *et al.* (eds), 2003, *Toward Adulthood: Exploring the Sexual Reproductive Health of Adolescents in South Asia*, Geneva: WHO, pp. 67–70.

25 *Kamasutra*, 3.2.5–6

26 This section is elaborated in greater detail in *The Inner World*, pp. 87–103.

27 Ramanujan, A. K., 'The Indian Oedipus', in E. Lowell and A. Dundes (eds), 1984, *Oedipus: A Folklore Casebook*, New York: Garland, p. 254.

28 Gore, M.S., 1961, 'The Husband-Wife and Mother-Son Relationship', *Sociological Bulletin*, 11, pp. 91–102.

29 Dube, S.C., 1967, *Indian Village*, New York: Harper & Row, pp. 190–7.

30 Asthana, S. and R. Oostvogels, 2001, 'The Social Construction of Male Homosexuality in India: Implications for HIV Transmission and Prevention', *Social Science & Medicine*, 52. See also Seabrook, J., 1999, *Love in a Different Climate: Men Who Have Sex with Men in India*, London: Verso.

31 Interview with Ashok Row Kavi, *http://gaytoday.badpuppy.com/garchive/interview/050399in.htm*

32 Vanita, R. and S. Kidwai (eds), 2000, *Same-Sex Love in India*, New York: St Martin's Press, pp. 28–30.

33 See Saleem Kidwai's Introduction to Part III of *Same-Sex Love in India*, pp. 107–22.

34 This is especially true of pre-colonial Urdu poets. See Rahman, T., 1990, 'Boy Love in Urdu Ghazal', *Annual of Urdu Studies*, 7, pp. 1–20; Naim, C.M., 'The Theme of Homosexual (Pederastic) Love in Pre-Modern Urdu Poetry', in M. U. Memon (ed.), 1979, *Studies in the Urdu Ghazal and Prose Fiction*, Madison: University of Wisconsin, pp. 120–42.

35 D. Shastri cited in Doniger and Kakar, *Kamasutra*, xxxv.

Psychobiography

Ramakrishna and the Mystical Experience*

OF THE MANY WAYS of inner transformation known to man, the mystical path is perhaps one of the most ancient, universal, and highly regarded, even when its practitioners have often lived in an uneasy truce, if not in frank antagonism, with the established religions of their societies.

The mystical path may be one but has many forks. Scholars of religion have distinguished them in various ways. Nathan Söderblom talks of 'mysticism of the infinite', an elevation of awareness where the unifying experience with the suprahuman eliminates perception of the concrete and abstract elements from the sensate world. He contrasts this to 'mysticism of personal life' where the experience is not rooted in ecstatic rapture, but in a meeting with God in the midst of life's problems and struggles, a meeting experienced at a deep level of faith within normal waking consciousness.[1] Martin Buber and John of the Cross would be two exemplars of Söderblom's mysticism of personal life. Of course, such distinctions are more signposts rather than sharp dividers since shades of both 'infinity' and 'personality' will exist in every mystic.

Mysticism of the 'infinite', my own focus of interest, has also been variously categorized—nature mysticism, theistic mysticism, and monistic or soul mysticism—although it is doubtful whether the categories are any different at the level of inner experience. Yet another distinction is the one made by William James between sporadic and cultivated mysticism, which

* From Sudhir Kakar, *The Annual of Psychoanalysis* 20: 215–34, 1992.

corresponds to Arthur Deikman's separation between untrained–sensate and trained–sensate mystical experiences.[2] Ramakrishna was of course, a 'career' mystic, and though his initial forays into mysticism may have been sporadic and untrained, the latter half of his life was marked by regular and frequent mystical experiences of the cultivated, trained–sensate kind.

A mystical experience may be mild, such as a contact with a 'sense of Beyond' among completely normal people, or it may be extreme with ecstasies and visions. We know from survey studies that more or less mild mystical experiences are widespread, even in countries without an active mystical tradition and where the intellectual climate is not particularly conducive to mystical thought. In the United States, for instance, 35 per cent of the respondents in a large sample study by Andrew Greeley in 1975 reported having mystical experiences, a finding which has been since confirmed by other, comparable studies. It is significant that those who had such experiences were more educated than the national average and in 'a state of psychological well-being' unmarked by any obvious neurotic difficulties.[3]

My focus here, though, is mysticism of the extreme variety and especially ecstatic mysticism. Most dramatically manifested in visions and trances, psychologically it is characterized by an expansion of the inner world, by a consciousness suffusing the whole of the body from inside. The expanding consciousness also fills the external world which appears to be pervaded by a oneness of existence.

The overwhelming feeling is of the object of consciousness, the world, having at last become transparent and more real than its conventional reality. All of this is accompanied by heightened intrapsychic and bodily sensations, culminating in a great feeling of pleasure which eliminates or absorbs all other experience.[4] Variously called cosmic consciousness, peak experience (Maslow), *mahabhava*, ecstatic mystical experience seems to differ from one where consciousness and its object, the world, become one and subject–object differentiations vanish. The *samadhi* of the Hindus, *satori* of Zen masters, and *fana* of the Sufis are some of the terms for this particular mystical experience. Again these distinctions are not either/or categories, the former often leading to the latter, as in the case of Ramakrishna, though not all mystics need to have spanned the whole gamut of mystical experience, each with its specific degree of ineffability and noesis—the conviction of knowing.

We must also remember that Ramakrishna was an heir to the Hindu mystical tradition which in spite of many similarities to the mysticism of other religious faiths, also has its own unique context. First, mysticism is the mainstream of Hindu religiosity, and thus Hindu mystics are generally without the restraints of their counterparts in monotheistic religious traditions such as Judaism, Islam, and to a lesser extent, Christianity, where mystical experiences and insights must generally be interpreted against a given dogmatic theology.[5] A Hindu mystic is thus normally quite uninhibited in expressing his views and does not have to be on his guard lest these views run counter to the officially interpreted orthodoxy. Second, God as conceived in the monotheistic religions does not have the same significance in two major schools of Hindu mysticism. Upanishadic mysticism, for instance, is a quest for spiritual illumination wherein a person's deepest essence is discovered to be identical with the common source of all other animate and inanimate beings. Yogic mysticism strives to realize the immortality of the human soul outside time, space, and matter. Through intensive introspection and practice of disciplines that lead to mastery of senses and mental processes, it seeks to realize the experience of one's 'soul' as an unconditioned, eternal being, distinct from the 'illusory' consciousness of the conditioned being. In both Upanishadic and Yogic mysticism there is no trace of love of or yearning for communion with God, which is considered the highest manifestation of the mystical mood in both Christian and Islamic traditions and without which no *unio mystica* is conceivable. In these two Hindu schools, mystical liberation is achieved entirely through the mystic's own efforts and without the intervention of divine grace. It is only in *bhakti* or devotional mysticism—Ramakrishna's preferred form—where love for the Deity creeps in, where the mystic's soul or 'self is finally united with God (or Goddess) in an ecstatic surrender, that Hindu mysticism exhibits a strong family resemblance to the mysticism of monotheistic faiths.

Let me state at the outset that given the theoretical uncertainties in contemporary psychoanalysis which threaten its basic paradigm, the earlier equation of the mystical state with a devalued, if not pathological, regression comparable to a psychotic episode is ripe for radical revision. Many analysts interested in the phenomenon would now agree that in spite of superficial resemblances, the mystical retreat is neither as complete nor as compelling and obligatory as psychotic regression. Moreover, in contrast to the psychotic, the mystic's ability to maintain affectionate ties remains unimpaired when it does not actually get enhanced. Given the analyst's commitment to Freud's dictum that the capacity 'to love and work' is perhaps the best outer criterium for mental health, then the mystic's performance on both counts is impressive—that is, if one can succeed in emancipating one's self from a circumscription of the notions of love and work dictated by convention. In short, the full force of the current flowing through the psyche that leads to short circuit in the psychotic may, and indeed does, illuminate the mystic.

Some of the more recent work in psychoanalysis recognizes that mystical states lead to more rather than less integration of the person.[6] The mystic's insight into the workings of his or her self is more rather than less acute. Although consciousness during the mystical trance may be characterized by 'de-differentiation' (to use Anton Ehrenzweig's concept),[7] that is, by the suspension of many kinds of boundaries and distinctions in both the inner and outer worlds, its final outcome is often an increase in the mystic's ability to make ever-finer perceptual differentiations. In other words, the point is not the chaotic nature of the mystical experience, if it is indeed chaotic, but the mystic's ability to create supreme *order* out of the apparent chaos. In fact, what I would like to do here is address the question Romain Rolland, in writing of Ramakrishna's initial trances, posed for 'physicians both of the body and of the mind', namely, 'There is no difficulty in proving the apparent destruction of his whole mental structure, and the disintegration of its elements. But how were they reassembled into a synthetic entity of the highest order?'[8] To put it differently, how does the mystic become master of his madness and of his reason alike whereas the schizophrenic remains their slave?

The timing of my attempt to formulate some kind of answers to these questions is not inopportune. Today, psychoanalysis is in a relatively better position of *adequatio* (adequateness) in relation to mystical phenomena as well as other states of altered consciousness, such as the possession trance. The adequatio principle, of course, states that the same phenomenon may hold entirely different sets of meaning for different observers.[9] To a dog, a book belongs to a class of object which can be played with but not eaten. To the illiterate, it may be just a book, ink markings on paper he cannot decipher. To the average educated adult, the book is an impenetrable scientific tome. To the physicist, the volume is a brilliant treatise on relativity which makes him question some of the ways he looks at the universe. In each case the level of meaning is a function of the adequatio of the observer. As far as mysticism is concerned, psychoanalysts today are neither dogs nor even illiterates but are, perhaps, just moving beyond the stage of the average educated adult.

The increase in the level of analytical adequatio has not come about because of any analyst's personal experience of training in the mystical disciplines (as far as I know). In part, this higher adequatio is due to the increased availability of analytically relevant information which is no longer limited to the writings or biographical and autobiographical accounts of a few western mystics such as Teresa of Avila and John of the Cross. In the last fifteen years, we have had access to psychodynamically informed interviews with members of mystical cults who have travelled varied distances on the mystical path and have experienced various states of altered consciousness, including the ecstatic trance.[10] In addition, we have at least two detailed case histories of intensive psychoanalytic therapy with patients who had both mystical proclivities and trance experiences.[11]

More than the availability of additional information, the greater adequatio of psychoanalysis in relation to mysticism stems from the work of many writers—Erik Erikson, Donald Winnicott, Wilfred Bion, and Jacques Lacan come immediately to my mind—who, in spite of their very different theoretical concerns, pursued a common antireductionistic agenda. The cumulative effect of their writings has been to allow the adoption of what Winnicott, in talking of transitional phenomena, called 'a particular quality in attitude', with which I believe mystical states should also be observed. In other words, my own enhanced feeling of adequatio reflects the presence of an unstated project in contemporary psychoanalysis in which the co-presence of different orders of experience is tolerated and no attempts are undertaken to explain one in terms of the other without reciprocity. As we shall see later, in their separate efforts to develop a phenomenology of creative experiencing, Winnicott, Lacan, and Bion are directly relevant for a reevaluation and reinterpretation of mystical phenomena.[12] Of the three, whereas Winnicott was more the poet, Lacan and Bion, in their explicit concern with questions of ultimate reality, its evolution and reflection in psychic life, may fairly be described as the mystics of psychoanalysis. (As someone who spent his childhood in India, it is quite appropriate that Bion is radically sincere in his approach to 'O', his symbol for ultimate reality, whereas Lacan, I like to think, as befitting a Frenchman talking of the Real, is more an ironic mystic.)

The psychoanalytic understanding of any phenomenon begins with the narrative, with the echoes and reverberations of individual history. The individual I have selected for my own explorations is the nineteenth century Bengali mystic Sri Ramakrishna. Together with Ramana Maharishi, Ramakrishna is widely regarded as the pre-eminent figure of Hindu mysticism of the last 300 years, whatever pre-eminence may mean in the mystical context. He is a particularly apt choice for a psychoanalytic study of ecstatic mysticism since Freud's observations on the mystical experience, on what he called the 'oceanic feeling', an omnibus label for all forms of extreme mystical experience, were indirectly occasioned by Ramakrishna's ecstasies.

It was the biography of Ramakrishna which Romain Rolland was working on at the time when he wrote of Freud in 1927, saying that though he found Freud's analysis of religion (in *The Future of an Illusion*) just, he would ideally have liked Freud to 'make an analysis of spontaneous religious feelings, or more exactly, religious sensations which are entirely different from religion proper and much more enduring.'[13] Rolland went to call this sensation oceanic, without perceptible limits, and mentioned two Indians who had such feelings and 'who have manifested a genius for thought and action powerfully regenerative for their country and for the world.'[14] Rolland added that he himself had all his life found the oceanic feeling to be a source of vital revival. Freud's response to Rolland, his analysis of the 'oceanic feeling,' was then spelled out in *Civilization and its Discontents.* It is highly probable that the term 'oceanic feeling', itself, is taken from Ramakrishna's imagery to describe the ineffable. For instance, one of Ramakrishna's oft-repeated metaphors is of the salt doll which went to measure the depth of the ocean: 'As it entered the ocean it melted. Then who is there to come back and say how deep is the ocean?'[15]

Of course, ocean as a symbol for boundless oneness and unity in which multiplicities dissolve and opposites fuse not only goes back to the Upanishads in the Hindu tradition, but is one of the preferred metaphors of devotional mystics for the melting of ego boundaries in the Buddhist, Christian, and Muslim traditions as well.[16] Christian mystics, for instance, have been greatly fond of the metaphor 'I live in the ocean of God as a fish in the sea.'

Freud's response to Ramakrishna, as generally to 'Mother India,' was of unease. Although of some professional interest, Ramakrishna's florid ecstasies were as distant, if not distasteful, to his sensibility as the jumbled vision of flesh, the labyrinth flux of the animal, human, and divine in Indian art. In his acknowledgement of Rolland's book about Ramakrishna, Freud writes,

I shall now try with your guidance to penetrate into the Indian jungle from which until now an uncertain blending of Hellenic love of proportion, Jewish sobriety, and Philistine timidity have kept me away. I really ought to have tackled it earlier, for the plants of this soil shouldn't be alien to me; I have dug to certain depths for their roots. But it isn't easy to pass beyond the limits of one's nature.[17]

We are, of course, fortunate that the last four years of Ramakrishna's life, from 1882 to 1886, were recorded with minute fidelity by a disciple, Mahendranath Gupta, or M as he called himself with modest self-effacement.[18] In the cases of most mystics throughout history, we have either had to rely on doctrinal writing that is formal and impersonal, or on autobiographical accounts from which intimate detail, considered trifling from transcendental heights, has been excised. M, on the other hand, with the obsessive fidelity of a Bengali Boswell, has left an enormously detailed chronicle of the daily life and conversations of Ramakrishna—his uninhibited breaking out in song and dance, his frequent and repeated ecstasies, his metaphysical discourses full of wisdom and penetrating insight, his parables, jokes, views, anxieties, and pleasures, the times he slept and ate and what he ate—which is rare in hagiographical literature. Let me then begin with the outer scaffolding of the story, a brief narration of events of Ramakrishna's early life. And though we can never know what *really* happened in his or anyone else's infancy and childhood, the former forever beyond the reach of memory, I have no hesitation in extending a qualified belief to Ramakrishna's own version of his life story. Yet, of course, it is not solely his version. As a re-teller of his tale, I cannot help but also bring to bear a psychoanalytic sensibility in the choice of events I emphasize and others that I must have underplayed. The biographies by his direct disciples, on the other hand, are shaped by the traditional Hindu religious idiom, while the narration by Romain Rolland is moulded by his more universalistic, spiritual concerns, in the sense of what Adlous Huxley called the 'perennial philosophy.'

Ramakrishna was born in 1836 in a Brahmin family in the village of Kamarpukur in Bengal. The parents were pious and very poor, but what I find exceptional about them in the context of nineteenth century village India is their ages at the time of Ramakrishna's birth. At a time when the average longevity was less than thirty years, maternal death during childbirth fairly common, and the sexually reproductive years of the woman over by her early thirties, Ramakrishna's father was sixty-one and his mother forty-five years old when he was born. In the family there was a brother thirty-one years older, a sister twenty-seven years older, and another brother eleven years older. Yet another sister was born when Gadhadhar (his given name) was four years old.

Ramakrishna later remembered his mother Chandra as a simple soul without a trace of worldliness who could not even count money. She said whatever came to her mind, without obfuscation or concealment, and people even called her a 'simpleton'. Devoted to her youngest son, the fruit of old loins, she was nevertheless, as elderly parents often tend to be, inordinately anxious about any harm befalling him when he was not within her ken. A curious and lively child, intent on exploring the world, Ramakrishna did not exactly help in allaying his mother's anxieties. She sought to master these by daily prayers to the family deity wherein she besought the continued welfare of her little boy. Perhaps Ramakrishna's later anxiousness whenever he was physically incapacitated, his almost hypochondriacal concerns at such times, can be directly traced to the elderly mother's anxieties about her youngest son.

The incident given as an example of the boy's wilfulness, which sometimes ignored the conventional rules of conduct, concerns his hiding behind a tree and peeping out at women while they washed clothes and bathed at the village tank. One of the women complained to Chandra who then admonished the boy that all women were the same as his mother. Shaming them was shaming her, insulting their honour was insulting hers. We are told that the mortified boy never again repeated his behaviour. To us post-Freudians, the incident embodies a child's natural sexual curiosity which the mother dampens by associating it with incestuous anxiety. Interestingly, in later life, Ramakrishna would use a mythological version of this personal experience, wherein the incestuous urgings and fears are much more explicit, to explain a part of his attitude towards women. One day, during his childhood, the god Ganesha saw a cat which, as some boys are apt to do, he proceeded to torture in various ways till the cat finally made its escape. When Ganesha came back home he saw to his surprise the bruises and marks of torture on his mother's, the goddess Parvati's body. The mother revealed to her son that all living beings in female form were part of her and whatever he did to any female he did unto his mother. On reaching marriageable age, Ganesha, lest he marry his mother, decided to remain a celibate forever. 'My attitude to women is the same,' was Ramakrishna's final comment.[19]

Khudiram, Ramakrishna's father, was a gentle man who is reported to have never scolded his son. He took a quiet pride in the boy's evident intelligence and phenomenal memory, which were further displayed to advantage when he started attending the village school at the age of five. However, though good at school (but bad at arithmetic), what the boy most enjoyed was painting pictures and spending time with the village potters learning how to make clay images of gods and goddesses. The artistic streak in Ramakrishna was strongly developed, and it seems appropriate that his first ecstasy was evoked by the welling up of aesthetic emotion; an episode of 'nature' mysticism, it was the consequence of an aesthetically transcendent feeling:

I was following a narrow path between the rice fields. I raised my eyes to the sky as I munched my rice. I saw a great black cloud spreading rapidly until it covered the heavens. Suddenly at the edge of the cloud a flight of snow white cranes passed over my head. The contrast was so beautiful that my spirit wandered far away. I lost consciousness and fell to the ground. The puffed rice was scattered. Somebody picked me up and carried me home in his arms. An excess of joy and emotion overcame me. ... This was the first time that I was seized with ecstasy.[20]

Ramakrishna's father, who had been ill for awhile, died when the boy was around eight years of age. The effect of the father's death was to make Ramakrishna withdrawn and fond of solitude. His attendance at school became fitful. He drew closer to his mother and spent much time in helping her with her household duties and her daily prayers to the gods. He became very fond of listening to discourses on spiritual matters and spent hours at a pilgrimage house where wandering ascetics found a bed for a night or two before they resumed their wanderings. The latter activity alarmed his mother who feared that her son might decide to leave home and embrace the renunciant's life.

There were other fainting spells, as on the way to the temple of a goddess or when acting the part of Shiva in a play he lost all external consciousness. He later attributed the states to spiritual stirrings although his family suspected a physical malady and refrained from forcing him to go to school which by now he quite disliked.

The gradually deteriorating condition of the family after Khudiram's death worsened with the marriage of Ramakrishna's second brother. With the advent of the new daughter-in-law, quarrels and bickering in the household increased markedly, a situation which the family's worsening economic circumstances, driving it to the edge of subsistence, did not help improve. The daily clamour and strife, I imagine, perhaps added its own impetus in pushing the sensitive and artistic boy more and more away from the distasteful discord of everyday reality and towards transcendental, spiritual matters and religious life. The latter too coursed through the village, as it does to great extent even today in rural India, in a powerful stream. There were the many rituals in which everyday life was embedded, frequent recitals from the Puranas, and the religious plays and festivals in which Ramakrishna participated by singing and dancing with fervid abandon. And, above all, there were the sudden inward, abstracted states, brought on at the oddest of times by outer stimuli such as listening to a song in praise of a god or to snatches of devotional music.

The young daughter-in-law died in childbirth when Ramakrishna was thirteen years old; and the burden of running the household once again fell on the aging shoulders of Ramakrishna's mother. To help alleviate the poverty, his eldest brother left for Calcutta to run a small Sanskrit school. His position as the head of the family now devolved on Ramakrishna's second brother who was temperamentally disinclined to take over responsibilities for his siblings and was in any case much too busy scrounging around for work.

Thus at the beginning of adolescence, Ramakrishna was left to his own devices, without the paternal guiding voice of his father or eldest brother. School became even more occasional. When he was not an enthusiastic participant in the village's religious life, he was at home with his mother, helping her with household tasks and sharing with her the rhythm of her woman's days. The village women who dropped in on his mother for a visit during the day seem to have adopted him as one of their own. They would ask him to sing—he had a very sweet singing voice—or to tell stories from the Puranas, of which he had an enormous stock. He performed scenes from popular plays for their amusement, playing all the parts himself. He listened to their secrets and woes and would attempt to lift the spirits of a dejected woman by acting out a rustic farce.

He loved putting on women's clothes and ornaments. Dressed thus, with a pitcher under his arm to fetch water from the tank like other village women, he would pass in front of the men and felt proud that no one suspected he was not a woman. Once, disguised as a poor weaver girl, he spent a whole evening in the closely guarded women's quarters of the village shopkeeper's house taking part in their conversation, without being discovered. In his mature years, talking to his disciples, there was a certain wry pride with which he related, and occasionally enacted to their surprised delight, incidents from his youth which showed his ability to mimic women's gestures and movements to perfection.

A fantasy from this period has Ramakrishna imagining that were he to be born again he would become a beautiful child widow with long black hair who would not know anyone else except Lord Krishna as a husband. The girl widow would live in a hut with an elderly woman as a guardian, a spinning wheel, and a cow which she would milk herself. During the day, after finishing household work, she would spin yarn, sing songs about Krishna, and after dusk ardently weep for the god, longing to feed him sweets made from the cow's milk. Krishna would come in secret, be fed by her and go away, his daily visits taking place without the knowledge of others.[21]

In the meantime, Ramakrishna's eldest brother Ramkumar was doing well in Calcutta, running his small school and performing religious services for some rich families. He called the seventeen-year-old Ramakrishna over to the city to assist him in his priestly duties. Soon after, a new opportunity opened up when a rich woman built and consecrated a temple to the goddess Kali outside Calcutta and employed Ramkumar as its full-time priest. Ramkumar, who had been ailing for some time, found the task arduous and handed over his duties to Ramakrishna, the younger brother. He died a year later.

Ramkumar's death was to have a profound effect on Ramakrishna. Thirty-one years older, he had looked after Ramakrishna like a father after Khudiram's death. 'Who can say,' Ramakrishna's disciple-biographer asks, 'how far his brother's death contributed to the kindling up of the fire of renunciation in the Master's pure mind, by producing in him a firm conviction about the transitoriness of the world?'[22] In any case, his behaviour changed markedly as he became more and more engrossed in the worship of the Mother Goddess. As her priest, he had to wake her up early in the morning, bathe and dress her, make garlands of flowers for her adornment. At nine he had to perform her worship, offer her food, and escort her to her silver bed at noon where she rested for the afternoon. Then came the evening worship. For Ramakrishna, these were no longer duties but heartfelt services. He became so absorbed in each one of them that he had to be reminded when it was time to go on to the next ritual.

After the closing of the temple at midday and midnight, Ramakrishna shunned all company and disconsolately roamed around in the jungle at the edge of which the temple was located. All he yearned for with all his soul, he was to later tell us, was a vision, the personal *darshan* of the Mother. The spiritual thirst, the clinician would observe, was embedded in all the signs of a full-fledged depression. There was a great restlessness of the body, sleepless nights, loss of appetite in which eating was reduced to the bare minimum, eyes that filled up often and suddenly with tears. The nephew who looked after him became alarmed for his sanity when at night he saw Ramakrishna sitting under a tree naked, having flung off his clothes and even the sacred thread of a Brahmin, or, when he saw him put the leavings from leaf plates from which beggars had eaten to his mouth and to his head.

But now, as we come to a culmination of his 'dark night of the soul', we need Ramakrishna's own words.

There was then an intolerable anguish in my heart because I could not have Her vision. Just as a man wrings a towel forcibly to squeeze out all the water from it, I felt as if somebody caught hold of my heart and mind and was wringing them likewise. Greatly afflicted by the thought that I might not have Mother's vision, I was in great agony. I thought that there was no use in living such a life. My eyes suddenly fell upon the sword that was in the Mother's temple. I made up my mind to put an end to my life with it that very moment. Like one mad, I ran and caught hold of it, when suddenly I had the wonderful vision of the Mother, and fell down unconscious. I did not know what happened then in the external world—how that day and the next slipped away. But in my heart of hearts, there was flowing a current of intense bliss, never experienced before. … It was as if the house, doors, temples, and all other things vanished altogether; as if there was nothing anywhere! And what I saw was a boundless infinite conscious sea of light! However far and in whatever direction I looked, I found a continuous succession of effulgent waves coming forward, raging and storming from all sides with great speed. Very soon they fell on me and made me sink to the abysmal depths of infirmity.[23]

Those familiar with mystical literature will recognize many elements in Ramakrishna's vision which are known to us from similar descriptions from all over the world, especially the feeling of being flooded by light. In the still controversial studies of near-death experiences, 'seeing the light' and 'entering the light' are said to be the deepest and most positive parts of that particular experience. The incident has not only universal but also cultural aspects. It is a very Hindu story of a man forcing the Goddess to appear by threatening to decapitate himself. This is an old theme, found both in religious and secular literature, for instance in the well-known story which has been so brilliantly retold for western readers by Thomas Mann in his *The Transposed Heads*.

Unlike similar accounts of the first vision in the lives of most mystics, this particular vision, to which we will come back later and to which all his boyhood experiences seem like forerunners, was not sufficient to take him out of the 'valley of the shadow of death'. Its aftertaste but whetted an appetite for repeated blissful salvings. Even for the pious visitors to the temple, accustomed to a wide range in manifestation of religious fervour, Ramakrishna's behaviour appeared bizarre. He would decorate his own person with the flowers and sandalwood paste brought for the worship of the goddess. He would feel the statue of the goddess breathing, try to feed her stony mouth, and carry on playful conversations as to who, the goddess or her priest, should eat first. Any diminution in the sense of her presence made him throw himself and roll violently on the ground, filling the temple with loud wailings at her absence. At such times his breath would almost stop, and he appeared to struggle for his very life. When he again received a vision of the goddess, he would beam with joy and become a different person altogether. The consensus of his employers and others was that he had become insane. Romain Rolland calls this a necessary period of hallucination, and even Ramakrishna referred to it as a passing phase of *unmada* (insanity), leaving it unambiguous—something he was not wont to do in respect of the visions in his later life—that the 'madness' was less divine intoxication than human disintegration, however necessary it may have been as a prelude to the former. Later in life, he would wonder at some of his behaviour during this phase—worshipping his own phallus as that of Shiva, being seized by ecstatic visions while he defecated, and so on.

The prescribed medical treatment for 'insanity' did not have the desired effect. Finally, he was taken to his village home where his worried mother had him ministered to by both an exorcist and an Ayurvedic doctor. Slowly, he regained his normal state of health. To safeguard the apparent gains the family arranged his marriage, a step, which I know from professional experience, is even today considered as the best antidote to threatened or actual psychic breakdown. Of course, as far as Ramakrishna was concerned, there was never any question of the marriage being consummated. From the very beginning, in relation to his girl bride, he saw himself either as a woman or, in his ecstatic state, as a child. In the former case, the husband and wife were both girlfriends (*sakhis*) of the Mother Goddess while, in the latter, the wife was envisioned as the Goddess herself.

At the age of twenty-four, Ramakrishna, now accompanied by his wife, returned to Calcutta to resume his priestly duties at the Kali temple. There was a relapse in his condition, though in an attenuated form. Whereas his initial visions had been untutored and spontaneous, intiated by the passionate intensity of his longing for darshan of the Goddess, during the next eight years he systematically followed the prescribed practices laid down by the different schools of Hindu mysticism. The disciplines were undertaken under the guidance of different gurus who were amazed at his natural facility and speed in reaching the goal of *samadhi*, a capability they themselves had acquired only after decades of strenuous effort.

First, there were the esoteric meditations of Tantra, fierce and fearful, under the tutelage of a female guru, Brahmani Bhairavi. This was followed by the non-dualistic way of Vedanta, of concentration and contemplation techniques which seek to discriminate the Real from the Non-Real, a discipline without the need for any divinity or belief in God, till in the attainment of the samadhi all distinctions between I and the Other vanish. Then there were the various ways of Vaishnava mysticism, full of love and devotion for Rama or Krishna, the incarnations of Vishnu, and of Shakta mysticism where the supreme deity is Shakti, the primordial energy and the great Mother Goddess. All of these, the Vaishnava and Shakta says, are essentially affective, and to which he felt personally most attuned. Whatever the discipline, his mystical genius was soon recognized by laymen and experts alike. Disciples gathered. Pandits—the theologically learned—came to visit and to partake of his clear insight into the whole gamut of Hindu metaphysics, a product of lived experience rather than scriptural proficiency; in any conventional sense, he was more or less illiterate. Ramakrishna would convey this experience simply yet strikingly through devotional songs, Puranic myths, analogies, metaphors, and parables fashioned out of the concrete details of the daily life of his listeners. Most of all, they were attracted by his riveting presence, even when he absented himself in ecstatic trances many times a day, with a few lasting for several days.

The samadhis did not now come unbidden but when his constantly receptive state crossed a certain threshold either in song or abandoned dance, in contemplation of a natural phenomena or absorption in the image of a divinity. He had become both a great teacher and a great mystic without losing his childlike innocence and spontaneity, which extended well into his final days. At the end of his life, dying of throat cancer, his disciples pleaded with him to ask the Mother Goddess for an easing of his disease so that he could eat some solid food rather than continue to subsist on a little barley water which had been his only nourishment for six months. Ramakrishna reluctantly agreed. On the disciples' inquiry as to the fate of their request, Ramakrishna answered: 'I said to the Mother, "I cannot eat anything on account of this (showing the sore in his throat). Please do something that I can eat a little." But the Mother said, "Why? You are eating through all these mouths (showing all of you)." I could speak no more for shame.'[24]

In my attempt to understand the meaning of Ramakrishna's inner states, let me begin with Ramakrishna's own version of his experience. Anthropologically speaking, I shall start with the 'native's point of view' on the phenomenology of mystical states.

Although Ramakrishna had successfully practised the 'higher' Vedantic disciplines of monotheistic, soul-mysticism his own personal preference was for devotional, theistic mysticism of the Vaishnava and Shakta varieties. Ultimately, of course, both roads lead to the same destination. The impersonal soul of the Vedantic seer and the God or Mother Goddess—the primordial energy—of the devotee are identical, like fire and its power to burn. At first one may take the '*neti, neti*' (not this, not this) road of discrimination in which only Brahman is real and all else is unreal. Afterwards, the same person finds that everything in the universe, animate and inanimate, is God himself—he is both the reality and the illusion of the *Maya*. The negation is followed by an affirmation.

Ramakrishna felt that the classical disciplines of yoga were very difficult to follow for most human beings since the identification of the self with the body, which these disciplines seek to undo, was too deeply embedded for any easy sundering. For those who could not get rid of the feeling of 'I', it was easier to travel on the devotional path where one could instead cherish the idea that 'I am God's servant' (or child, or friend, or mother, or lover, as the case may be). He illustrated this point through the example of the monkey god Hanuman, symbol of *dasa* (servant) devotionalism, who when asked by Rama, by God, how he looked at Him, replied, 'O Rama, as long as I have the feeling of "I", I see that you are the whole and I am a part; you are the Master and I am your servant. But when, O Rama, I have the knowledge of truth, then I realize that You are I and I am You.'[25]

Even the passions—lust, anger, greed, inordinate attachment, pride, egoism—which have been traditionally held as obstacles to spiritual progress, do not need to be vanquished in devotional mysticism. The *vairagya*, the renunciation or rather the de-passioning, can take place equally well by changing the object of these passions, directing them towards God rather than the objects of the world.

Lust for intercourse with the soul. Feel angry with those who stand in your way towards God. Be greedy to get Him. If there is attachment, then to Him; like *my* Rama, *my* Krishna. If you want to be proud, then be like Vibhishana [Ravana's brother in the epic of *Ramayana*] who says, "I have bowed before Rama and shall not bow to anyone else in the world."[26]

Devotional mysticism does not demand an elimination of a sense of individual identity, of I-ness, which can instead be used to progress along the spiritual path. Thus in *vatsalya* devotionalism, the attitude of a mother towards God, Ramakrishna gives the example of Krishna's mother as the ideal to be emulated.

Yashoda used to think, "Who will look after Gopala (Krishna's name as child) if I do not? He will fall ill if I do not look after him." She did not know Krishna as God. Udhava said to Yashoda, "Mother, your Krishna is God Himself. He is the Lord of the Universe and not a common human being." Yashoda replied, "O who is talking about your Lord of the Universe? I am asking how *my* Gopala is. Not the Lord of the Universe, *my* Gopala."[27]

Ramakrishna's preferred mystical style did not need ascetic practices, yogic exercises, or a succession of ever more difficult meditations. What it required of the aspirant was, first, a recovery of a childlike innocence and freshness of vision, a renunciation of most adult categories.

To my Mother I prayed only for pure devotion. I said "Mother, here is your virtue, here is your vice. Take them both and grant me only pure devotion for you. Here is your knowledge and here is your ignorance. Take them both and grant me only pure love for you. Here is your purity and here is your impurity. Take them both Mother and grant me only pure devotion for you. Here is your *dharma* (virtue) and here is your *adharma.* Take them both, Mother, and grant me only pure devotion for you."[28]

And at other place, 'Who can ever know God? I don't even try. I only call on him as Mother. … My nature is that of a kitten. It only cries "Mew, mew." The rest it leaves to the Mother.'

Being like a child in relation to the Divinity does not mean being fearful, submissive, or meek, but of existing in the bright-eyed confidence of continued parental presence and *demanding* its restoration when it is felt to be lacking or insufficient. 'He is our Creator. What is there to be wondered if He is kind to us? Parents bring up their children. Do you call that an act of kindness? They must act that way. Therefore we should force our demands on God. He is our Father and Mother, isn't He?'[29] Being a child, then, meant the joy of total trust, of being in the hands of infinitely powerful and infinitely beneficient forces. The power of this total trust is tremendous; its contribution to reaching the mystical goal vital. One of Ramakrishna's illustrative stories went that Rama who was God Himself had to build a bridge to cross the sea to Lanka. However, the devotee Hanuman, trusting only in Rama's name, cleared the sea in one jump and reached the other side. He had no need of a bridge.

Nevertheless, perhaps the most important requirement of devotional mysticism, in all its varieties, was the intensity of the aspirant's yearning to be with God, whether in the dyad of mother–child, or as friend or as servant, or as lover. The longing had to be so intense that it completely took over body and mind, eliminating any need for performing devotions, prayers, or rituals. Ramakrishna illustrated this, his own yearning, through the parable of a guru who took his disciple to a pond to show him the kind of longing that would enable him to have a vision (darshan) of God. On coming to the pond, the guru pushed the disciple's head underwater and held it there. After a few seconds he released the disciple and asked, 'How do you feel?' The disciple answered, 'Oh, I felt as if I was dying! I was longing for a breath of air!' 'That's exactly it,' said the guru.[30] Like other kinds of mysticism, affective mysticism too has its developmental stages. Devotion (*bhakti*) matures into (*bhava*), followed by *mahabhava*, *prema*, and then attainment of God in the *unio mystica.* Since the distinctions between bhava, mahabhava, and prema seem to me to lie in their degrees of intensity rather than in any fundamental qualitative difference, let me try to understand the nature of only one of the three states, bhava, a term which Ramakrishna uses constantly to describe states of consciousness which preceded his visions and ecstatic trances.

Literally translated as 'feeling', 'mood', bhava in Vaishnava mystical thought means a state of mind (and body) pervaded with a particular emotion. Basing his illustrations on Hindu ideals, Ramakrishna lists the *bhava*s in relation to God as *shanta*, the serenity of a wife's devotion to her husband, *dasya*, the devoted submissiveness of the servant, *sakhya*, the emotion of friendship, *vatsalya*, the feeling of mother towards the child, and *madhurya*, the romantic and passionate feelings of a womam towards her lover. Ramakrishan felt that the last, symbolized in Radha's attititude towards Krishna, included all the other bhavas. Indeed, the discourse of passionate love is conducted in many bhavas. At times idealizing the lover makes 'me' experience the loved one as an infinitely superior being whom I need outside myself as a *telos* to which or whom 'I' can surrender and obey in dasya. At other times, there is the contented oneness of vatsalya as the lover becomes as a babe on the breast, not in quiescence, a complacence of the heart, but in voluptuous absorption and repose. At yet other times, there is the serene tranquillity of shanta, the peace of the spouses in an ineffable intimacy, a state which the eighth century Sanskrit poet Bhavabhuti lets Rama, with Sita asleep across his arm, describe as 'this state where there is no two-ness in response of joy or sorrow / where the heart finds rest; where feeling does not dry with age / where concealments fall away in time and essential love is ripened.'[31] Besides the compulsions of possessive desire, all these bhavas too are at the core of man's erotic being.

Vaishnava mysticism, being a mysticism of love, does not consider awe as a legitimate bhava in relation to the Divine. Thus there are no feelings of reverence, of the uncanny, or of mystery. Nor are there the degrees of fear associated with awe where, in extremity, terror and dread can reign. Awe is perhaps the central bhava of what Erich Fromm called authoritarian religion. Vaishnava devotionalism, on the other hand, would consider awe as an obstacle in the mystical endeavour. It distances and separates rather than binds and joins.

I am aware that Ramakrishna's immersion in the various bhavas at different times in which he even adopted their outward manifestations can make him appear an outrageous figure to unsympathetic and prosaic observers. Practising the madhurya bhava of Radha towards Krishna, he dressed, behaved, and lived as a girl for six months. At another time, going through the dasya bhava of Hanuman, he attached an artifical tail to his posterior in an effort to resemble the monkey god. When living in the motherly bhava of Yashoda towards Krishna, he had one disciple, who felt like a child towards him, lean against his lap as if suckling at his breast while the mystic talked or listened to the concerns of his other disciples.

I have mentioned mahabhava and prema as the higher, more intense states of bhava which most aspirants never manage to reach. Mahabhava shakes the body and mind to its very foundations, and Ramakrishna compared it to a huge elephant entering a small hut. Prema, on the other hand, which makes visions of the Divine possible, was in his analogy a rope by which one tethered God. Whenever one wanted a darshan, one had merely to pull the rope, and He appeared.

Psychologically speaking, I would tend to see bhavas as more than psychic looseners that jar the soul out of the narcissistic sheath of normal, everyday, self-limiting routine. They are experiences of extreme emotional states which have a quality of irradiation wherein time and space tend to disappear. We know of these feeling states from our experience of passionate love where, at its height, the loved one's beauty is all beauty, the love cannot be conceived as not being eternal, and where the memories of all past loves dim so precipitately as to almost merge into darkness. We also know bhava from our experience of grief which, beginning with a finite loss, irradiates all the world at its height. The world becomes empty, and all that is good is felt to be lost forever. We even know of the quality of bhava from states of extreme fear when the smallest sound, the minutest changes of light and shade, the quivering shapes of objects in the dark, all take on an air of extreme menace. The threat becomes eternal, with nary a thought that it might ever end.

Bhava, then, is a way of experiencing which is done 'with all one's heart, all one's soul, and all one's might.' The bhava fills the ecstatic mystic, as it did Ramakrishna, to the brim. He is not depleted, and there is no need for that restitution in delusion and hallucination that is the prime work of insanity. In a bhava, Ramakrishna rekindled the world with fresh vision, discovering or rather endowing it with new-found beauty and harmony. Bhava animated his relation with nature and human beings, deepened his sensate and metaphysical responsiveness.

Bhava, then, is creative experiencing, or rather the ground for all creativity—mystical, artistic, or scientific. The capacity for bhava is what an ideal analysis strives for, an openness towards experiencing; a capacity for 'experiencing experience' as Bion would call it. All the other gains of analysis—insight into one's conflicts, the capacity to experience pleasure without guilt, ability to tolerate anxiety without being crippled, development of a reliable reality testing, and so on—are secondary to the birth of the analytic bhava. Of course, the analytic bhava, the total openness to the analytic situation manifested in the capacity to really *free*-associate, is not simply a goal to be reached at the end of analysis, but a state to strive for in every session. In the language of the traditional drive–defence analytic model, if we divide defences into creative and uncreative, the latter by definition pathological, then the capacity for bhava is perhaps the most creative of defences and needs a place of honour beside and even beyond sublimation.

From bhava, the ground of mystical creativity, let us turn to darshan, vision, the mystic's primary creative product, his particular non-material creation or mystical art. Ramakrishna's explanation of visionary experience is simple, heartfelt, and sensuous. 'God cannot be seen with these physical eyes. In the course of spiritual discipline (*sadhana*) one gets a love's body endowed with love eyes, love ears, and so on. One sees God with these love eyes. One hears His voice with these love ears. One even gets a penis and a vagina made of love. With this love body one enjoys intercourse with the soul.'[32]

In my own explorations, I prefer to use the religious term vision rather than its psychiatric counterpart hallucination for the same reason that I have talked of mystical *ecstasy* rather than of euphoria, namely the connotations of psychopathology associated with psychiatric categories. The distinction between the two, though, is not very hard and fast, their boundaries constantly shifting. Both can be produced by severe depression or manic excitement, toxic psychosis due to exhaustion or starvation or sensory deprivation or simply a febrile illness. What is important in distinguishing them is their meaning and content and not their origin.

Visions are like hallucinations in that they too are images, such as flashes of light, which are visually perceived without the external stimulation of the organ of sight. They are, however, not hallucinations in that they occur during the course of intense religious experience rather than during a psychotic episode. They are thus less bizarre and less disorganized. Visions belong more to the realm of perceptions that take place say, during a dream, while falling asleep (hypnagogic) or when awakening (hypnopompic). None of these can be called a consequence of psychic impairment. Visions are, then, special kinds of dreams which find their way into waking life. To have vision is in itself as much a manifestation of mental disorder as is the corresponding process of real events being drawn across the barrier of sleep into the formation of dreams. Freud recognized the special nature of visions when, in an aside on the psychology of the mystic, he remarked, 'It is easy to imagine, too, that certain mystics may succeed in upsetting the normal relations between the different regions of the mind, so that, for instance, perception may be able to grasp happenings in the depths of the ego and in the id which were otherwise inaccessible to it.'[33] Ramakrishna's visions, as perhaps those of other mystics, do not constitute a unitary phenomenon. They span the whole range from what can be fairly described as hallucinations in the psychiatric sense, through more or less conscious visions, to what I would call 'unconscious visions' (or 'visions of the unconscious'?) which cannot be described since the observing ego is absent. These are the ineffable 'salt doll' visions which comprise a small, though perhaps the most striking part of the total mystical repertoire.

Before we discuss the various kinds of visions, let us note their central common feature: the intense affect they generate, an affect that endows them with their characteristic sense of noesis. The affect, so strong that it is experienced as *knowing* partakes of some of the quality of the symbiotic state in infancy when the child knew the mother through an interchange of their feelings, when affect and cognition were not differentiated from one another.[34]

The affects are also manifested in the body, and Ramakrishna's visions had certain well-defined physical correlates. At times, he would shudder while tears of joy streamed unchecked down his cheeks. At other times, his eyes would become half closed and unfocussed, a faint smile playing around the mouth while his body became completely rigid and had to be supported by a disciple lest he fall and hurt himself. The accompaniment to certain other trance states was a flushed chest or a strong burning sensation all over the body. Ramakrishna reports that once when in such a state, Brahmani, his tantric guru, tried to lead him to his bath. She could not hold his hand, so hot was his skin, and she had to wrap him in a sheet. The earth that stuck to his body while he was lying on the ground became baked. Then there is the feeling of being famished—one wonders, spiritual receptivity with a bodily analogue (or is it vice versa)? Or there are the bouts of gluttony in which he consumed enormous quantities of food, generally sweets. The craving for a particular dish or a sweet would come upon Ramakrishna unexpectedly, at any time of night or day. At these moments, Ramakrishna would be like a pregnant woman who is dominated by her obsession and cannot rest till the craving is satisfied.

From inside the tradition, all these manifestations are some of the nineteen bodily signs of the mystical experience. To the analyst, however, they are a further confirmation of the mystic's access to a period in early life—'oral' in the classical nomenclature—when the boundary between psyche and soma was much more porous than is the case in adulthood. His is the reclamation of a truly dialogical period wherein engendered affects were discharged through the body while physical experience found easy expression in affective states. Ramakrishna's longing for the Mother, accompanied by breathlessness of a kind where he feels he is about to die, for instance, is akin to a certain type of asthmatic bodily manifestation of dammed-up urge for the mother's succour.

Coming back to the various types of visions, the hallucinations, unbidden and unwelcome, belong to his period of insanity (unmada): 'I would spit on the ground when I saw them. But they would follow me and obsess me like ghosts. One day after such a vision I would have a severe attack of diarrhoea, and all these ecstasies would pass out through my bowels.'[35]

These hallucinations, or better, nightmarish visions, are not alien but perhaps as much a part of Ramakrishna's personality as are his artistic sensibility or his more elevated, mystical visions. Their essential linkage may be better understood if we take recourse to Ernst Hartmann's work on nightmares.[36]

In his study of non-psychiatric volunteers who suffered from nightmares since childhood, Hartmann found that these subjects were usually sensitive people with a strong artistic bent and creative potential. More important, they demonstrate what he calls 'thin boundaries of the mind,' a permeability between self and object, waking/sleeping, fantasy/reality, adult/child, human/animal, and other such boundaries, which are relatively fixed for most people. The thin boundary of the mind, Hartmann tries to show, is at the root of both their artistic sensibility and potential for nightmares. It is tempting to speculate that Ramakrishna, and perhaps most other mystics, have a *genetic* biological predisposition, reinforced by some early experiences to which we will come later, to thin boundaries, also between nightmarish and ecstatic visions.

The second class of visions are the conscious ones. Welcomed by a prepared mind, they fall on a receptive ground. Conscious visions may be symbolic representations of an ongoing psychic process, the symbols taken from the mystic's religious and cultural tradition. This is true, for instance, of Ramakrishna's vision of his 'enlightenment', which he 'saw' in the traditional yogic imagery of *Kundalini*, the coiled serpent energy rising through the different centres (*chakras*) of his body and opening up the 'lotuses' associated with these centres, a specifically Hindu metaphor for mental transformation and the opening up of the psyche to hitherto inaccessible psychic experience.

> I saw a 22, 23-year-old, exactly resembling me, enter the Sushumna nerve and with his tongue 'sport' (*raman*) with the vuvla-(*yoni*) shaped lotuses. He began with the centre of the anus, through the centres of the penis, navel, and so on. The respective four-petaled, six-petaled, and ten-petaled lotuses which had been dropping, rose high and blossomed. I distinctly remember that when he came to the heart and sported with it with his tongue, the 12-petaled lotus which had been dropping rose high and opened its petals. Then he came to the 16-petaled lotus in the throat and the two-petaled one in the forehead. And last of all, the 1000-petaled lotus in the head blossomed.[37]

This particular vision, in which self-representation is split into observing and participating aspects, can also be seen through psychiatric glasses as a heutroscopic depersonalization which occurs particularly among individuals with tendencies towards self-contemplation and introspection. Yet in the absence of any associated painful or anxious affect and the fact that this kind of vision was only one among Ramakrishna's vast repertoire of visions with very different structures and qualities, I would tend to see its ground in creativity, akin to the heightened fantasy of an artist or a writer, rather than in pathology. Goethe and Maupassant are two instances of creative writers who also experienced the phenomenon of their doubles.[38]

Other conscious visions are visual insights, images full of conviction and sudden clarity, couched either in a universal–mystical or in a particular, cultural–historical idiom. Some examples of the former would be seeing the universe filled with sparks of fire, or glittering like a lake of quicksilver, or all its quarters illuminated with the light of myriad candles. Such visions of light, we mentioned earlier, have been reported by mystics throughout the ages, and, indeed, seeing the divine light has been a central feature of many mystical cults, including seventeenth century Quakerism. Another visual insight of the universal variety is seeing everything throbbing with consciousness: 'Sometimes I see the same consciousness playing in small fish that is animating the world. Sometimes I see the world soaked with consciousness in the same way as the earth is soaked with water during the rains.'[39]

The full import of the more culturally constituted visions, on the other hand, can only be appreciated if we keep in mind that Ramakrishna was a Hindu Brahmin living at a time—the nineteenth century, and place—rural Bengal—in which the ideas of pollution and polluting substances were strong, caste taboos strict, and the threatened loss of caste a horror of the first magnitude. Visions dissolving religious distinctions and caste taboos, such as the ones on touching forbidden substances or taking food from forbidden persons, were thus primarily expressed in a cultural imagery relevant to Ramakrishna's community. For instance, 'Then I was shown a Muslim with a long beard who came to me with rice in an earthen plate. He fed other Muslims and also gave me some grains to eat. Mother showed me there exists only one and not two.'[40] 'Another day I saw excrement, urine, rice, vegetables, and other foods. Suddenly the soul came out of my body and, like a flame, touched everything: excrement, urine, everything was tasted. It was revealed that everything is one, that there is no difference.'[41] Or, when on the repeated egging on by his nephew, he asked the Goddess for occult powers and saw a middle-aged prostitute come up, squat on her haunches with her back to him, and proceed to evacuate. The vision revealed that occult powers were the shit of that whore.

There is another class of visions, or strictly speaking, mystical illusions, since these rest on a transmutation of external stimuli into creations which are nearer to those of the artist. Thus the way an English boy leans against a tree is transformed into a vision of Krishna; a prostitute walking towards him is changed into a vision of the Mother Goddess—both images irradiate his body and mind with beneficence. In Blake's words, these illusions are 'auguries of innocence' enabling the mystic 'to see a world in a grain of sand, and a heaven in a wild flower.'

And finally, there are the indescribable, unconscious visions. Ramakrishna once said to his disciples,

'You see, something goes up creeping from the feet to the head. Consciousness continues to exist as long as this power does not reach the head; but as soon as it reaches the head, all consciousness is completely lost. There is no seeing or hearing anymore, much less speaking. Who can speak? The very idea of "I" and "You" vanishes. While it (the serpent power) goes up, I feel a desire to tell you everything—how many visions I experience, of their nature, etc. Until it comes to this place (showing the heart) or at most this place (showing the throat) speaking is possible, and I do speak. But the moment it goes up beyond this place (showing the throat) someone forcibly presses the mouth, as it were, and I lose all consciousness. I cannot control it. Suppose I try to describe what kind of vision I experience when it goes beyond this place (showing the throat). As soon as I begin to think of them for the purpose of description the mind rushes immediately up, and speaking becomes impossible.[42]

His feelings during these visions could then only be expressed in metaphors—'I feel like a fish released from a pot into the water of the Ganges.' Ramakrishna, however, does not seem to have been overly enamoured of these states which have been so often held as the apex of the mystical experience. He consciously tried to keep a trace of the observing ego—a little spark of the big fire—so as not to completely disappear, or disappear for a long time, into the *unio mystica* with its non-differentiation of 'I and the 'Other.' 'In *samadhi*, I lose outer consciousness completely, but God generally keeps a little trace of the ego in me for the enjoyment [here he uses a deliberately sensual metaphor, *vilas*] of intercourse. Enjoyment is only possible when "I" and "You" remain.' As he maintained, 'I want to taste sugar, not become sugar.' Yet in spite of himself he was often the salt doll that went into the ocean.

The unconscious visions, irreducible to language, are different from other visions which are ineffable only in the sense that their description can never be complete. The unconscious visions are a return to the world before the existence of language, visions of 'reality' through the destruction of language that the particular mystical act entails. As Octavio Paz puts it, 'Language sinks its roots into this world but transforms its juices and reactions into signs and symbols. Language is the consequence (or the cause) of our exile from the universe, signifying the distance between things and ourselves. If our exile were to come to an end, languages would come to an end.'[43] The salt doll ends exile, writes a *finis* to language.

The vicissitudes of separation have been, of course, at the heart of psychoanalytic theorizing on mysticism. The yearning to be reunited with a perfect, omnipotent being, the longing for the blissful soothing and nursing associated with the mother of earliest infancy (perhaps as much an adult myth as an infantile reality), has been consensually deemed the core of mystical motivation. What has been controversial is the way this longing has been viewed and the value placed on it by different analysts.

The traditional view, initiated by Freud, sees this yearning as reactive, a defence against the hatred directed towards the Oedipal father. For writers influenced by Melanie Klein, the longing for the blissful 'good' mother is a defensive denial of her terrifying and hated aspects.[44] Given the limitation that Ramakrishna did not spend any time on the couch (but, then, neither have other theorists had mystics as patients), I can only say that there is no evidence in the voluminous record of his conversation, reminiscences, and accounts of his visions which is remotely suggestive of any strong hostility towards the Oedipal father. The evidence for the denial of the dreaded aspects of the mother is slightly greater, namely through a plausible interpretation of some elements of his vision in the Kali temple when he had taken up a sword to kill himself. However, seen in the total context of a large number of visions of the Mother Goddess, the ambiguous evidence of one particular vision is not enough to compel an acceptance of the Kleinian notions on mystical motivation.

Paul Horton has advanced a more adaptive view of mystical yearning and mystical states, especially during adolescence.[45] He sees them as a consequence of the pangs of separation in which the felt reality of being utterly and agonizingly alone is *transiently* denied. The mystical experience is then a transitional phenomenon which soothes and reassures much as a baby is soothed by a blanket, a child by a stuffed toy or fairy-tale, an adult by a particular piece of music—all these various creations, material and nonmaterial, providing opportunities for the controlled illusion that heals.

There is much to be said for the hypothesis that experiences of separation and loss spurred Ramakrishna onto the mystical path. We know that Ramakrishna's first quasi-mystical ecstasy when he became unconscious at the sight of white cranes flying against a background of dark clouds took place in the last year of his father's final illness (according to one place in Ramakrishna's reminiscences, two years after his father's death), that is, at a time of an impending loss. And I have described the marked change that came over Ramakrishna is not unlike some of the Christian mystics in whose lives too, as David Aberbach has demonstrated, one could hypothesize a link between personal loss and their mystical calling.[46] Teresa of Avila's life in the church began with the death of her mother when Teresa was twelve years old. The loss of a parent or parent–surrogate may also be an early one, heightening a later sense of abandonment and the subsequent search for the 'eternal Thou,' as perhaps in the examples of St John of the Cross, whose father died a few months after his birth, or of Martin Buber, whose mother deserted him when he was three.

The mystical path is then also a way of lessening the agony of separation, mitigating the grief at loss, reducing the sadness of bereavement. In my own interviews with members of a mystical cult in India, loss was the single most important factor in their decision to seek its membership. The very embarkation on the mystical path had a therapeutic effect by itself, while any experience of a mystical state had a further marked effect in altering the person's dysphoric state of mind.[47] In contrast to the person's previous feelings of apathy and depression, the turn to mysticism had the consequence of his dealing with grief in a more orderly and more detached, though in a more transcendent, manner. Perhaps T.S. Eliot is correct in observing that 'A man does not join himself with the universe so long as he has anything else to join himself with.'[48]

Of course, Ramakrishna's two actual experiences of loss are not sufficient to explain the totality of his mysticism, the intensity of his yearning throughout life to end the state of separation from the Divine, and the acuteness of his distress at the absence of the Mother. The motivational skein of mysticism, as of any other psychic phenomenon, is composed of many strands. One could speculate that the advanced age of his mother at his birth, his family's poverty and thus his mother's added preoccupations with household tasks, the birth of another sibling when he was four, may have led to the emotional unavailability of the mother at a phase of the child's development when his own needs were driving him closer to her. In other words, the suggestion is that in the crucial 'rapprochement' phase (which occurs later in India than in psychoanalyst Margaret Mahler's timetable), the mother was unavailable at a time when his anxiety about separation, and its convergent depression, were at their apex. This would fix separation and its associated anxiety as the dominant theme of his inner life. Each feared or actual loss would reactivate separation anxiety together with a concomitant effort at combating it by reclaiming in fantasy an adored and adoring intimacy with the maternal matrix. The unity Ramakrishna aimed for is, then, not the merger like states of the infant at the breast, though these too prefigured his trances, but the ending of separation striven for by the toddler. It is a state in which both mother and child have boundaries in relation to each other while another boundary encloses their 'double unit' from the rest of the world. Here the enjoyment of the mother's presence is deeply sensuous, almost ecstatic, and informs Ramakrishna's selection of words; images and metaphors that describe his experiences.

Together with the speculated impact of early mother–child interaction in Ramakrishna's psychic life, admittedly a construct derived from analytic theory rather than a reconstruction based on compelling psychobiographical evidence, I would tend to attribute his acute sensitivity to the theme of separation to the mystical gift (or curse) of a specific kind of creative experiencing. This can be understood more clearly, if we take recourse to some ideas of the 'metaphysical' analysts mentioned earlier.

Lacan, for instance, has postulated that man's psychic life constantly seeks to deal with a primordial state of affairs which he calls the Real. The Real itself is unknowable, though we constantly create myths as its markers. Perhaps the principal myth involves the rupture of a basic union; the separation from the mother's body, leaving us with a fundamental feeling of incompletion. The fantasies around this insufficiency are universal, governing the psyche of both patients and analysts alike. In the psyche, this lack is translated as desire, and the human venture is a history of desire as it ceaselessly loses and discovers itself in (what Lacan calls) The Imaginary and, with the advent of language, The Symbolic order. Born of rupture, desire's fate is an endless quest for the lost object; all real objects merely interrupt the search. As the Barandes put it, 'It is the task of the *néoténique* [that is, immature, even foetalized being] being separated from its original union by its fall into life and into time, to invent detours for itself, deviations of object as well as means and aims. Its condition is inexorably perverse—if perversions must be.'[49] The mystical quest seeks to rescue from primal repression the constantly lived contrast between an original interlocking and a radical rupture. The mystic, unlike most others, does not mistake his hunger for its fulfilment. If we are all fundamentally perverse in the play of our desire, then the mystic is the only one who seeks to go beyond the illusion of The Imaginary and, yes, also the maya of The Symbolic register.

One of Ramakrishna's more 'private' visions attempts to paint the issue of separation with crude yet compelling brushstrokes. As Bion would say, here he is like the analyst who knows that emotional truth is ineffable, available only in intimations and approximations. Like the Bionian analyst, the mystic too is compelled to use terms from sensuous experience to point to a realm beyond this experience.

> Let me tell you a very secret experience. Sitting in a pine grove, I had the vision of a small, hidden [literally 'thief's door'] entrance to a room. I could not see what was inside the room. I tried to bore a hole with a nail file but did not succeed. As I bored the hole it would fill up again and again. And then suddenly it made a big opening.

He kept quiet and then started speaking again. 'These are all higher matters. I feel someone is closing my mouth. I have seen God residing in the vagina. I saw Him there at the time of sexual intercourse of a dog and a bitch.'[50]

Ramakrishna's vision, followed by an associative sequel, does not need extended analytic gloss. The small secret opening to a room into which he cannot see and which he tries to keep open, the seeing of God in the genitals of a bitch in intercourse, do not encode the mystical preoccupation with opening a way back to the self-other interlocking in any complex symbolic language. This interlocking, the mystical unity, is not unitary. As we saw in Ramakrishna's case, it extends in a continuum from the foetalized being's never having known separation from the mother's insides, an expulsion from her womb, through the satiated infant's flowing feelings of merger at the breast, to the toddler being pulled back to the mother as if held at one end of an invisible string.

What I am emphasizing, however, is not the traditional analytic agenda of pathological, defensive, or compensatory uses of these various degrees of dyadic unity in mystical experiencing. As Michael Eigen has elaborated in a series of papers, for Freud, ideal experiencing, that is, states or moments of beatific (or horrific) perfection, in which I would include the mystical states, usually involved something in disguise—mother, father, sex, aggression and so on.[51] Lacan, Winnicott and Bion (and implicitly also Erikson), on the other hand, look at ideal experiencing in its own right, as a spontaneously unfolding capacity for creative experiencing. This capacity can be deployed defensively as has been spelled out in detail in the Freudian literature, but it is not coterminous with defence.

All these authors emphasize the positive, regenerative aspects of this experiencing not as idealists but as empirical analysts who chart out its developmental vicissitudes from early infancy onward. The experiencing itself, they maintain, should not be confused with the introjection of the mother and father images or functions. These only foster or hamper this capacity.

If one reads these authors carefully, one discovers that the *primary object of creative experiencing is not mother or father but the unknowable ground of creativeness as such.* Winnicott, for example, emphasizes that what is at stake in transitional experiencing is not mainly a self or object (mother) substitute, but the creation of a symbol, of symbolizing experiencing itself. The subject lives through and towards creative immersion (including phases of chaos, unintegration, waiting).[52]

What we should then pay equal attention to is not only the conflicts of the mystic that threaten to deform or disperse his creative experiencing, but the experiencing itself—its content, context, and evolution.

Most of us harbour tantalizing 'forgotten' traces of this kind of experiencing, an apperception where what is happening outside is felt to be the creative act of the original artist (or mystic) within each of us and recognized as such with (in Blake's word) *delight.* For in late infancy and early childhood we did not always see the world as something outside ourselves, to be recognized in detail, adapted, complied with, and fitted into our idiosyncratic inner world, but often as an infinite succession of creative acts.

Mystical experience, then, is one and—in some cultures and at certain historical periods—the pre-eminent way of uncovering the vein of creativity that runs deep in all of us. For some, it is the throes of romantic love that gives inklings of our original freshness of vision.

Others may strive for creative experiencing in art or in natural science. In the West, the similarities between mystics and creative artists and scientists have been pointed out since the beginning of the century. Evelyn Underhill in her path-breaking work on mysticism emphasized the resemblance between artistic geniuses and mystics—though one should hesitate to use the terms as interchangeable—while James Leuba pointed out the similarity at a more mundane level in creative phenomena of the daily kind and at a lower level of intensity.[53] In China, we know that it was the mystical Taoists stressing spontaneity, 'inaction,' 'emptying the mind,' rather than the rational Confucians, who stimulated Chinese scientific discovery. In India, too, in different epochs, the striving for mystical experience through art, especially music, has been a commonly accepted and time honoured practice. And Albert Einstein writes of his own motivations for the scientific enterprise, 'The most beautiful, the most profound emotion we can experience is the sensation of the mystical. It is the fundamental emotion that stands at the cradle of true art and science.' Einstein goes on to say that there is a need 'to escape from everyday life with its painful crudity and hopeless dreariness, from fetters of one's own shifting desires.' Instead the scientist and the artist creates his own reality, substituting it for the world of experience and thus overcoming it: 'Each makes his own cosmos and its construction the pivot of his emotional life, in order to find in this way peace and security which he cannot find in the narrow whirlpool of personal experience.'[54] Here it seems to me that Einstein is not talking as some who is depressed but with a creative individual's clear-sighted and inevitable response to the world as it is. When Buddha, as the young Siddhartha confronted with illness, old age, and death proclaims '*Sabbam dukham* (All is suffering)', he too is not depressed but in perfect attunement with the reality principle. To see the world with a creative eye but a sober perspective is perhaps our greatest adaptation to reality—a state where Buddha, Freud, and Ramakrishna come together.

Sexuality and the Mystical Experience

Ramakrishna was one with other Vaishnava mystics in his insistence that sexuality, by which he meant male sexuality, phallic desire, constituted the biggest obstacle to mystical experiencing. This is a formulation with which psychoanalysts will not have any quarrel. For both male and female infants, the differentiation between self and object is achieved and ego boundaries constituted by a gradual detachment from the mother. The presence of the father is vital for this process. Whereas the masculinity of the father makes it possible for the boy to overcome his primary femininity, the presence of the paternal phallus also helps to protect the little girl from fusional tendencies with the mother. Male sexuality and male desire may thus be viewed as obstacles in the path of fusion, the phallus as the prime symbol of boundaries the mystic seeks to transcend.

The renunciation of adult masculinity is not only a feature of Hindu devotional mysticism but is also a feature of Christian emotional mysticism of medieval and early modern Europe. Affective prayer or Bernardine mysticism, as it has often been called after the influential sermons of the eleventh century saint Bernard of Clairvaux, possesses a striking affinity to its Hindu counterpart. Femininity pervades both. In the case of medieval Europe, most of the practising mystics were women. But even the outstanding male mystics—St John of the Cross, Francois de Sales, Fenelon—show strong feminine identifications and produced their most important ideas under the direct influence of women.[55] The psychological stance of Christian ecstatics towards Divinity, paralleling that of the Vaishnava mystics, is either that of the infant towards a loving maternal parent, or of a woman towards a youthful lover. Like the Hindus, the Christian mystics too disavowed or overthrew the paternal phallus as they divested the Judeo–Christian God of much of his original masculinity and sternness, virtually relegating him to the role of a grandfather. The message of the European emotional mystics seems to be the same as that of Ramakrishna: the actual gender of the mystic is not important for his practice. It is, however vital that the mystic accept and cultivate his or her femininity to the point that the female-self part becomes dominant in his or her inner psychic reality.

Of the many mystical disciplines, the one Ramakrishna could never practise was the 'heroic' one of Tantra where, at its culmination, God as a female is sought to be pleased—or perhaps I should say, pleasured—as a man pleases a woman through intercourse. In his own Tantric training, he had escaped the demand for ritual sex by going into an ecstatic state just before he had to actually 'perform'. He repeatedly warned his disciples against *kamini–kanchani* (literally, woman and gold), and his advice to novices on the mystical path was to avoid the female sex altogether, the whirlpool in which even Brahma and Vishnu struggle for their lives. For a renunciant, he felt, to sit with a woman or talk to her for a long time was a kind of sexual intercourse of which there were eight kinds. Some of these were to listen to a woman, to talk to her in secret, to keep and enjoy something belonging to a woman, to touch her, and so on. Given the fact that a vast majority of widely known mystics, at least in medieval Christian and devotional Hindu traditions, have been celibates, one wonders whether celibacy, with its profound influence on hormonal balance, is not an important physiological technique for mystical ecstasy.

The prescribed avoidance of women was only for beginners. Once mystical knowledge was gained, sexual differentiation too vanished: 'Then you don't have much to fear. After reaching the roof you can dance as much as you like, but not on the stairs.' Yet, though Ramakrishna constantly reiterated that he looked at the breasts of every woman as those of his mother, that he felt as a child or as another woman with women, his male awareness of women as sexual beings, and of the dangers of a desire that separates and bifurcates, never quite disappeared as his biographers would have us believe. He felt uncomfortable with female devotees sitting in his room and would ask them to go and visit the temple as soon as he could decently get rid of them. Being touched by a woman was not a matter of unconcern but evoked strong physical reactions. 'If a woman touches me, I fall ill. That part of my body aches as if stung by a horned fish. If I touch a woman my hand becomes numb; it aches. If in a friendly spirit I approach a woman and begin to talk to her, I feel as if a curtain has come down between us.'[56] However minimal his sexual conflict, even a great mystic seems to retain at least a vestigial entanglement with the world of desire. In his normal non-ecstatic state, Ramakrishna too was never quite free of the sexual maya, free from the delight, wisdom, beauty, and pain of the 'illusion' which so beguiles the rest of us.

Ramakrishna's attempted renunciation of male sexual desire is the subject of one vision, although as someone who claimed to never having even dreamt of intercourse with a woman, the *conscious* promptings of desire could not have been too peremptory. 'During the *sadhanas*, I vividly perceived a heap of rupees, a shawl, a plate of sweets and two women. "Do you want to enjoy any of these things?" I asked my mind. "No," replied the mind. I saw the insides of those women, of what is in them; entrails, piss, shit, phlegm and such things.'[57] We can, of course, try to understand the contents of this vision in biographical terms. Money, shawl, and sweets embody overpowering temptations for a boy who grew up in a poor family whose dire financial straits allowed but the most spartan of fare. Similarly, one possible cause for the hankering after sexual purity in his youth could be a deep feeling of shame he associated with the sexual act. In a country and at a time where women not infrequently became grandmothers in their late twenties, where sexual activity has always been considered a prerogative of the young—sexual desire of older men and women occasioning derisive laughter—Ramakrishna's birth itself (followed by that of the sister) is the sign of a tainted and deeply mortifying sexuality of his old parents. We have already seen how Ramakrishna's enduring wish to be a woman, expressed variously in dressing and moving his limbs like one, his fantasy of being a girl widow who secretly trysts with Krishna every evening, fitted in well with a tenet of Vaishnava mysticism that all mankind is female while God alone is male. Ramakrishna would approvingly cite the opinion that irrespective of biological gender everyone with nipples is a female. Arjuna, the heroic warrior of the Mahabharata, and Krishna are the only exceptional males since they do not have nipples. In the madhurya bhava, Ramakrishna had even tried to engender in himself female erotic feelings. Moved by an intense love for Krishna, 'such as a woman feels for her lover,' he had stretched out his arms to embrace the Lord's stone idols.

Just as the writings of medieval European female mystics, wherein they wax rhapsodic over their ecstatic union with Jesus, portrayed as an exceedingly handsome and loving bridegroom of the human soul, have been analyzed as expressions of a pathological, hysterical sexuality, it would not be difficult to diagnose Ramakrishna in traditional Freudian terms as a secondary transsexual. He would seamlessly fit in with Robert Stoller's description of the secondary transsexual as being someone who differs from his primary counterpart in that he does not appear feminine from the start of any behaviour that may be classed in gender terms.[58] Under the surface of masculinity, however, there is the persistent impulse towards being feminine, an urge which generally manifests itself in adolescence. The most obvious manifestation of these urges is the wish for the actual wearing of women's clothes. Though these urges may gather in strength and last for longer and longer periods, the masculine aspects of identity are never completely submerged.

Ramakrishna's open espousal and expression of his feminine identifications as a boy, however, also have to do with the greater tolerance of his community and its culture towards such identifications. His urge towards femininity did not meet an unyielding opposition or strenuous attempts at suppression by an enforced participation in masculine play. Any transsexual or homosexual labels may obscure his sense of comfort and easy familiarity with the feminine components of his self. It may hide the fact that the freeing of femininity from repression of disavowal in man and vice versa in a woman may be a great human achievement rather than an illness or a deviation. The deviation may actually lie, as in one view of the etiology of homosexuality, in the *inability* to come to terms with the opposite sexual personality in one's self.[59]

Summarizing, I would say that the male-self part of Ramakrishna's personality was split off in early childhood and tended to grow, if at all, rather slowly. In contrast, the female-self part of his personality dominated his inner psychic reality. Ramakrishna's girl-self was neither repressed nor disassociated but could mature to an extent where psychically he could even possess female sexual equipment and enjoy female sexual experience.

Yet, even a celebratory avowal of secondary femininity in a male mystic may not be enough to exhaust the mystery of the link between sexuality and mysticism. For if, together with 'infant-likeness,' secondary femininity and female bodily experience—breast pride, absence of male external genitalia, the presence of vulva and womb—are important for affective mysticism, then women will be seen as having a head start in this particular human enterprise. They naturally are what male aspirants must become. This may be true though it has yet to be demonstrated that gender makes a substantial difference in the making of a mystic. What is perhaps essential in mysticism is not the presence of secondary but of 'primary' femininity—the 'pure female element' (not the female person) in Winnicott's sense of the term. In his theory of the life of male and female elements in a person, the purely male element, in both man and woman, presupposes separateness and tracks in terms of active relating, or being passively related to, and is backed by the whole apparatus of instinctual drives.[60] The female element, on the other hand, relates to the other—the breast, the mother (both with a small and capital 'm')—in the sense of an identity between the two. When this element finds the other, it is the self that has been found. It is the female element that establishes the simplest, the most primary of experiences, the experience of *being*. Winnicott remarks, 'Psychoanalysts have perhaps given special attention to this male element or drive aspect of object relating and yet have neglected the subject–object identity to which I am drawing attention here, which is at the basis of the capacity to be. The male element *does* (active–passive) while the female element *is* (in males and females) and concludes 'After being—doing and being done to. But first *being*.'[61]

Looking at Ramakrishna's sexuality in relation to his mystical experience in terms of oral, anal, and phallic stages of development or of identifications with mother, father and so on, as in classical analytic discourse, is then to forget that this discourse itself may be based on the life of the male element. Our psychology has still little to say of the distilled female element, the primary femininity, at the heart of emotional mysticism. The pure female element, in both men and women, continues to testify to the category of mystery as a basic dimension in which we all, and especially the mystic, live. As analysts, however, we cannot look at mystery as something eternally beyond human comprehension, but as a phenomenon to which we repeatedly return to increase our understanding. As our perspectives change, our earlier views do not get replaced but are subsumed in an ever-widening set of meanings.

Notes and References

1 Söderblom, N., *Till mystikens belysning* (Lund, 1985), cited in H. Akerberg, 'The Unio Mystica of Teresa of Avila,' in N.G. Holm (ed.), *Religious Ecstasy*, 1981, Stockholm: Almqvist and Wiksell, pp. 275–9.

2 James, William, 1902, *The Varieties of Religious Experience*, New York: Longmans, Green.

3 Greeley, Andrew M., 1975, *The Sociology of the Paranormal: A Reconnaissance*, Beverly Hills: Sage Publications, p. 62.

4 For a psychological description of the structure of mystical experience see Committee on Psychiatry and Religion, 1976, *Mysticism: Spiritual Quest or Psychic Disorder*, New York: Group for Advancement of Psychiatry. See also Hof, H., 'Ecstasy and Mysticism', in Holm, *Religious Ecstasy*, pp. 243–9.

5 Zaehner, R.C., 1960, *Hindu and Muslim Mysticism*, London: Athalone Press, 1960. The authoritative work on Hindu mysticism remains Dasgupta, S.N., 1927, *Hindu Mysticism*, Delhi: Motilal Banarsidas.

6 See Committee on Psychiatry and Religion, *Mysticism*, especially pp. 782–6. For specific psychoanalytic contributions stressing the ego-adaptive aspects of the mystic experience see Horton, Paul C., 1974, 'The Mystical Experience: Substance of an Illusion', *Journal of the American Psychoanalytic Association*, 22, pp. 364–80; Aberbach, David, 1987, 'Grief and Mysticism', *International Review of Psychoanalysis*, 14, pp. 509–26.

7 Ehrenzweig, Anton, 1967, *The Hidden Order of Art*, London: Weidenfeld and Nicolson.

8 Rolland, Romain, 1986, *The Life of Ramakrishna*, Calcutta: Advaita Ashram, p. 38.

9 For the arguments against a psychoanalytic, 'scientific' study of mysticism, see Walsh, Roger N., 1980, *et al.*, 'Paradigms in Collision', in R.N. Walsh and F. Vaughan (eds), *Beyond Ego: Transpersonal Dimensions in Psychology*, Los Angeles: Tarcher, pp. 36–52.

10 See Buckley, Peter and Marc Galanter, 1979, 'Mystical Experience, Spiritual Knowledge, and a Contemporary Ecstatic Experience', *British Journal of Medical Pyschology*, 52, pp. 281–9.

11 For the case histories see Horton, P.C., 'Mystical Experience', and Committee on Psychiatry and Religion, *Mysticism*, pp. 799–807.

12 For a comprehensive comparison of the three see Eigen, Manfred, 1981, 'The Area of Faith in Winnicott, Lacan and Bion', *International Journal of Psychoanalysis*, 62, pp. 413–34.

13 Cited in Harrison, Irving B., 1979, 'On Freud's View of the Infant-Mother Relationship and of the Oceanic Feeling—Some Subjective Influences', *Journal of the American Psychoanalytic Association*, 27, p. 409.

14 Ibid.

15 J.M. Masson suggests a different passage from the writings of Ramakrishna as the source for the term 'oceanic feeling'; see his 1980, *The Oceanic Feeling: The Origins of Religious Sentiment in Ancient India*, Dordrecht: Reidel, p. 36.

16 Pajin, Dushan, 1989, 'The Oceanic Feeling: A Reevaluation', Belgrade, manuscript.

17 Letter to R. Rolland, 19 January 1930, in *The Letters of Sigmund Freud* (edited by E. Freud), 1960, New York: Basic Books, p. 392.

18 Gupta, Mahendranath, 1988, *Sri Ramakrishna Vachanamrita* (translated into Hindi by Suryakant Tripathi 'Nirala'), 3 vols., Nagpur: Ramakrishna Math.

19 Swami Saradananda, 1983, *Sri Ramakrishna, The Great Master*, 2 vols., Mylapore: Sri Ramakrishna Math, vol. 1, pp. 276–7.

20 Rolland, *Life of Ramakrishna*, pp. 22–3.

21 Saradananda, *Sri Ramakrishna*, vol. 1, pp. 276–7.

22 Ibid. p. 156.

23 Ibid, pp. 162–3.

24 Saradananda, *Sri Ramakrishna*, vol. 1, p. 424.

25 Gupta, *Vachanamrita*, vol. 1, p. 71.

26 Ibid., p. 301.

27 Ibid., p. 320.

28 Ibid., pp. 135–6.

29 Ibid., p. 41.

30 Ibid., vol. 2, p. 241.

31 Bhavabhuti, 1964, *Uttara Rama Charita*, in *Six Sanskrit Plays*, Bombay: Asia, p. 368.

32 Gupta, *Vachanamrita*, vol. 1, p. 90.

33 Freud, S., 1933, *New Introductory Lectures, Standard Edition*, vol. 22, pp. 79–80.

34 Ross, Nathaniel, 1975, 'Affect as Cognition: With Observation on the Meaning of Mystical States', *International Review of Psychoanalysis*, 2, pp. 79–93.

35 Gupta, *Vachanamrita*, vol. 3, pp. 238–89.

36 Hartmann, Ernst, 1984, *The Nightmare: The Psychology and Biology of Terrifying Dreams*, New York: Basic.

37 Gupta, *Vachanamrita*, vol. 3, p. 289.

38 Damas Mora, J.M.R. *et al.*, 1980, 'On Heutroscopy or the Phenomenon of the Double', *British Journal of Medical Psychology*, 53, pp. 75–83.

39 Gupta, *Vachanamrita.* vol. 1, p. 388.

40 Ibid., vol. 3, p. 109.

41 Ibid., vol. 1, p. 431.

42 Saradananda, *Sri Ramakrishna*, vol. 1, p. 417.

43 Paz, Octavio, 1981, *The Monkey Grammarian* (Helen Lane, trans.), New York: Seaver Books, p. 133.

44 For representative statements of the classical Freudian view see Salzman, L., 1953, 'The Psychology of Religious and Ideological Conversion', *Psychiatry*, 16, pp. 177–87. For the Kleinian view see Harrison, Irving B., 1975, 'On the Maternal Origins of Awe', *The Psychoanalytic Study of the Child*, 30, pp. 181–95.

45 Horton, P.C., 'Mystical Experience'.

46 For a detailed discussion of the link and parallels between the process of mourning and mysticism see Aberbach, 'Grief and Mysticism', pp. 509–26.

47 Kakar, S., 1982, *Shamans, Mystics and Doctors*, New York: Knopf, chap. 5. See also Buckley and Galanter, 'Mystical Experience', p. 285; Horton, P.C., 1973, 'The Mystical Experience as a Suicide Preventive', *American Journal of Psychiatry*, 130, pp. 294–6.

48 Cited in Aberbach, 'Grief and Mysticism', p. 509.

49. Barande, I. and R. Barande, 'Antinomies du concept de perversion et epigenese del' appetit de excitation', cited in Leavy, S.A., 1985–6, 'Male Homosexuality Reconsidered', *International Journal of Psychoanalytic Psychotherapy*, 11, p. 163.

50 Gupta, *Vachanamrita*, vol. 1, p. 388.

51 Eigen, 1979, 'Area of Faith', 'Ideal Images, Creativity and the Freudian Drama', *Psychocultural Review*, 3, pp. 278–98; 1981, 'Creativity, Instinctual Fantasy and Ideal Images', *Psychoanalytic Review*, 68.

52 Eigen, 'Area of Faith', p. 431.

53 Underhill, E., 1961, *Mysticism* , New York: E.P. Dutton; Leuba, J.H., 1925 *The Psychology of Religious Mysticism*, New York: Harcourt, Brace.

54 Einstein, A., 1954, *Ideas and Opinions*, New York: Crown Publishers, p. 75.

55 Moller, Herbert, 1965, 'Affective Mysticism in Western Civilization', *Psychoanalytic Review*, 52, pp. 259–67. See also McDonnel, E.W., 1954, *The Beguines and Beghards in Medieval Culture*, New Brunswick: Rutgers University Press, pp. 320–32.

56 Gupta, *Vachanamrita*, vol. 3, pp. 535–6.

57 Ibid., p. 107.

58 Stoller, Robert, 1979, 'The Gender Disorders', in *Sexual Deviation*, (I. Rosen, ed.), New York: Oxford University Press, pp. 109–38.

59 Wisdom, J.O., 1983, 'Male and Female', *International Journal of Psychoanalysis*, 64, pp. 159–68.

60 Winnicott, D.W., 1971, 'Creativity and its Origins', in *Playing and Reality*, London: Tavistock, pp. 72–85.

61 Ibid., p. 85.

Childhood of a Spiritually Incorrect Guru—Osho*

I FIRST MET RAJNEESH, later known as Bhagwan ('Blessed One', 'Incarnation of God') and still later as Osho, in 1971 in the rapturous accounts of a visit to his Poona ashram by a young German woman who had been in psychotherapy with me for six months. She had been 'spiritually transformed' by what she had experienced there, she declared, and was unsure whether she needed to continue therapy. I was curious and envious, not necessarily in that order. Over the next decades, I followed the meteoric rise and fall of perhaps one of the best known, and certainly the most notorious gurus in the spiritual bazaar of the nineteen seventies and eighties.[1]

Rajneesh's Poona ashram was at the centre of a spiritual movement that had successfully spread to Europe, North America, Australia, and Japan. At one time, his Western disciples, primarily from a social and cultural elite—members of European aristocracy, lawyers, doctors, writers, artists, academics, and other professionals outnumbered by far the Indians that came for enlightenment to the 'sex guru' or the 'guru of the Rich', as Rajneesh had come to be known. By 1981, over forty thousand had been initiated as '*sanyasins*.' These were not the traditional Indian sanyasins who renounce the world, leave their families, and take vows of non-possession while they devote themselves to their spiritual search. The

* From *Mad and Divine: Spirit and Psyche with Modern World*, Delhi: Viking-Penguin, 2008.

commitment demanded of the Rajneeshis, as his disciples were called, was limited to using the new names Rajneesh gave them at the time of the initiation, dressing in 'sunrise' colors (orange-red at first but later, pink), wearing a necklace with 108 beads and a locket containing a picture of Rajneesh, and continuing an appropriate practice of meditation.

Rajneesh loved to shock the media which, in turn, loved to be shocked by this bright eyed, high-domed, lushly bearded imp, whose admirers considered him to be one of the wisest men of the age. Lurid stories circulated about his large, sprawling ashram in Koregaon Park in Poona. There were reports of a widespread use of drugs and rampant prostitution by Western female sanyasins. Orgies of group sex were said to be on the daily menu in the ashram. A deeply conservative Indian society was scandalized by the unrestrained sexual goings-on as much as by Rajneesh's mockery of the Indian establishment and his ridiculing of Indian icons. Moraji Desai, the puritan Prime Minister and the self-confessed daily imbiber of his own urine, who came to power in 1976, was an easy target for Rajneesh's barbs. Rajneesh's followers, successful and intelligent people who, like their guru, had little interest in ideology and no respect for authority, might have enjoyed his descriptions of Gandhi as a 'masochist,' a 'pervert', and a 'Hindu chauvinist,' or of Mother Teresa as a 'charlatan' and 'hypocrite,' a religious politician hiding behind the façade of helping the poor.[2] However, many Indians and, more importantly, the Indian government was not amused. Hefty tax arrears were slapped on the commune and dark hints were thrown out on investigations that had been or were soon going to be launched into its financial affairs.

Rajneesh's response was to pack up and move the ashram to a small town in Oregon in the United States which he renamed Rajneeshpuram. His mission, he proclaimed, was to lead his followers to the higher states of consciousness and transform the world. Freed from the distorting conditioning of society, families, and politics would become obsolete in the new world. Living in harmony and pursuing spiritual aims, the Rajneeshis would become the nucleus of a new race of human beings that would emerge after the nuclear holocaust he predicted would take place at the end of twentieth century.

Rajneesh's Oregon stay was a disaster. The guru became more and more withdrawn, taking drugs, inhaling nitrous oxide, watching videos in his darkened room and emerging only occasionally to ride in one of the ninety two Rolls Royces donated by his followers. His few trusted lieutenants who ran the Oregon commune became increasingly paranoid in the unsympathetic environment of the American West. Listening devices were planted in the quarters of those suspected of disloyalty, weapons were hoarded, obsessive and bizarre measures to protect against AIDS were taken and, finally, a campaign to poison suspected traitors inside the group and those outside who were thought to be hostile to the ashram, was initiated. Rajneeshpuram was shut down when these illegal activities came to light. Rajneesh tried to flee the country but was arrested while boarding his flight. He was finally allowed to leave after pleading guilty to two felony charges. Some of his closest associates who had run the Oregon ashram were sent to prison. Rajneesh finally returned to Poona after his efforts to set up the ashram at other locations failed because of the world-wide notoriety he and his movement had acquired. Suffering from various allergies and chronic asthma, Rajneesh died in Poona in 1991. He was fifty-nine.

Rajneesh can be regarded as a pioneer in the globalization of spirituality and Rajneeshism as one of the first global brands in the spiritual marketplace. There have been other Indian gurus before him who took their spiritual wares to the West but their 'product' had remained recognizably Indian, comparable, say, to the export of traditional Indian handicrafts to a specialized niche market. Rajneesh's 'product', though inspired by Hindu and Buddhist *tantra* which attaches spiritual significance to sex, was crafted through techniques that were eclectic in nature. It owed as much to the healing practices of American Indian shamans and the middle-eastern Sufi orders as to New Age psychotherapy techniques of transpersonal psychology which were coming into vogue in Europe and especially in the United States.

Rajneesh was not a 'sex guru' although, like Michael Foucault, he, too, believed that a person's sexuality revealed his or her essence, or as he put it, '... the attitude towards sex is a very symbolic attitude; it shows everything about your whole life.'[3] It would also be doing him injustice to believe that the attraction of his movement lay in the provision of orgiastic sex under the garb of spiritual striving. At the time of a flourishing 'counter-culture' movement in the West, the 'Age of Aquarius', 'flower power', marijuana and LSD, one did not have to spend a fortune to travel to India, risk diarrhea and other infections, just to get laid. By itself, sex was 'stupid', Rajneesh maintained; its spiritual significance lay in producing mindlessness or the silence of the mind that made true meditation possible. The orgasm was a door into silence, into 'the secret that there is no secret.'[4] It was the stillness and meditation after the intercourse which was the real object of the feast although Rajneesh's critics insisted on mistaking the appetizer for the main course. His other appellation, 'the guru of the rich' was more deserved. Rajneesh was definite in maintaining that only those who were comfortably off, who did not need to toil to fulfil their material needs, were receptive to their spiritual nature; or to adapt a well-known quote from the German playwright and poet Bertold Brecht 'Erst kommt das Fressen, dann kommt die Moral (Food first, then spirituality).'

Rajneesh's 'religionless religiousness', a spirituality without adherence to any creed, demanded a de-programming or de-conditioning of the mind. It required a transcendence of the personal past through an erasing of the markings on the black board which had been scribbled over again and again in the course of growing up by such cultural institutions as the family, the school, and official religions. Rajneesh's philosophy of liberation emphasized a rejection of all conventional values. It highlighted direct, ecstatic experience, a knowing through intense feelings (hence, the importance of sex), and acting in the world according to the dictum 'Be absolutely selfish' or, in other, somewhat more palatable words, 'The most basic and the most fundamental commitment is to love oneself'.[5] This is a far cry from most other spiritual trends. One of the most visible icons of contemporary spirituality, the Dalai Lama, states flatly, 'Paying attention to one's own needs is a producer of suffering; cherishing others a giver of happiness.'[6] The mansion of spirituality indeed has many rooms.

Rajneesh used various techniques for de-conditioning the mind. The primary one with which he began his mission in 1971 was Dynamic Meditation. This involved letting one's body go without restrictions, in a group setting and in the presence of the guru. To the accompaniment of pulsating music, disciples let their bodies dance and gyrate in any manner they liked. They shouted, laughed, sobbed, rolled on the ground till a coordinated climax with strong sexual overtones was reached.[7] This was followed by communal breathing exercises and sitting quietly in meditation. Modern minds cannot be quieted by old meditative procedures requiring silence and immobility, Rajneesh asserted. The unstill mind needs to be exploded, an explosion that lets out all pent up emotions. Only after such an active release, could modern man reach a state of natural silence.

Over the years, other techniques to foster the disintegration of social constraints and personal identity were added to the repertoire offered at the ashram. Western psychotherapists of varied persuasions—practitioners of Reichian Body Work, Gestalt therapy, Primal Screaming, Past Life Regression, and other 'humanistic' therapies that were being developed in the counter-culture of the West of 1970s and 1980s—joined

Rajneesh and were given free rein to search for ever more effective ways to uncover the 'true, inner self.' Inevitably, 'therapy intensive' groups involving group sex became a part of the repertoire. Often, with the removal of the lid from the cauldron of instincts, overt violence and untrammelled sexuality ran riot in these quasi-therapeutic groups where physical injury and psychological trauma were not uncommon.

However, more than Rajneesh's philosophy or their experiences in therapy groups, his followers held that it was Rajneesh's presence that had the power to give them the ecstasy of transcending all boundaries. His ability to induce euphoric states in his disciples carried a conviction of his divinity that was impervious to scepticism and disbelief.

There is little doubt that Rajneesh was a fascinating, charismatic figure. It was a charisma infused with great charm, an irresistible combination. For whereas charisma fascinates and awes, charm, connected (also etymologically) to magic and spells, seduces. Almost everyone, disciples and non-believers alike, who attended his discourses, testify to his charisma that carried them—the sceptics perhaps only temporarily—to a plane of enchantment beyond the common place reality of ordinary lives. Warm, playful, humorous, Rajneesh's voice and especially his eyes are most often described as 'hypnotic'. In a study of Rajneesh's charisma, the sociologist Charles Lindholm has given a vivid description of the effect he had on his audience:

> His performances were expressive improvisations which moved, without pause or doubt, from highly abstract philosophical reflections to obscene jokes and racist remarks that were designed to shock his audience. They were also caught up in the exhilaration of his rapidly changing moods, his intonations and dramatic pauses, his potent rhetoric ... As he caressed the audience with his voice, shifted emotions and rhetoric with fluidity, and used his expressive hands to counterpoint his remarks, Rajneesh gave the faithful a sense of being carried onto a higher level of existence, both immediate and transcendent.[8]

It is also true that Rajneesh self-consciously prepared for his public appearances as does an actor for his role. In later life, he would use make up, wear rich robes that accentuated his broad shoulders and jewel-studded caps that hid his baldness. The setting for his discourse was as carefully prepared as was the selection of music and his dramatic entry and exit at the venue in one of his Rolls Royces.

The contradiction between authenticity and theatricality in Rajneesh's character is not the only one in a man teeming with contradictions. He is described by his followers as incredibly warm but also remote, as someone capable of great empathy but also of complete detachment and indifference. He could be bitingly cruel, as we saw in his comments on Gandhi and Mother Teresa, but, on rare occasions, he was also capable of magnanimity and genuine admiration. The 'masochist' Gandhi, for instance, had a beautiful smile and 'an immense capacity to feel the pulse of millions of people together.'[9] And Krishnamurti, whose hyper intellectuality induces a migraine headache in everyone who listens to him is also the author of *First and Last Freedom*, 'one of the greatest books ever written.'[10]

Rajneesh's own books, over four hundred of them, compiled by disciples from his talks, showcase a vast and eclectic erudition. They are highly readable, often poetic. Studded with some striking insights, illustrated by dramatic parables, they also display his talent as a gifted story teller. At the same time, his books have many ideas borrowed from philosophers and spiritual teachers of the world which Rajneesh blithely appropriates without attribution. They also contain some outlandish assertions: for instance, that Hindus had been to North and South America long before Columbus and that Arjuna, the famous archer of the epic Mahabharata, was married to a Mexican girl.[11]

There are many other contradictions: the guru who rejects all authority and preaches complete freedom, himself exercises totalitarian control over his disciples; the messiah of sexual love who exalts intercourse between man and woman as the highest manifestation of life force was himself, as reported by many who were in a position to observe him at close quarters, a voyeur who liked to watch couples, especially two women, make love and preferred to masturbate aspiring female disciples, preferably those with large breasts.[12] Rajneesh was indeed of the same stamp as the individuals William James writes about, in whom there is a fusion of superior intellect and 'psychopathic temperament', creating geniuses who 'do not remain mere critics and understanders with their intellect. Their ideas possess them, they inflict them, for better or worse, upon their companions or their age.'[13]

Rajneesh was, of course, supremely aware of his contradictions and indeed revelled in them. Consistency for him was the mark of fools and Rajneesh may have been outrageous, but rarely foolish. Yet, if there was one trait in his personality that seemed to be without its attendant shadow, then it was a truly inordinate self-regard, an astonishing grandiosity, at least in his public pronouncements and persona. Normally, we feel repulsed by the boastfulness, self-aggrandizement, and disdainful dismissal of others in which exaggerated narcissism manifests itself in a person. A braggart irritates us because we feel his insensitivity, his lack of connection with us as he goes into raptures of self-infatuation.

We feel, and rightly so, that he is using us only as a mirror to keep the image of an idealized self intact, an admired self-representation he needs for his feelings of well-being. Rajneesh, on the other hand, remained acutely aware of his audience and what they were eager or willing to believe. Many of his improbable claims and fantastic stories about his past and his 'previous lives', as we shall see below, were first narrated in the small circle of his closest devotees who believed that 'Bhagwan (Rajneesh) … has traveled all the paths, all the highways and byways open to any man through the aeons of time. He has played all the roles, has seen through all the games, done everything, been everywhere, and now He is a living statement of total fulfillment.'[14] The claims of such grandiosity in someone of average talent most often leads to bitterness and whining complaints of having been denied his due by 'society', 'enemies', 'fate', or whatever else. The exuberant grandiosity of someone like Rajneesh, though, who is endowed with superior gifts and what appears to be unshakeable self-belief, can be vital for his accomplishment in becoming a messianic figure.[15]

Grandiosity had been a part of Rajneesh since early childhood and remained with him, undiminished, till the end of his life. ('But I had nothing to be modest about!' I can hear Rajneesh protest with a glint of mischief in his eyes). Let us take only one example, Rajneesh's account of his birth and his 'previous lives'.

In his last birth, seven hundred years ago, Rajneesh was a great spiritual master. Seekers from all over the known world flocked to him. Three days before he was to die or rather be finally liberated from the cycle of births and deaths, he was assassinated by a disciple. (The man was once again to be his *sanyasin* in the ashram). Rajneesh was in deep meditation when he died the last time around.

> I died consciously, hence I had the great opportunity to be born consciously. I chose my mother and father.
>
> Thousands of fools are making love around the earth, around the clock. Millions of unborn souls are ready to enter into any womb, whatsoever. I waited seven hundred years for the right moment, and I thank existence that I found it. Seven hundred years are nothing compared to the millions and millions of years ahead … I chose this couple, just simple villagers. I could have chosen kings and queens. It was in my hands. All kinds of wombs were available, but I am a man of simple tastes: I am always satisfied with the best.[16]

Rajneesh's other lives, too, were no less distinguished. Another seven hundred years earlier, he had been great friends with Bodhidharma, the famed seventh century Budddhist monk who brought Buddhism to China and Japan. The two travelled together for three months and though Bodhidharma had pleaded with him to stay, Rajneesh had left him to go his own way. 'Bodhidharma could not believe it. He had never invited anyone before. This was the man who had even refused Emperor Wu—the greatest emperor of those days, with the greatest empire—as if he was a beggar.'[17] His followers are the luckiest people on earth, Rajneesh said, since 'Jesus can be found again very easily. People are becoming enlightened all the time. But to find a man like me—who has traveled thousands of ways, in thousands of lives, and has gathered the fragrance of millions of flowers like a honeybee—is difficult.'[18]

If I now turn to Rajneesh's early childhood to understand the major themes in the inner world of this fascinating man who marched to his own ethical drum beat, a *homo spiritus* in spite of his many contradictions, tall tales, and affronts to conventional morality, then it is not out of any psychoanalytic reflex. Rajneesh, himself, would have agreed that his particular genius cannot be understood without recapturing the quality of his earliest experiences. 'The first seven years are the most important in life, never again will you have that much opportunity,' he says. 'Those seven years decide your seventy years, all the foundation stones are laid in those seven years.'[19] Or, at another place, 'unless you understand the seed you will miss the tree and the flowering, and perhaps the moon through the branches.'[20] Yet, as a psychoanalyst, the kind of a biographer who is more interpretive than historical, who is concerned with the hidden meanings of childhood experiences, I must also remain true to my professional *dharma* of going beyond the facts of his life into the heart of the man. The search for a psychoanalytic 'truth' does not compromise my memorial admiration of Rajneesh which, though, is without the idealization and reverence of a follower. Respecting his religious genius yet aware of his human shortcomings, I am heedful of Nietzsche's warning to the scholar of religion in a secular age, namely the 'boundlessly foolish naïveté' involved in the 'belief of the scholar in his superiority, in the good conscience of his tolerance, in the unsuspecting simple certainty with which his instinct treats the religious man as a lower and less valuable type, beyond, before and ABOVE which he himself has developed.'[21]

Rajneesh's reminiscences of his childhood, *Glimpses of a Golden Childhood,* are compiled from notes of his talks in 1981. These were informal, rambling talks within the small circle of four or five of his most intimate and trusted associates, whom he affectionately called his

'Noah's Ark'. Since the reminiscences are compiled from the spoken rather than written word, they are not as well organized and edited at the source (that is, by Rajneesh) than is normally the case with written communication. Indeed, often they have the quality of free-association: 'That's how I am speaking. I do not know what the next sentence is going to be or whether it is going to be at all. Suspense is beautiful.'[22] As the psychoanalyst George Morartis observes, speech tends to be more repetitive and loosely associative than writing and has a greater chance of bringing concealed thoughts into forms.[23] We see this, for instance, in the frequent repetition of the number seven at various places, even in the first fifty pages of the text, as if this number is forcing itself on Rajneesh's consciousness and into his speech. The follower who had killed Rajneesh *seven* hundred years ago in a previous incarnation confessed that he had come to kill him again in his present one, *seven* years after he had been a sanayasin. (p.15). Rajneesh's father was a poor man who had only *seven* hundred rupees when he was born (p.18). The famous astrologer who came to their village refused to make his birth chart because he did not think the child would survive his *seven*th birthday (p. 25). Above all, the reason, I would speculate, why the number seven held a special meaning for Rajneesh and inserted itself in *Glimpses of a Golden Childhood* in different contexts, is its association with the death of his beloved grandfather when he was *seven* and which brought an end to a golden childhood that had lasted for *seven* years.

As an infant, Rajneesh was handed over by his parents to his maternal grandparents who had expressed a wish to bring up their first-born grandson, a not uncommon occurrence in the Indian context. His *nana* and *nani* were thus the only father and mother he knew for the first years of his life; in fact, later in life, imitating his father's younger brothers, he would always address his biological mother as *bhabhi*—sister-in-law, the place of the mother in his heart and mind occupied by his remarkable grandmother.

There is an elegiac quality to Rajneesh's memories of his years with his grandparents and of the village in which he grew up. Although many factual details are inconsistent with each other—Rajneesh was never a slave to the tyranny of facts—the narrative has a ring of emotional truth. It transcends any irritation caused by the play of his imagination which invents highly improbable incidents and encounters that could not have taken place. An autobiography is a myth we create about ourselves and would like others to believe in. Not that an autobiographer does not struggle to be truthful. It is only that his striving for truth is undermined by the unconscious power of human narcissism. The highest commandment that rules autobiographical forays into the past seems to be that the memories of our life must not do any real damage to our feelings of self-worth. Notwithstanding a few admirable exceptions, this is the unacknowledged secret of all autobiography … and of neurosis. If Rajneesh's memories of his life diverge from those of many others in their relentless self glorification, then it is only because of the implacability of this commandment in his case which forbids him taking even the slightest risk that might be a threat to self esteem. An inner censor keeps a strict watch that memories that may compromise a lifelong project of maintaining a magnificent self intact are turned away at the gate of consciousness.

My childhood was golden. Again, I am not using a cliché. Everybody says his childhood was golden, but it is not so. People only think that their childhood was golden because their youth is rotten; then their old age is even more rotten … But my childhood was certainly golden—not a symbol, absolutely golden; not poetically, but literally, factually … Those years are unforgettable. Even if I reach Dante's paradise I will still remember those years.[24]

The village of Kuchwada in Madhya Pradesh where Rajneesh grew up was small and remote, without a railway station, post office, school, or doctor. It had a few straw huts and its only brick house belonged to Rajneesh's grandparents. Through the golden haze of his memory, it appears as an ideal world, free of conflict and turmoil. 'The village was beautiful,' he says, 'I have traveled far and wide but I have never come across that same beauty … Things come and go, but it is never the same.'[25] Surrounded by small hills the village had an ancient pond with hundreds of years old trees around it.

Nobody could describe that pond except Basho. Even he does not describe the pond, he simply says,

The ancient pond

Frog jumps in

Plop!

… and certainly the frogs jumped; day in and day out you could hear 'plop', again and again. The sound of frogs jumping really helped the prevailing silence. That sound made the silence richer, more meaningful … But the silence of that ancient pond stays with me.[26]

Raja ('King'), as the little boy was called by his adoring grandparents, was an emperor in this small world. Rajneesh remembers that his birthdays were celebrated in the same fashion as that of a king. His grandfather would hire an elephant from a nearby town and fill two big bags, hanging on either side of the elephant, with silver coins. The small boy would then ride the elephant through the village, throwing silver rupees to an awed populace. In every possible way, Raja was given 'the idea that I belonged to some royal family.'[27]

Rajneesh does not remember little Raja ever being disciplined, irrespective of the mischief he got up to, which was considerable.

> The whole day he [grandfather] would sit on his *gaddi*—as the seat of a rich man is called in India—listening less to his customers, and more to the complainers. But he used to say to them, 'I am ready to pay for any damage he has done, but remember, I am not going to punish him' … Once in a while I would say, 'Nana, you can punish me. You need not be so tolerant.' And, can you believe it, he would cry! Tears would come into his eyes, and he would say, 'Punish you? I cannot do that. I can punish myself but not you.'[28]

Raja was a lonely child. He did not play with other children of the village who were regarded by his grandparents as 'dirty' and socially inferior. 'So for seven years nobody tried to corrupt my innocence; there was nobody. Those three old people who lived in the house, the servant and my grandparents, were all protective in every possible way that nobody should disturb me.'[29] And the most fiercely protective, or rather indulgent, was his grandmother. Sensitive, beautiful, and strong—some would say, headstrong—the nani insisted that Raja be left alone and be allowed to be his natural self, uninfluenced by any adult. For a short while, a private tutor was engaged, but in a pattern that continued through the years of his growing up, the child would first expose and then become teacher to the man. At the end of every such encounter, Raja's uniqueness and superiority was recognized and celebrated rather than sought to be moulded by the adult—revered Jaina monks, schoolteachers, professors, the vice chancellor of the university—who initially presumed to exercise authority over the boy. 'That is how,' he says, 'without knowing it at all, I came to have the taste of Tao. Lao Tzu says, "Tao is the watercourse way. The water simply flows downwards wherever the earth allows it". That is how those early years were. I was allowed. I think every child needs those years. If we could give those years to every child in the world we could create a golden world.'[30]

If Rajneesh remembers his grandfather as a paragon of unconditional though passive love, the love of his nani was active and energetic, '… my grandmother helped me immensely. My grandfather loved me, but could not help me much. He was so loving, but to be of help more is needed—a certain kind of strength. He was always afraid of my grandmother. He was, in a sense, a henpecked husband.'[31] His nani was the reigning monarch of his soul, an extremely beautiful, 'strong woman, very strong.' The grandfather, affable and totally indulgent, was the queen's consort in the background who nonetheless represented an enclave of calmness, the quiet pole in the psyche of the little boy, a needed refuge from the fierce power of the beautiful nani: 'Beauty is always so, courageous and dangerous.'[32]

Simple, uneducated, yet independent, his grandmother had married at the age of twenty-four and from love, both aspects unheard of in India at the beginning of twentieth century when girls got married at nine or ten to husbands selected by their family. Rajneesh relates many incidents where she encouraged him to be rebellious, to dare all: for instance, to show a venerable Jaina monk the door if the child so wanted. She told the boy that when he was older he must visit Khajuraho, her birthplace and the site of temples with erotic carvings that still have the power to shock a sexually conservative society. When Rajneesh was in his teens, she provided him money to smoke, drink, and visit prostitutes if he wanted to. Experience every experience without fear, seemed to be her message to the child, exhorting him to seek, in the words of the poet Ernest Dowson, 'madder music, stronger wine'. She held before the child the vistas of his future greatness: 'Perhaps she could see something in me of which I was not aware in those days. Perhaps that's the reason she loved me so much … I can't say.'[33] In turn,

I never saw a more beautiful woman than my Nani. I myself was in love with her, and loved her throughout her whole life. When she died at the age of eighty, I rushed home and found her lying there, dead … To put the fire to her body was the most difficult task I have ever done in my life. It was as if I was putting fire to one of the most beautiful paintings of Leonardo or Vincent van Gogh. Of course to me she was more valuable than the Mona Lisa, more beautiful to me than Cleopatra. It is not an exaggeration. All that is beautiful in my vision somehow comes through her. She helped me in every way to be the way I am. Without her I may have been a shopkeeper or perhaps a doctor or engineer …[34]

The striking nani, then, gifted her adored Raja, 'the king of my heart' with (in Nabokov's phrase) 'unreal estate', where nothing would ever go wrong and where, in an artistic elaboration of the child's mental state,

You were carried and you were enveloped in the amplitude of sure protection, like a king on his throne, with his faithful bodyguards many ranks deep about him; and the landscape beyond, with its motley episodes, became the most entertaining of spectacles, where everything was unexpected and exciting, yet where nothing could go wrong; as if your mother herself had been telling you a story, and these pictures were only the illustrations to it which painted themselves on your listening mind.[35]

Nothing could go wrong, except that everything did. Rajneesh's grandfather died when he was seven and the golden childhood came to an abrupt and traumatic end. The child returned to live with his parents in their small town and in a large, extended family with its inevitable conflicts and clamour, not to speak of the demands made on the child by school and other institutions of society to conform to their norms. For instance,

I was forced almost violently to go to school. And it was not a one-day affair, it was an everyday routine. One of my uncles, or whosoever, would take me there, would wait outside until the master had taken possession of me—as if I was a piece of property to be passed from one hand to another, or a prisoner passed from one hand to another.[36]

At school,

It was a daily routine, almost the usual practice, that I was sent to the headmaster to be punished. The captain of the class would take me to the headmaster, who used to then ask me what I had done that day. But by and by the headmaster stopped asking. I would go there and he would punish me, slap me on the face, and that was all. He did not even ask what wrong I had done.[37]

What helped the child save his battered soul from irreversible damage was the refuge he could find with his nani. After the grandfather's death, nani left Kuchwada and moved into a small house in the town so that she could be close to her Raja. Rajneesh would spend the nights with her so that she was 'not alone and by herself' and, perhaps more important, though unacknowledged, that neither was he. She soothed the hurts of his day, mirrored the grandiose self now under violent attack from reality, helping him salvage the early psychological buoyancy and creativity of the child and carry them into adulthood.

I will not belabour the obvious psychoanalytic inference that Rajneesh's childhood experience led to the formation of a highly narcissistic personality, hyperempathic to his own needs and with an inordinate need to maintain the conscious experience of a grandiose self. All small children go through a phase of heightened narcissism but, if they are lucky, also move away from it in a gradual, non-traumatic manner, carrying away with them some of the uplifting triumphs of this stage: humour, creativity, aesthetic pleasure, optimism. It is only when parental indulgence and mirroring has been intense, and the exile from the symbiotic nest sudden and traumatic, as in Rajneesh's case, that there is a strong probability of developmental arrest at this early stage of life. The longing for the lost paradise of childhood where a great self existed in a symbiosis with ideal parents, becomes the central motif in the psyche, the theme song of the person's unconscious life ever after. Rajneesh's more or less conscious stance, 'I am great. I walk alone. I need no one. Others need me,' which provided a template for his later relationships with others; he not only desperately needed disciples and followers to reassure him that its fictions were true but also became vulnerable to bouts of regressive longing. At the time when he was sharing memories of his childhood with his close disciples, he constantly played one old song by Noorjahan, a famous singer of the 1930s and early 1940s. He would listen to this particular song again and again, morning and night. The song (in Rajneesh's translation):

Whether you remember or not,
Once there was passionate love between us.
You used to tell me,
'You are the most beautiful woman in the world,'
Now I don't know if you will recognize me or not,
Perhaps you do not remember, but I still remember.
I cannot forget the passionate love, and the words you said to me,
You used to say your love was impeccable,
Do you still remember?
Perhaps not—but I remember,
Not in its totality, of course,
Time has done much harm.
I am a dilapidated palace,
But if you look minutely,
I am still the same.
I still remember the passionate love and your words,
That passion love that once existed between us,
Is it still in your memory or not,
I don't know about you,
But I still remember.[38]

There is heartbreak, longing and hints of betrayal of old promises in the song that Rajneesh sings silently, again and again, through the haunting voice of Noorjahan. Is this a song to his nani? To his lost childhood? To the transience of love? Or perhaps to all of them? Here, we can sense the presence of a deeply sad and deprived core in his psyche that is split off from consciousness. Strong defenses guard against the emergence of this depressed core which, however, sometimes breaks through the fortifications. On occasion, it even takes over the personality, as it did during periods of psychic breakdown in youth, especially the long stretch of psychic disintegration that preceded his spiritual enlightenment at the age of twenty-one.

In contrast to the endearing narcissism of the child and its demands to be at the centre of attention, the grandiose self of the adult arrested at the stage of infantile narcissism is infused with heightened aggression. In Rajneesh's case, this was expressed in his disdain, arrogance, and frequent devaluation of others, especially of other religious teachers and spiritual preceptors. To Rajneesh, they were all worthless, 'bullshitters', not holy men but 'holy dung'. Swami Muktananda, a contemporary Indian guru with a large following, was an 'Idiotananda'.

Identifying with a grandiose self and its sense of manifest destiny, growing up without playmates or peers and hence never learning to compromise with the needs of others, bathed in parental overindulgence which rendered the internalization of 'no' impossible, was bound to lead to a lack of any self discipline. Rajneesh was thus relatively free of restraints that would check his psyche's expansiveness and sometimes manic exuberance. Feelings of guilt and pangs of conscience that serve to regulate the behaviour of normal mortals were conspicuously absent. It is essentially the recapture of a 'remembered' total state of freedom which he elaborated in his spiritual message and philosophy with erudition, rhetoric giftedness and, above all, conviction; for Rajneesh had himself been *there*.

> So don't be worried about what you are doing; remember only one thing: what you are being. This is a great question, about doing and being. If your being is right, and by right I mean blissful, silent, peaceful, loving, then whatever you do is right. Then there are no other commandments for you, only one: just be. Be so totally that in the very totality no shadow is possible. Then you cannot do anything wrong. The whole world may say it is wrong, that does not matter; what matters is your own being.[39]

The death of his grandfather at the age of seven that marked the end of a golden childhood, was not only decisive for the course of Rajneesh's psychic life but its trauma; it provided the glue that cemented the grandiose self firmly in his psyche, and was also vital in awakening and giving form to his spiritual strivings. Rajneesh returns to the deeply traumatic experience again and again.

I was so attached to him that his death appeared to be my own death ... In the very first attack of death upon my grandfather, he lost his speech. For twenty-four hours we waited in the village for something to happen. However, there was no improvement. I remember a struggle on his part in an attempt to speak something but he could not speak. He wanted to tell something but could not tell it. Therefore, we had to take him towards the town in a bullock cart. Slowly, one after another, his senses were giving way. He did not die all at once, but slowly and painfully. First his speech stopped, then his hearing. Then he closed his eyes as well. In the bullock cart I was watching everything closely and there was a long distance of thirty-two miles of travel.

Whatsoever was happening seemed beyond my understanding then. This was the first death witnessed by me and I did not even understand that he was dying. But slowly all his senses were giving way and he became unconscious. While we were nearby the town he was already half dead. His breathing still continued, but everything else was lost. After that he did not resume consciousness but, for three days, he continued breathing. He died unconsciously.

The slow losing of his senses and his final dying became very deeply engraved in my memory.[40]

How traumatic the grandfather's demise must have been for the child and how his psyche struggled to master its attendant anxiety and the radical restructuring the death required, is evident from Rajneesh's extraordinary reactions to the event. Now there is a consensus among psychoanalysts that children do not pass through the same mourning process as adults in whom a gradual and painful emotional detachment from the inner images of the person who has passed away takes place. In children, the reaction to parental death in childhood is not mourning but rather a complex series of defensive phenomena aimed at denying the reality of the event. An unconscious denial, a screening out of feelings of sadness and loss ('It can't be bad if I don't feel bad!'), and other responses, such as glorification and idealization of the dead parent and unconscious fantasies of a reunion, are some of the more common.[41] Rajneesh's reactions, however, went much beyond these normal responses. As an older child and youth, it was his practice to follow dead bodies that were being carried to the cremation ground. Watching people die became a hobby: 'The moment I would hear that somebody was on his deathbed, I would be there ... and I would sit and watch.'[42]

He would imitate the state of death, go to cremation grounds at night, and lie there as motionless as a corpse for hours at a stretch, trying to achieve, the analyst would say, a reunion with the grandfather.

Seven years later, at the age of fourteen, convinced he himself was about to die, he took *seven* days leave from the school. He went to an old isolated temple at the outskirts of the town and lay there 'being dead'. Spiritually, his reactions to his grandfather's death may be seen as so many efforts at detachment and, indeed, this is how Rajneesh interprets them: 'His death freed me forever from all relationships … whenever my relationship with anyone began to become intimate, that death stared at me.'[43] Indeed, St John of the Cross holds such radical detachment to be essential for travel on the spiritual path: 'The soul cannot be possessed of the divine union, until it has divested itself of the love of created beings.'[44] In line with a more modern, sceptical sensibility, the poet T.S. Eliot avers that detachment is not a choice but the only option available when human relationships have failed: 'A man does not join himself with the Universe so long as he has anything else to join himself with.'[45]

Spiritually, the most important episode of Rajneesh's life took place another *seven* years later when he was twenty one and went through a prolonged period of psychological breakdown, his 'dark night of the soul'. It was a time of what he calls 'nervous breakdown and breakthrough' that was to be the midwife for his emergence as a spiritual Master.

> For one year it was impossible to know what was happening … just to keep myself alive was a very difficult thing, because all appetite had disappeared. Days would pass and I would not feel any hunger, days would pass and I would not feel any thirst. I had to force myself to eat, force myself to drink. The body was so non-existential that I had to hurt myself to feel that I was still in the body. I had to knock my head against the wall to feel whether my head was still there or not. Only when it hurt would I be a little in the body … For one year it persisted. I would simply lie on the floor and look at the ceiling and count from one to a hundred then back from a hundred to one. Just to remain capable of counting was at least something.[46]

The dreams of flying, through which the grandiose self often exhibits its perfection,[47] gave way to those of falling, that reflected the disintegration of this self just as Icarus hurtling down from the heights, its wings burnt to cinder:

> My condition was one of utter darkness. It was as if I had fallen into a deep dark well. In those days I had many times dreamt that I was falling and falling and going deeper into a bottomless well. And many times I … awakened from

a dream full of perspiration, sweating profusely, because the falling was endless without any ground or place anywhere to rest my feet ... My condition was full of tension, insecurity and danger.[48]

And then, as in accounts of so many mystics all over the world, at the worst point of the breakdown, after 'seven days [that] I lived in a very hopeless and helpless state', the spiritual dawn breaks through. There is 'the presence of a totally new energy, a new light and new delight, [that] became so intense that it was almost unbearable, as if I was exploding, as if I was going mad with blissfulness.'[49]

Spiritual transformation thoroughly shakes up the body–mind entity yet does not completely re-arrange the psychic furniture. Our psyche that has been developing since birth and is physiologically embedded deep in the neuronal networks of the brain cannot be wiped out by even the most powerful mystical experience. The latter may create new neuronal pathways without, however, erasing the old ones. In a myriad anxious, stressful moments of daily life, and especially during long periods of psychological stress, there is an automatic regression to earlier ways. Rajneesh's 'anniversary reactions' to his grandfather's death, for instance, did not disappear with his enlightenment. The psychological effect of this death accompanied him throughout his life, demonstrating the force of its impact. There were other 'anniversary reactions' at the end of seven year cycles, of which perhaps the best documented is the one in 1981—the year he reminisces about his childhood in such detail. This was the year when, at the age of forty-nine, he moved the ashram from Poona to the United States. Before the move, he had become more and more withdrawn, rarely showed himself in public, while his physical condition—diabetes, asthma, and various allergies—worsened.

I am aware that given his reputation as a highly gifted fabulist, there will be many who will doubt Rajneesh's account of his spiritual journey. Instead, they would prefer to believe that large swathes of it are probably fabricated out of a voracious reading in mystical literature harnessed in service of a lively imagination and using the many devices of fiction, such as suspense and coincidence. Personally, I have little difficulty in holding incompatible convictions about Rajneesh's spiritual enlightenment. In other words, as a novelist fascinated with the spiritual destiny of his fictional characters, I believe what I have difficulty believing as a psychoanalyst, namely that Rajneesh *did* pass through his valley of the shadow of death before emerging into spiritual light, while at the same time the sceptical psychoanalyst in me wonders whether it was not merely a period of extended clinical depression that ended with a hypomanic episode.

Today, as we gain a more intimate knowledge of lives of saints and spiritual masters than was provided by hagiographies, we can say that the spirit, when it soars, often pulls up the psyche in its wake. Nevertheless, we also know that the spirit never completely escapes the gravitational pull exerted by the forces of narcissism, aggression, and desire in the psyche. What may be essential for our gaze, however, is to attend to the vision of the spirit's soaring, not the oft-repeated tragedy of its fall.

Notes and References

1 The literature on the Rajneesh movement is vast. It includes accounts by his followers or those who broke with him, as also by scholars of sociology and new religious movements. In the latter category see, especially, Urban, Hugh B., 1999, 'Zorba the Buddha: Capitalism, Charisma and the Cult of Shree Rajneesh', *Religion*, 26, pp. 161–82; Carter, Lewis F., 1987, 'The New Renunciates of the Rajneesh Shree Rajneesh: Observations and Identification of Problems of Interpreting New Religious Movements', *Journal for the Scientific Study of Religion*, 26(2), pp. 148–72; Lindholm, C., 2003, 'Charisma and Consciousness: The Case of the Rajneeshee', *Ethos*, 30:3, pp. 1–19.

2 For the remarks on Gandhi see, for instance, Feuerstein, G., 1991, *Holy Madness: The Shock Tactics and Tactical Teachings of Crazy Wise Adepts, Holy Fools and Rascal Gurus*, New York: Paragon House, p. 26; for the remarks on Mother Teresa see, Mullan, B., 1983, *Life as Laughter*, London: Routledge, Kegan Paul, p. 25.

3 Ma Amrit Chinmayo, 1981, *Sex: Quotations from Rajneesh*, Shree Rajneesh Foundation, Woodland Hills, CA: Lear Enterprises, p. 52.

4 Cited in Urban, 'Zorba and Buddha', p. 170.

5 Cited in Mullan, 'Life as Laughter', p. 43.

6 Dalai Lama in a Workshop on Buddhism held in New Delhi, 21–3 December 2006.

7 One of Rajneesh's close female disciples describes her experience of dynamic meditation:

Dancing wildly, carried along by the pulsating rhythm of the music and the energy of Rajneesh's presence, the top of my head suddenly exploded with the most powerful orgasm I had ever experienced. It flooded every recess of my body; I fell to the ground, people dancing over me and around me. I was stepped on, kicked; it didn't seem to matter. I was 'off' somewhere. Ecstatic, in bliss. (cited in Franklin, S.B., 1992, *The Promise of Paradise*, New York: Station Hill Press, p. 52).

8 Lindholm, 'Charisma and Consciousness', pp. 19–20.

9 Rajneesh, 1985, *Glimpses of a Golden Childhood*, Rajneeshpuram, OR: Rajneesh Foundation International, p. 664.

10 Rajneesh, 1985, *Books I have Loved*, Rajneeshpuram, OR: Rajneesh Foundation International, p. 175.

11 Rajneesh, *Glimpses*, pp. 74–5.

12 Franklin, *Promise of Paradise*, pp. 279, 325; Milne, H., 1987, *Rajneesh: The God That Failed*, New York: St Martin's Press, p. 186.

13 James, W., 1997 (1902), *The Varieties of Religious Experience*, New York: Touchstone, p. 37.

14 Swami Devgeet in his introduction to Rajneesh, *Glimpses*.

15 As the psychoanalyst and theorist of narcissism, Heinz Kohut has shown, for someone with an 'ego of average endowment', the delusional claims of a grandiose self can be highly disruptive. In a person of superior gifts, though, it is precisely this grandiosity that fuels their ambition and pushes them to outstanding achievement. See Kohut, H., 1971, *The Analysis of the Self*, New York: International Universities Press, pp. 108–9.

16 Rajneesh, *Glimpses*, 15–18. The phrase 'I am a man of simple tastes ...' is Oscar Wilde's.

17 Ibid., p 77.

18 Ibid., p. 45.

19 Osho (Rajneesh), 2000, *Autobiography of a Spiritually Incorrect Mystic*, New York: St Martin's Press, p. 20.

20 Rajneesh, *Glimpses*, p. 106.

21 Nietzsche, *Beyond Good and Evil*, Aphor. p. 58.

22 Rajneesh, *Glimpses*, p. 8

23 Moraitis, G., 'The Ghost in the Biographer's Machine', in J.A. Winer and J.W. Anderson (eds), 2003, *Psychoanalysis and History*, Hillsdale, NJ: Analytic Press, p. 105.

24 Rajneesh, *Glimpses*, p. 20.

25 Ibid., p. 8.

26 Ibid., pp. 11–12.

27 Osho, *Autobiography*, p. 20.

28 Rajneesh, *Glimpses*, p. 60.

29 Osho, *Autobiography*, p. 6.

30 Rajneesh, *Glimpses*, p. 37.

31 Osho, *Autobiography*, p. 9.

32 Rajneesh, *Glimpses*, p. 52.

33 Ibid., p. 126.

34 Ibid., pp. 83–4.

35 Santayayana, 'The Last Puritan', quoted in Tolpin, M., 1974, 'The Daedalus Experience: A Developmental Vicissitude of the Grandiose Fantasy', *Annual of Psychoanalysis*, 2, p. 216.

36 Rajneesh, *Glimpses*, p. 265.

37 Rajneesh, *Books I Have Loved*, p. 116.

38 Rajneesh, *Glimpses*, p. 88. Although Rajneesh translates *karar* as 'trust' at this particular place, he later (p. 114) holds 'passionate love'—the word used here for *karar*—to be more appropriate.

39 Ibid., p. 111.

40 Cited in the authorized biography by Joshi, V., 1982, *The Awakened One*, San Francisco: Harper & Row, pp. 22–3. In Rajneesh's other accounts of the event, the grandfather is not in a coma but, with his head in the boy's lap as the bullock cart rattles along, carries out long philosophical discussions on death and attachment. (Rajneesh, *Glimpses*, p. 79ff.). Wendy Doniger, in a personal communication, notes that the scene is also very much like the Upanishadic description of the *pranas* and then the senses leaving one by one.

41 See Menes, J.B., 1971, 'Children's Reactions to the Death of a Parent: A Review of the Psychoanalytic Literature', *Journal of American Psychoanalytic Association*, 13, 697–719; see also, Wolfenstein, M., 1966, 'How is Mourning Possible?', *Psychoanalytic Study of Child*, 21, pp. 93–123.

42 Milne, *Rajneesh*, p. 96. See also the confirmatory account by Joshi, p. 31.

43 Fitzgerald, F., 1986, 'Rajneeshpuram-I', *The New Yorker*, 22 September, p. 86.

44 Aberbach, D., 1987, 'Grief and Mysticism', *International Review of Psychoanalysis*, 14, p. 509.

45 Ibid.

46 Joshi, *Awakened One*, pp. 52–3.

Religion and Psyche

Religious Conflict in the Modern World*

OUR TIMES ARE WITNESS to a worldwide wave of religious revival. Islam, Hinduism, Buddhism, the new religions in Japan, born-again Christians in the United States, and the Protestant sects in Latin America are undergoing a resurgence which is regarded with deep distrust by all the modem heirs to the Enlightenment. Although a secular humanist might find most manifestations of the current religious zeal personally distasteful, he or she is nonetheless aware that the revitalization of religion at the end of the twentieth century constitutes a complex attempt at the resacralization of cultures beset with the many ills of modernity. As Andrew Samuels reminds us, this fragmented and fractured attempt at resacralization to combat the sense of oppression and a future utterly bereft of any vision of transcendent purpose is not only a part of the new religious fundamentalisms but also integral to the so-called left-leaning, progressive political movements.[1] One can discern the search for transcendence even in concerns around ecological issues and environmental protection where at least some of the discourse is comprised of elements of nature mysticism.

However, if we look closely at individual cases around the world, we will find that the much-touted revival is less of religiosity than of cultural identities based on religious affiliation. In other words, there may not be any great ferment taking place in the world of religious ideas, rituals, or any

*From *The Colours of Violence*, Delhi: Viking-Penguin, 1995; University of Chicago Press, 1996.

marked increase in the sum of human spirituality. Where the resurgence is most visible is in the organization of collective identities around religion, in the formation and strengthening of communities of believers: what we are witnessing today is less the resurgence of religion than (in the felicitous Indian usage) of communalism where a community of believers not only has religious affiliation but also social, economic, and political interests in common which may conflict with the corresponding interests of another community of believers sharing the same geographical space. Indeed, most secular analysts and progressive commentators have traditionally sought to uncover factors other than religion as the root cause of an ostensibly religious conflict. This has been as true of the anti-Semitic pogroms in Spain in the fourteeth century, of sixteenth-century Catholic–Protestant violence in France, of anti-Catholic riots in eighteenth-century London, as of twentieth-century Hindu–Muslim riots in India.[2] The 'real' cause of conflict between groups in all these instances has been generally identified as a clash of economic interests; the explanation embraces some version of a class struggle between the poor and the rich.

The danger to the material existence of an individual can indeed be experienced as an identity threat which brings a latent group identity to the forefront. This heightened sense of identity with the group provides the basis for a social cohesiveness which is necessary to safeguard the individual's economic interests. But there are other threats besides the economic one which too amplify the group aspect of personal identity. In an earlier chapter, I described the identity–threat which is being posed by the forces of modernization and globalization to peoples in many parts of the world. Feelings of loss and helplessness accompany dislocation and migration from rural areas to the shanty towns of urban megalopolises, the disappearance of craft skills which underlay traditional work identities, and the humiliation caused by the homogenizing and hegemonizing impact of the modern world which pronounces ancestral, cultural ideals and values as outmoded and irrelevant. These, too are conducive to heightening the group aspects of identity as the affected (and the afflicted) look to cultural–religious groups to combat their feelings of helplessness and loss and to serve as vehicles for the redress of injuries to self-esteem.

The identity threat may also arise due to a perceived discrimination by the state, that is, a disregard by the political authorities of a group's interests or disrespect for its cultural symbols. It can also arise as a consequence of changing political constellations such as those which accompany the end of empires. If Hindu–Muslim relations were in better shape in the past, with much less overt violence, it was perhaps also because of the kind of polity in which the two peoples lived. This polity was that of empire, the Mughal Empire followed by the British one. An empire, the political scientist Michael Walzer observes, is characterized by a mixture of repression for any strivings for independence and tolerance for different cultures, religions and ways of life.[3] The tolerance is not a consequence of any great premodern wisdom but because of the indifference, sometimes bordering on brutal incomprehension, of the imperial bureaucrats to local conflicts of the peoples they rule. Distant from local life, they do not generally interfere with everyday life as long as things remain peaceful, though there may be intermittent cruelty to remind the subject peoples of the basis of the empire—conquest through force of arms. It is only with self-government, when distance disappears, that the political questions—'Who *among* us shall have power here, in these villages, these towns?' 'Will the majority group dominate?' 'What will be the new ranking order?'—lead to a heightened awareness of religious–cultural differences. In countries with multireligious populations, independence coincides with tension and conflict—such as we observe today in the wake of the unravelling of the Soviet empire.[4]

The identity–threats I have outlined above do not create a group identity but merely bring it to the fore. The group aspect of personal identity is not a late creation in individual development but exists from the beginning of the human lifecycle. Although Freud had no hesitation in maintaining that from the very first individual psychology is a social psychology as well, psychoanalysts, with their traditional emphasis on the 'body-in-the-mind', have tended to downplay the existence of the 'community-in-the-mind'.[5] They have continued to regard the social (*polis*) aspects of man's being as an overlay which compromises the wishes and needs of the self or, in the case of the crowd is destructive of individual self and identity. Erikson has been one of the rare psychoanalysts who has called for a revision of this model that differentiates so starkly between an individual-individual and the individual-in-mass who has no individuality at all: 'Yet that a man could ever be psychologically alone; that a man 'alone' is essentially different from the same man in a group; that a man in a temporary solitary condition or when closeted with his analyst has ceased to be a 'political' animal and has disengaged himself from social action (or inaction) on whatever class level—these and similar stereotypes demand careful revision.'[6]

Such revisions would begin with the idea that the inner space occupied by what is commonly called the 'self—which 1 have been using synonymously with 'identity'—not only contains mental representations of one's bodily life and of primary relationships within the family but also holds mental representations of one's group and its culture, that is, the group's configuration of beliefs about man, nature, and social relations (including the view of the Other). These cultural propositions, transmitted and internalized through symbols have a strong emotional impact on those who grow up as members of a particular cultural group. The self, then, is a system of reverberating representational worlds, each enriching, constraining, and shaping the others, as they jointly evolve through the lifecycle. A revision of psychoanalytic notions of the self, identity, and subjectivity would also acknowledge that none of these constituent inner worlds is 'primary' or 'deeper', that is, there is no necessity of identity or an 'archaeological' layering of the various inner worlds, although at different times the self may be predominantly experienced in one or other representational mode. It is not only the brain that is bicameral.

At some point of time in early life, like the child's 'I am!' which heralds the birth of individuality, there is also a complementary 'We are!' which announces the birth of a sense of community. 'I am' differentiates me from other individuals. 'We are' makes me aware of the other group (or groups) sharing the physical and cognitive space of my community. The self-assertion of 'We are' with its potential for confrontation with the 'We are' of other groups, is *inherently* a carrier of aggression, together with the consequent fears of persecution, and is thus always attended by a sense of risk and potential for violence. (The psychological processes initiated by an awareness of 'We are', I suggest, also provide an explanation for the experimental findings of cognitive psychologists that the mere perception of two different groups is sufficient to trigger a positive evaluation of one's own group and a negative stereotyping of the other).

The further development of the social-representational world or the group aspect of identity has some specific characteristics which I have discussed in detail at various places in this book in the context of Hindu–Muslim relations. To abstract briefly: this aspect of identity is powerfully formed by the processes of introjection, identification, idealization, and projection during childhood. On the one hand, the growing child assimilates within itself the images of the family and group members. He or she identifies with their emotional investment in the group's symbols and traditions and incorporates their idealizations of the group which have served them so well—as they will serve the child—in the enhancement of self-esteem for belonging to such an exalted and blessed entity. On the other hand, because of early difficulties in integrating contradictory representations of the self and the parents—the 'good' loving child and the 'bad' raging one; the good, caretaking parent and the hateful, frustrating one—the child tries to disown the bad representations through projection. First projected to inanimate objects and animals and later to people and other groups—the latter often available to the child as a preselection by the group—the disavowed bad, representations *need* such 'reservoirs', as Vamik Volkan calls them. These reservoirs—Muslims for Hindus, Arabs for Jews, Tibetans for the Chinese, and vice versa—are also convenient repositories for subsequent rages and hateful feelings for which no clear-cut addressee is available. Since most of the 'bad' representations arise from a social disapproval of the child's 'animality', as expressed in its aggressivity, dirtiness, and unruly sexuality, it is pre-eminently this animality which a civilized, moral self must disavow and place in the reservoir group. We saw this happening in the Hindu image of the dirty, aggressive, and sexually licentious Muslim, and we encounter it again and again in both modern and historical accounts of other group conflicts. Thus in sixteenth century France, Catholics 'knew' that the Protestants were not only dirty and diabolic but that their Holy Supper was disordered and drunken, a bacchanalia, and that they snuffed out the candles and had indiscriminate sexual intercourse after voluptuous psalm singing. Protestants, on their part, 'knew' that Catholic clergy had an organization of hundreds of women at the disposal of priests and canons who, for the most part, were sodomites as well.[7]

The psychological processes involved in the development of 'We are' not only take recourse to the group's cultural traditions—its myths, history, rituals, and symbols—to make the community a firm part of personal identity but also employ bodily fantasies as well as family metaphors to anchor this aspect of identity in the deepest layers of individual imagination. The 'pure' us versus a 'dirty' them, the association of a rival group with denigrated, often anal, bodily parts and functions, representations of one's group in metaphors of a body under attack or as a 'good' son of the mother(land) while the rival group is a 'bad' son, are some of the examples from Hindu and Muslim discourse which I have discussed in earlier chapters.

We must, however, also note that there are always some individuals whose personal identity is not overwhelmed by their religious or cultural group identity even in the worst phase of violent conflict. These are persons capable of acts of compassion and self-sacrifice, such as saving members of the 'enemy' group from the fury of a rampaging mob even at considerable danger to their own physical safety. There are yet others—the fanatics—whose behaviour even in times of peace and in the absence of any identity-threat seems to be exclusively dictated by the 'We are' group aspect of their identity. What the social and psychological conditions are that make one person wear his or her group identity lightly whereas for another it is an armour which is rarely taken off is a question to which the answers are not only of theoretical interest but also of profound practical importance and moral significance.

Religious Identities and Violence

The development of religious identity follows the same lines through which the more global aspects of individual and group identities are also constructed. The individual track, which may be called religious selfhood, is an incommunicable realm of religious feeling which quietly suffuses what D.W. Winnicott termed 'the isolated core of the true self requiring isolation and privacy, a core which 'never communicates with the world of perceived objects [and] must never be communicated with.'[8] In an integrated state, religious selfhood is a quiet self-experience, marked by a calmness of spirit that comes from being alone in the presence of the numinous. With its access to preverbal experience which can link different sensory modalities of image, sound, rhythm, and so on, religious selfhood deepens religious feeling and consolidates religious identity. In a state of fragmentation or threatened disintegration, religious selfhood is prey to a variety of dysphoric moods. For a few, the saints, whose religious identity constitutes the core of their being, the dysphoria can extend to the state of utter despair, the 'dark night of the soul.'

Together with religious selfhood, the 'I-ness' of religious identity, we have a second track of 'We-ness' which is the experience of being part of a community of believers. Religious community is the interactive aspect of religious identity. In contrast to the quietness of religious selfhood, the individual's experience of religious community takes place in an alert state. Optimally, this facet of religious identity expands the self and creates feelings of attunement and resonance with other believers. A threat to the community aspect of religious identity, however, gives birth to communalism, intolerance, and the potential for social violence. In the communal phase, the feeling of intimacy and connectedness characterizing the religious community are polluted by an ambience of aggression and persecution. Whereas both the selfhood and community facets of religious identity are only partially conscious, the change from community to communalism is accompanied and, indeed, initiated by a heightened awareness of 'We-ness', making the community aspect of religious identity hyperconscious. This awareness can be put in the form of declarations similar to the ones Oscar Patterson suggests take place in the inner discourse of an individual who, as a consequence of a shared threat, is in the process of self-consciously identifying with his or her ethnic group.[9] First, I declare to all who share the crisis with me that I am one with them—a Hindu, a Muslim. Second, from my multiple identities I choose the identity of belonging to my religious community though (paradoxically) I have no other choice but to belong. Third, this is my most basic and profound commitment and the one which I am least likely to abandon.

Communalism as a state of mind, then, is the individual's *assertion* of being part of a religious community, preceded by a full *awareness* of belonging to such a community. The 'We-ness' of the community is here replaced by the 'We are' of communalism. This 'We are' must inevitably lead to intolerance of all those outside the boundaries of the group. The intolerance, though, is not yet religious conflict since it can remain a province of the mind rather than become manifest in the outer, public realm; its inherent violence can range from a mild contempt to obsessive fantasies around the extermination of the enemy–'other' rather than find explosive release in arson, rioting, and murder. The psychological ground for violence, however, has now been prepared. In mapping the sequence of religious violence from the inner to the outer terrain, I do not mean to give group psychology primacy but only precedence. Riots *do* start in the minds of men, minds conditioned by our earliest inner experience of self affirmation and assertion.

For the outbreak of violence, the communal identity has to swamp personal identity in a large number of people, reviving the feelings of love connected with early identifications with one's own group members and the hate towards the outgroup whose members are homogenized, depersonalized, and increasingly dehumanized. For social violence to occur, the threat to communal identity has to cross a certain threshold where the persecutory potential becomes fully activated and persecutory anxiety courses unimpeded through and between members of a religious group. Amplified by rumours, stoked by religious demagogues, the persecutory anxiety signals the annihilation of group identity and must be combated by its forceful assertion. Acting demonstratively in terms of this identity as a Hindu or Muslim, though, threatens members of the rival community who too mobilize their religious identity as a defence. The spiral of threats and reactive counter threats further fuels persecutory anxiety, and only the slightest of sparks in needed for a violent explosion.

The involvement of religious rather than other social identities does not dampen but, on the contrary, increases the violence of the conflict. Religion brings to conflict between groups a greater emotional intensity and a deeper motivational thrust than language, region, or other markers of ethnic identity. This is at least true of countries where the salience of religion in collective life is very high. Religious identity, for instance, is so crucial in the Islamic world that no Muslim revolutionary has been able or willing to repudiate his religious heritage.[10] To live in India is to become aware that the psychological space occupied by religion, the context and inspiration it provides for individual lives, and its role in fostering the cultural identity and survival of different groups—Hindus, Muslims, Sikhs, Christians, Parsis—is very different from the situation, say, in the United States. An Indian atheist cannot go along with an American counterpart's casual dismissal of religion as 'important, if true' but must amend it to 'important, even if not true'.

With its historical allusions from sacred rather than profane history, its metaphors and analogies having their source in sacred legends, the religious justification of a conflict involves fundamental values and releases some of our most violent passions. Why this is so is not only because religion is central to the vital, 'meaning-making' function of human life, causing deep disturbance if the survival of all that has been made meaningful by our religious beliefs is perceived to be under attack. Religion excites strong emotions also because it incorporates some of our noblest sentiments and aspirations—our most wishful thinking, the sceptic would say—and any threat to a belief in our 'higher' nature is an unacceptable denuding of self-esteem. Our wishful construction of human nature—that 'man is naturally good or at least good-natured; if he occasionally shows himself brutal, violent or cruel, these are only passing disturbances of his emotional life, for the most part provoked, or perhaps only consequences of the inexpedient social regulations he has hitherto imposed on himself,'[11]—is matched by our equally wishful constructions around religion. Religion, we like to believe, is about love—love of God, love of nature, and love of fellow man. Religion, we feel, is essentially about compassion and strives for peace and justice for the oppressed. Indeed, freedom from violence, an enduring wish of mankind, is reflected in various religious visions of heaven.

This construction is confronted with the reality that violence is present in all religions as a positive and even necessary force for the realization of religious goals. Religious violence has many forms which have found expression in the practice of animal or human sacrifice, in righteous and often excruciatingly cruel punishment envisaged for sinners, in the exorcism of spirits and demons, killing of witches or apostates, and in ascetic violence against the self.[12] The point is, as John Bowker has vividly demonstrated, that every religion has a vision of divinely legitimized violence—under certain circumstances.[13] In the Semitic religions, we have the Holy War of the Christians, the Just War of the Jews, and the Jehad of the Muslims where the believers are enjoined to battle and destroy evildoers. In other religions such as Hinduism and Buddhism, with their greater reputation for tolerance and nonviolence, violence is elevated to the realm of the sacred as part of the created order. In Hinduism, for instance, there is a cycle of violence and peacefulness as the Kali Age is followed by the Golden Age. Buddhist myths talk of Seven Days of the Sword where men will look on and kill each other as beasts, after which peace will return and no life is taken. Although Islam (especially in its current phase) and medieval Christianity have had most violent reputations, the question as to which religions have unleashed the greatest amount of violence is ultimately an empirical one.[14] In any event, fundamentalists can unleash any violence contained in a religion even if the religion is rarely perceived to have a violent potential, as amply demonstrated by our experience of Buddhist violence in Sri Lanka and Hindu violence in India. Moreover, as Natalie Davis has observed of Catholic–Protestant violence in 16th-century France and as we saw in the case of the Hyderabad riots, so long as rioters maintain a given religious commitment they rarely display guilt or shame for their acts of violence.[15]

Rhythms of religious ritual, whether in common prayer, processions, or other congregational activities, are particularly conducive to breaking down boundaries between members of a group and thus, in times of tension and threat, forging violent mobs. I have called these instruments of the community's violence 'physical' groups since the individual's experience of group identity here is through unconscious bodily communication and fantasies rather than through the more consciously shared cultural traditions. Physical groups seem to come into existence more effortlessly in religious than in other kinds of conflict.

Histories and Futures

In this book, I have attempted to contribute a depth-psychological dimension to the understanding of religious conflict, especially the tension between Hindus and Muslims. I am aware that this may be regarded by some as 'psychologizing' an issue which demands social and political activism and which could well do without the introduction of psychological complexities, that 'pale cast of thought', which can only sow doubt and sap the will for unself-conscious action. In retrospect, I realize I have gone about this task in consonance with my professional identity as a clinician, though not as a psychoanalyst with an individual patient but more akin to the psychotherapist with a family practice who is called upon for assistance in a disintegrating marriage. I looked at the history of the Hindu–Muslim relationship, made a diagnostic assessment of what has gone wrong, and considered the positive forces in the relationship which were still intact. At the end, it is time to weigh the possible courses of action.

The awareness of belonging to either one community or the other—being a Hindu or Muslim—has increased manifold in recent years. Every time religious violence occurs in India or in some other part of the subcontinent, the reach and spread of modem communications ensure that a vast number of people are soon aware of the incident. Each riot and its aftermath raise afresh the issue of the individual's religious–cultural identity and bring it up to the surface of consciousness. This awareness may be fleeting for some, last over a period of time for others, but the process is almost always accompanied by a preconscious self interrogation on the significance of the religious–cultural community for the sense of one's identity and the intensity of emotion with which this community is invested. For varying periods of time, individuals consciously experience and express their identity through their religious group rather than through traditional kinship groups such as those of family and caste. The duration of this period, or even whether there will be a permanent change in the mode of identity experience for some, depends on many factors, not the least on the success of revivalist and fundamentalist political and social groupings in encouraging such a switch. They do this by stoking the already existing persecution anxiety—its combination of aggression and fear weakening the individual sense of identity. The needed support to a weakened personal identity is then provided by strengthening its social, group aspect through an invitation to the person to identify with a grandiose representation of his or her community. The shared 'contemplation' and growing conviction of the great superiority of Hindu or Muslim culture and ways is then the required tonic for narcissistic enhancement and identity consolidation around the religious–cultural community as a pivot.

As for the future, there is more than one scenario for the likely evolution of Hindu–Muslim relations. The Hindu nationalist, who views the conflict as a product of Hindu and Muslim cultural and institutional traditions, believes the only way of avoiding future large-scale violence is a change in the Muslim view of the community's role, traditions, and institutions so that the Muslim can 'adapt'—the word meaning anything from adjustment to assimilation—to the Hindu majority's 'national' culture. To ask the Muslims to recognize themselves in the Hindu nationalist history of India, to expect them to feel their culture confirmed in Hindu symbols, rituals, and celebrations is asking them to renounce their cultural identity and to erase their collective memory so that they become indistinguishable from their Hindu neighbours. To be swamped by the surrounding Hindu culture has been historically the greatest fear of the Indian Muslim, articulated even by some medieval Sufis who are commonly regarded as having been closest to the Hindu ethos. Such an assimilation is feared precisely because it is so tempting, holding the promise of a freedom from fear of violence and an active and full participation in the majority culture and life, especially now when the majority is also politically dominant. The Hindu nationalist's dilemma is that the Muslims continue to decline an offer the nationalist believes they cannot refuse. The nationalist finds that the Muslim is too big to be either swallowed or spit out. Even if the Muslim was willing to undertake the exercise in assimilation voluntarily, a highly improbable scenario, the task would involve the immensely difficult understanding of how religious–cultural traditions are transmitted and internalized and how those processes can be effectively interfered with and halted.

The secularist, who views the conflict as rooted in social–structural considerations, especially economic, is more sanguine on the future of Hindu–Muslim relations. In the long run, the secularist believes, the inevitable economic development of the country will alter social–structural conditions and thus assign the conflict, as the cliché would have it, 'to the dust heap of history' as religious identities fade and play less and less of a role in private and public life. A sceptical note on the belief in the primacy of political and economic structures in the shaping of consciousness, however, needs to be sounded. Cultural traditions—including the ideology of the Other—transmitted through the family can and do have a line of development separate from the political and economic systems of a society. This is strikingly apparent if one takes the case of Germany where recent studies indicate that, after living for forty years under a radically different political and economic system, the political orientation and values of the young in relation to the family in eastern Germany are no different from those of their counterparts in the western part of the country; cultural socialization patterns within the family have survived the change in political systems relatively untouched and are stronger than the logic of the political superstructure.[16]

The optimistic realist, a breed with which I identify, believes that we are moving towards an era of recognition of Hindu–Muslim differences rather than pursuing their chimerical commonalities. We are moving towards multiculturalism, with majority and minority cultures, rather than the emergence of a 'composite culture'. Such multiculturalism is neither harmful nor dangerous but necessary, since it enables different religious groups to deal with the modernizing process in an active way rather than making them withdraw in lamentation at the inequities of modernization or endure it as passive victims. The problem is to ensure that one identity, Hindutva, does not dominate or assimilate other religious-cultural identities which are also embarked on the same quest as the Hindus. I can understand the validity of the nationalist call to the Hindus to find new meaning in customs, practices, and symbols of Hindu culture. By the same logic, why should this be denied to the Muslims who, too, are engaged in the same struggle to find meaning in the modern world? The realist would say that the solution is to build a state which protects the equal rights of Hindus and Muslims to be different. He believes that we must work towards building a polity which respects the beliefs of both Hindus and Muslims however odd or perverse they may seem to each other and however scornful they may be of the other community in private. Being a sceptic, he is also aware that the creation of such a public realm may be a long drawn-out affair accompanied by much tension and open conflict between the communities which will strain the social and political fabric of the country.

This realist agrees with the Hindu nationalist that clouds of violence loom over the immediate future of Hindu–Muslim relations. He is convinced, though, that achieving the desired goal of a truly multicultural polity will ultimately generate much less tension than the permanent discord which is the probable consequence of the nationalist vision. I can only hope that the violence is short-lived and that it will hasten the creation of a common, tolerant public realm. Our experience of needless suffering and cruelty can sometimes have the effect of jolting us out of accustomed ways of interpreting the world and making us more receptive to fresh ideals and new social–political arrangements. When stress and anxiety are at their greatest there is perhaps enough survival need in humans to suddenly make them reasonable. I hope the poet Theodore Roethke is right that 'In a dark time, the eye begins to see.'[17] This realist is not a cynic since unlike the latter, he still has hope. And even if the hope turns out to be illusory, he knows that, in the words of the Mahabharata, 'Hope is the sheet anchor of every man, When hope is destroyed, great grief follows, which is almost equal to death itself'. This applies not only to individuals but also to communities and nations.

Notes and References

1 Samuels, Andrew, 1993, *The Political Psyche*, London: Routledge, Kegan and Paul, pp. 11–12.

2 See Wolff, Phillipe, 1971, 'The 1391 Pogrom in Spain: Social Crisis or Not?' *Past and Present*, 50, pp. 4–18; Rude, George, 1964, *The Crowd in History: A Study of Popular Disturbances in France and England, 1848*, New York; Estebe, Janine, 1968, *Tocsin pour un massacre*, Paris. For the 'clash of economic interests' theory of religious-ethnic conflicts in South Asia see, Veena Das (ed.), 1990, *Mirrors of Violence*, Delhi: Oxford University Press.

3 Walzer, Michael, 1982, 'Nations and Minorities', in C. Freud (ed.), *Minorities: Community and Identity*, Berlin: Springer-Verlag, pp. 219–27.

4 The leading proponent of the theory that the international environment, especially the ending of colonial rule, is responsible for ethnic conflict is D. Horowitz; see Horowitz, 1985, *Ethnic Groups in Conflict*, Berkeley and Los Angeles: University of California Press.

5 Freud, Sigmund, 1921, 'Group Psychology and the Analysis of the Ego' *Standard Edition*, vol. 18.

6 Erikson, Erik H., *Identity: Youth and Crisis*, p. 46. See also Puget, Janine, 1991, 'The Social Context: Searching for a Hypothesis', *Free Associations*, 2 (1).

7 Davis, pp. 156–60.

8 Winnicott, D.W., 1963, 'Communicating and Not Communicating Leading to a Study of Certain Opposites', in his *The Maturational Process and the Facilitating Environment*, New York: International Universities Press, p. 187. For a succinct discussion of contemporary psychoanalytic thinking on self and relatedness, see Soref, Alice R., 1992, 'The Self, in and out of Relatedness', *The Annual of Psychoanalysis*, 20, pp. 25–48.

9 Patterson, Orlando, 'The Nature, Causes and Implications of Ethnic Identification', in Charles Fried (ed.), *Minorities: Community and Identity*, Berlin: Dahlen Konferenzen, Springer-Verlag, pp. 25–50.

10 Rapoport, David, 'Comparing Militant Fundamentalist Movements', in Marty and Appleby, *Fundamentalisms and the State: Remaking Polities, Economies, and Militance*, Chicago: University of Chicago Press, p. 443.

11 Freud, Sigmund, 1993, 'New Introductory Lectures', *Standard Edition*, vol. 22, p. 104.

12 See von Stietencorn, Heinrich, 1979, 'Angst und Gewalt: Ihre Funktionen und ihre Bewältigung in den Religionen', in Stietencorn (hrg.), *Angst und Gewalt: Ihre Präsenz und Ihre Bewaltigung in den Religionen*, Düsseldorf: Patmos Verlag, pp. 311–37.

13 Bowker, John W., 1986, 'The-Burning Fuse: The Unacceptable Face of Religion', *Zygon*, 21 (4), pp. 415–38; see also Boulding, Elise, 1986, 'Two Cultures of Religion as Obstacles to Peace', *Zygon*, 21 (4), pp. 501–18.

14 Rapoport, 'Comparing Militant Fundamentalist Movements'.

15 Davis, p. 165.

16 Bertram, Hans, 1994, 'Germany—One Country with Two Youth Generations?', paper presented at the Seminar on Childhood and Adolescence, Goethe Institut, Colombo, Sri Lanka, February, pp. 17–21.

17 Cited in Makiya, Kanan, 'From Cruelty to Toleration', unpublished paper read at the conference on *Religion and Politics Today*, organized by the Rajiv Gandhi Foundation, New Delhi, 30 January–2 February, 1994.

The Resurgence of Imagination*

OUR TIMES SEEM POISED to witness the resurgence of the romantic vision of human life, a view that underlines the importance of the spiritual by conceiving of life as a quest. In such a view, there are many obstacles and difficulties along the way, but if the seeker persists, then he or she will be rewarded by a union with a higher power or the Spirit. In contrast, the rationalist vision is sceptical of all higher powers and exalted aims of life and likes to show that all gods have clay feet. The romantic vision also emphasizes an intimate connection between humankind and universe, between self and not-self, while the rationalist insists on an enduring separation between the two. He looks down at the romantic view as a scientifically wrong and philosophically confused reaction to the objective rift between mind and nature. For the rationalist, the romantic is engaged in a futile and regressive revolt against the 'bad news' of the Enlightenment: Separateness.[1]

As a broader intellectual and social current, the romantic resurgence is more characteristic of Western societies than of most non-Western ones where the romantic vision never lost its ascendancy over the rational. Or, to put it more accurately, the *Ur*-romantic vision of non-Western societies generally remained oblivious of separateness and thus differs from the Western post-enlightenment romantic sensibility which has been struggling to overcome the rift even as it has remained exquisitely

*Revised version of an essay first published in *Harvard Divinity Bulletin*, 39:1, 2009.

aware of it. In fact, with the spread of modern scientific and technical education in the non-Western world, the movement seems headed in an opposite direction as educated professionals in these countries enthusiastically embrace the rationalist vision of Western Enlightenment. This trend is perhaps most visible in China. To a lesser degree, it also holds true for modern India where the romantic view, including its excrescences of occultism and superstition, still holds considerable sway over the Indian imagination.

It is instructive to remember that even in the West, in spite of the attacks by the rationalists and the scientific and technological successes of the post-Enlightenment world, the romantic vision did not completely disappear but continued to persist in embattled enclaves. In philosophy, one can think of Kant versus Hume, in science, of Einstein versus Watson. In my own discipline, psychoanalysis, Ferenzci and Jung and, more recently Kohut, can be said to represent the romantic position against a rationalist Freud. In anthropology, the divide cuts through each anthropologist. The participant anthropologist, identifying with and often idealizing the culture he is studying, struggles against the empiricist and detached observer within himself, seeking a balance which, depending on his life experience, is apt to be skewed in one or the other direction.[2]

I am, of course, aware of the oversimplification involved in the use of such binaries as romantic and rational. The romantic and the rational are not necessarily oppositional. A complex mind will be guided by both visions, the romantic one enlivening and lending a 'poetic' sensibility and sentiment to reason, while the rational vision guards against the sentimental excesses to which the romantic is all too susceptible. Since differentiation precedes integration, it may well be that the Enlightenment's project to differentiate itself from its past by rejecting romanticism is due for a revision that will begin to integrate the two views.

What are some of the signs of this romantic resurgence? Recent developments in social neurosciences and evolutionary psychology highlight an innate altruism in human beings, and seem as supportive of Rousseau's view of man as intrinsically good, a 'noble savage', as the research that leans towards Hobbes's darker vision of man as being basically self-centered. I will not go into detail about the now familiar research which suggests that empathy and altruistic behaviour that are motivated by empathy may be wired into our brains. I will only emphasize here that the call of the great *homini religiosi* of the world to place primacy on empathic altruism in social life may indeed not be a utopian dream but an evolutionary reality. Even economic theory, based on the premise of *homo economicus* acting rationally out of self-interest, which used to be as uneasy with altruistic behaviour as was sociobiology with its belief in the 'selfish gene', is becoming more uncertain about its basic assumption.

My own discipline, psychoanalysis, has also been deeply suspicious of altruistic behaviour. Just as sociobiology allows a limited altruism in the animal kingdom—more in the sense of self-sacrifice that benefits the kin group rather than empathy-driven human altruistic acts—psychoanalysis, too, exempts the 'proto-altruism' of maternal and paternal caretaking[3] from its general view that altruism essentially rests on a pathological base. Otherwise, altruism, when it is not driven by psychotic delusions that lead to bizarre acts of self-sacrifice, is regarded as a sub-category of masochism. In psychoanalytic thought, altruistic behaviour in the individual is usually a defense against his strong aggressive strivings and envy, and is also a super-ego driven need to suffer and be a victim. Even in less conflicted cases, psychoanalysis tends to view altruism as the by-product of a 'healthy narcissism' which is essential for mental well-being, maintaining that a person can love others only if he first loves himself. For a psychoanalyst, a person acting on the Golden Rule and doing good is nevertheless deriving a secret narcissistic satisfaction of being a do-gooder.

However, what if this dichotomy between narcissism and altruism is false? It can be argued that altruistic empathy and egotistic prudence are not in conflict but complementary to each other. Doing good to others is also doing good to yourself. In other words, acting on the Golden Rule, present in various forms in all the world's religions, may not only be vital for an individual's spiritual progress but for his psychological happiness. Research increasingly shows that this is not only a moral exhortation but an empirical fact.

The quickening of the altruistic impulse is also evident in the wider social arena. The flourishing of NGOs, including some on a global scale, such as *Medecins sans Frontier*, Oxfam and Amnesty International, and the unprecedented rise in charitable giving which is not limited to one's own community but embraces the whole of humanity, are some other signposts on this road.[4]

In Western societies (and in Westernized enclaves of non-Western societies around the world), there is also a widespread and very visible quest for 'authenticity', a notion closely associated with Rousseauan romanticism. As the anthropologist, Charles Lindholm, has shown, the search for personal and collective authenticity has become omnipresent in modern life. Indeed, in such diverse areas as art, music, religious life, or even in travel and cuisine,[5] it is what we look for. In Western art, of course, the romantic impulse did not weaken as much as in other areas. Metaphysical questions maintained their significance for artists from Wassily Kandinsky to Francis Bacon, from Joseph Beuys to Damien Hirst. Kandinsky believed that painting represented 'pure art in the service of the divine'.[6] As is evident from the catalogue of the exhibition, *Traces of the Spiritual*, that began in the Centre Pompidou in Paris and is currently in Haus der Kunst in Munich, to touch, 'refine and enrich' the 'soul', the 'spirit', has become a central concern for many artists today.

What are the implications of the romantic revival and the probable integration of the romantic and rational for the pre-eminently Western discipline of psychoanalysis? Let me begin to answer this question with an anecdote.

In 1994, I was honoured with an invitation from the Foundation for Universal Responsibility, which was set up by the Dalai Lama from his Nobel Peace Prize award in order to have a dialogue with His Holiness in New Delhi. The subject of the dialogue was Buddhist and Western psychology and I, as a psychoanalyst, was asked to represent the viewpoint of Western psychology.

What I remember most vividly about the dialogue is an exchange when the topic of hatred came up. I gave the orthodox psychoanalytic view: there is something wrong with the person if he cannot hate. There is also something wrong if the person cannot stop hating. A mature person should be able to hate but also be capable of transcending hatred.

'No, No!' the Dalai Lama exclaimed. 'This is not true of Buddhist psychology.'

He then proceeded to tell the story about his friend, a spiritually advanced Lama who was incarcerated in a prison in Tibet and tortured by the Chinese. After many years, the Lama managed to escape and reach Dharamshala, the home of the Dalai Lama in India.

'How was it?' the Dalai Lama asked his old friend about his long years of imprisonment.

'Oh, twice it was very bad,' the Lama replied.

'Were you in danger of losing your life?' the Dalai Lama expressed his concern.

'No. Twice I almost *hated* the Chinese!'

Of course, the psychoanalytic gloss on hatred applies to a Tibetan as much as it does to a Westerner. And yet, the aspect of Buddhist psychology which the Dalai Lama had brought into the discussion introduced the spiritual into the purely psychological.

Spirituality, like culture, has many definitions. Originally, spirituality and mysticism were terms created by elite nineteenth-century Western intellectuals, poets, and scholars, mostly of a Whitmanian or Emersonian orientation, then later became part of a variety of Quaker, theosophical, human potential, and New Age lineages. I am not quite comfortable with these terms myself, but will use them because they are current in English language discourse. For me, the spiritual incorporates the transformative possibilities of the human psyche: total love without a trace of hate, selflessness carved out of the psyche's normal self-centredness, a fearlessness that is not a counter-phobic reaction to the fear that is an innate part of the human psyche. Yet, spiritual transformation is not a once and forever achievement even in the case of enlightened spiritual masters and saints. It remains constantly under threat from the darker forces of the psyche. One is never *not* human—'Twice I almost hated the Chinese.' For me, 'spirit' is not the 'luminous cloud' of the mystic that floats ethereally in mysterious regions of the human stratosphere, but one that swirls among the crags of human passions—above all, desire and narcissism.

A spirituality that does not take into account and engage with the complexities and dynamic nature of the psyche will fail to touch people who are not incurably romantic. It will remain experience-distant rather than experience-near. Equally, a psychology that refuses to recognize the potentialities of the psyche, of its possible extension into the realm of the spirit, a psychology which contents itself with Freud's healing offer of replacing hysterical misery with common unhappiness, does not provide enough emotional sustenance to modern man.

To describe the relationship between the spirit and the psyche, I must take recourse to metaphors which comprehend the body, psyche, and spirit as intimately related entities with fuzzy boundaries that flow into each other. I envision the psyche as a large lake. The waters of this lake are warm, heated by the energy of sexuality, aggression and, above all, narcissism, that comes pouring in from the surrounding earth and the body, and keeps the waters in turbulence. Ripples can become waves which may assume frightening proportions. At the bottom of the lake, there flows the cool stream of the spirit, its water fed by the subterranean spring of loving connection, which is kept apart from the upper layers by the difference in temperature between the two. Spiritual adepts dive often and deep into this stream, although there is perhaps none among them who does not also dwell in the shallower reaches of the lake, sharing the joys, sorrows and circumstances of our common humanity.

We ordinary mortals are not cut off from the spiritual stream. The cool water often surges up to the surface in trickles, though rarely in flood. These are perceptible moments of elation felt in presence of nature, the thrill felt in front of a work of art, the ineffable intimacy with the beloved after the sexual embrace when the bodies have separated and are lying together side by side, or the moments of communion between the mother and the baby on her breast. There are many other such minor epiphanies, fleeting moments stamped with the seal of eternity, which may escape our conscious awareness because we expect the spiritual to be an exception rather than a rule in human life.

The spiritual quest, except for those rare people who have set their sights on the summits of spirituality, is not so much a search but a *recognition* of the many instances when the spirit touches the psyche. The touch may be barely noticeable, like the wing of a butterfly whispering against the cheek. The quest is not to catch and hold the butterfly, which will die and become desiccated if captured. The challenge is to be aware of the spiritual moments as we travel through life, to look around and see again with the innocent eye. There is a story about the Zen monk who had been meditating for many years in a cave. When he became old and felt the approach of death, he expressed his desire to finally visit the fabled valley of flowers of which he had heard so much when he was a child. 'It is beyond that yonder range of mountains,' he was told. The monk started climbing, his gaze fixed on the mountain peaks. When he reached the top of the range, he asked another monk going in the opposite direction how far the valley of flowers still was. 'Look behind you,' he was told. When he looked back, the monk found he had walked through the valley of flowers without seeing it.

An invaluable ally for 'seeing' is imagination, which the romantics have always considered to be the basis of reality. Today, we usually think of imagination as the ability to make images, although the capacity to access and elaborate on early memories is equally important. Indeed, it is a complex and often a playful combination of the two which characterizes a bold leap of imagination. As we now know, the area of the brain activated in remembering the past and visualizing the future is the same.

Imagination, which in the words of the psychoanalyst Gilbert Rose 'propels one beyond prosaic reasonableness into a less tangible world of emotions, dreams, suggestions, and impressions where there is no rigid separation between self and not-self,'[6] is not opposed but complementary to reason. Even the eighteenth century English poet John Keats, that most eloquent partisan of imagination, visualized a smoothly working partnership between the two as an ideal, holding that a truly complex mind would be 'one that is imaginative and at the same time careful of its fruits' and would exist 'partly on sensations and partly on thought.'[7] The enemy of imagination is not reason but its overbearing, over-critical form that disparages the illogical and the incongruent, smothers spontaneity and feeling, banishes the poetical, excludes all tendencies towards symbol and metaphor, and acknowledges the primacy of only the statistical and the quantifiable. If the pathological form of imagination is delusion, then that of reason is obsession.[8]

However, imagination also has a spiritual dimension; the English poet Samuel Coleridge called it 'primary imagination' and John Keats called it 'unitive imagination'.[9] A spiritual more than a psychological category, primary imagination has been viewed by romantics as the basis of reality. Kant held it to be the basis for all productive knowledge. Einstein agreed when he asserted that 'I am enough of an artist to draw freely upon my imagination. Imagination is more important than knowledge. Knowledge is limited. Imagination encircles the world.'[10] Writers and poets have concurred with this judgment, explicitly attributing this mysterious source of their creativity to the 'spiritual'. Saul Bellow, in his Nobel prize acceptance speech, articulates the position of many elite intellectuals and creative writers on the problematic nature of spiritual realities.

The sense of our real powers, powers we seem to derive from the universe itself, also comes and goes … We are reluctant to talk about this because there is nothing we can prove, because our language is inadequate, and because few people are willing to risk talking about it. They would have to say that there is a spirit, and that is taboo.[11]

Even V.S. Naipaul, that most rationalist of writers who values the conscious, thinking mind so much that he speaks of his detestation of music (widely regarded as the most spiritual of art forms), calling it 'the lowest art form, too accessible, capable of stirring people who think little,' admits that 'when the work is good I am not responsible.'[12] He tells his biographer that in such a phase 'the material seemed to be given to him from nowhere' as he moved into that 'determined stupor' out of which great books are written.[13]

In nineteenth century India, Mirza Ghalib, the great Urdu poet, had no such difficulty: *Aate hain ghaibse ye / mazamiin khyal mein / Ghalib sareer e khama / navaye sarosh hai* (My thoughts come to me / From somewhere Beyond / When Ghalib is attuned / To the music of the stars).[14] Artists have called the spirit their Muse and it is a rare artist, whether agonistic or atheist, who does not believe in the existence of the Muse or does not have his own magical techniques of invoking and controlling it.[15]

Perhaps the most passionate advocate of the spiritual basis of imagination was Keats, who went beyond the psychology of imagination—the use of condensation, displacement, symbolism—into its spiritual dimension by highlighting the imaginative process as a union between the knower and the known. In his description of this 'unitive' imagination, he writes, 'No sooner am I alone than shapes of epic greatness are stationed around me' and 'according to my state of mind I am with Achilles shouting in the trenches, or with Theocritus in the Vales of Sicily.'[16] Likewise, Gustave Flaubert, while writing *Madame Bovary*, confides to a friend,

> It is a delicious thing to write, to be no longer yourself but to move in an entire universe of your own creating. Today, for instance, as a man and woman, both lover and mistress, I rode into a forest of an autumn afternoon under the yellow leaves, and I was also the horses, the leaves, the wind, the words my people uttered, even the red sun that made them close their love-drowned eyes.[17]

I would call the spiritual dimension of imagination *connective* rather than unitive, with the latter constituting an end point of a spectrum, accessible only to individuals with extraordinary spiritual gifts. Just as an altruistic act is spiritual only if there is a vision of love behind it, imagination is spiritual only when it is connective. Connective imagination is not only limited to literary works and creation of images in painting and sculpture, but it is the essence of many religious forms. I am especially thinking of Tibetan-Buddhist and Hindu Tantra which have the visualization of the deities and the devotee's union with these mind-created forms as their central spiritual practice. Here, let me mention only one of the many tantric techniques, *nyasa*, in which a Tantrik visualizes the goddess and then interjects her into the various parts of his body by touching them. The imaginative world created by the Tantrik is not the personal one of the artist (nor is it the world of the psychotic), but, instead, it is both shared and public. It is based upon, guided and formed by the symbolic, iconic network of his religious culture.

Another example of religious practice where connective imagination manifests itself is in the daily ritual *puja* of an orthodox Hindu who gets the gods to dwell in the various limbs and parts of his body before he begins to chant his prayers. This is also true of the Muslim *namaz* or the Catholic Mass. Indeed, a great attraction of religious practices may well lie in the opportunity they afford the believer to release and exercise his capacity for connective imagination.

Connective imagination, then, is not only the basis of much great art and some visions of science and philosophy, but is also the underlying principle of many religious rituals and spiritual disciplines. Perhaps the time has come that connective imagination also receives serious attention in psychological disciplines concerned with the apprehension of the world and empathy, as a singular mode of understanding other human beings, assumes its rightful place at the head of the psychotherapy table. However, is the romantic veneration of imagination universal, or is it limited to the Western world? Here, I will only discuss traditional Indian thought with the caveat that I am not a scholar of Indian philosophical systems but merely a curious student.

My major impression is that Indian thought shares the Western romantic belief in the omnipotence of imagination but has regarded this fact with ambivalent feelings. The Nyaya and Advaita schools both agree that we live in an imagined world and, as the great seventh century philosopher, Shankara, put it, we are wrapped in this imaginary world as a moth in its cocoon.[18] Shankara even argued that dreams are real because they have real effects on waking life; a man bitten by an imaginary snake can die from the imaginary venom.[19] The spiritual goal of both of these schools is a direct perception of reality (*nirivikalpa pratyksha*), which is only possible at birth since reality becomes veiled by the operation of imagination as life takes hold and changes our apprehension of the world into a *svaikalpa pratyksha*. Imagination, then, is a hindrance to reaching the spiritual goal of life and needs to be combated. In other words, the status of imagination in Hindu thought has varied with the corresponding status of *maya* of which imagination is an integral part. In Vedic times, when maya was viewed as the creative power of the gods and defined as 'incomprehensible insight, wisdom, judgment and power enabling its possessor to create something or to do something, ascribed to mighty beings',[20] the status of imagination was high. Gradually, as maya came to mean illusion, the power of imagination remained beyond doubt but, as we saw from Shankara's views, it began to be seen as inimical to spiritual strivings.

Perhaps only a few, rare saints can reach the summit of connective imagination, expressed in the Upanishadic ideal of 'he who sees all beings in his own self and his own self in all beings'. Most of us can consider ourselves fortunate if we can catch a glimpse of the peak from the base camp of an all-encompassing compassion. Personally speaking, I am keenly aware of the power of human passions of desire, aggression, and narcissism to shape our beliefs, thoughts, and behaviour, and equally conscious of our supreme human capacity to deceive ourselves with regards to our motives. As a result, I will be satisfied to reach the starting point of this spiritual expedition, namely a wide-ranging tolerance which the late philosopher Ramachandra Gandhi defined, minimally, as giving the benefit of doubt to others.[34] If one wants to go anywhere spiritually, tolerance is a good place to start.

Notes and References

1 See Klugman, David, 2001, 'Empathy's Romantic Dialectic: Self Psychology, Intersubjectivity and Imagination', *Psychoanalytic Psychology*, 18, pp. 684–704.

2 Lindholm, Charles, 2008, *Culture and Authenticity*, Malden, MA: Blackwell, pp. 141–2.

3 Seelig, Beth J. and Lisa S. Rosof, 2001, 'Normal and Pathological Altruism', *Journal of the American Psychoanalytic Association,* 49, pp. 933–59.

4 In a talk at a conference on 'Emerging Images of Humanity', *Fetzer Institute and Eranos Foundation,* Ascona, 5–11 August 2007, the religious scholar Ursula King called these organizations part of 'the global quest for spiritualities'.

5 Lindholm, *Culture and Authenticity*.

6 Rose, Gilbert J., 1996, *Necessary Illusion: Art as 'Witness',* Madison, CT: International Universities Press, p. 58.

7 Cited in Leavy, Stanley A., 1970, 'John Keats's Psychology of Creative Imagination', *Psychoanalytic Quarterly*, 39(2), p. 176.

8 Ibid., p. 174.

9 Britton, Ronald, 'Reality and Unreality in Phantasy and Fiction', in Ethel Person, Servulo Augusto Figueira, and Peter Fonagy (eds), 1995, *On Freud's 'Creative Writers and Day-dreaming',* New Haven: Yale University Press, p. 94.

10 Calaprice, Alice (ed.), 2000, *The Expanded Quotable Einstein*, Princeton: Princeton University Press, p. 10.

11 Cited in Knight, James A., 1987, 'The Spiritual as a Creative Force in the Person', *Journal of American Academy of Psychoanalysis,* 15, p. 365.

12 Cited in French, Patrick, 2008, *The World is What it is: The Authorized Biography of V. S. Naipaul*, London: Picador, p. 403.

13 Ibid., p. 389.

14 Personal communication from Abid Hussain, Shimla, 14 September 2007.

15 Knight, 'The Spiritual as a Creative Force', p. 368.

16 Leavy, 'John Keats's Psychology', p. 178

17 Gustave Flaubert cited in Margulies, Alfred, 1993, 'The Empathic Imagination', *Journal of American Academy of Psychoanalysis,* 21, p. 516.

18 Personal Communication from Anand Paranjpe.

19 Shankara's Commentary on the Vedanta Sutras 2.1.4, cited in O'Flaherty, Wendy Doniger, 1984, *Dreams, Illusion and Other Realities*, Chicago: University of Chicago Press, p. 286.

20 Gonda, J., *Four Studies in the Language of the Veda*, cited in O'Flaherty, *Dreams*, p. 118.

Childhood

and

Identity

Mothers and Infants*

THE FIRST MONTHS OF HUMAN life are a period of wordless oblivion which is of root significance for individual development. At once timeless and fleeting, infancy is the foundation for all later psychological experience. Moreover, the nature of an individual's first relationship—with his mother—profoundly influences the quality and 'dynamics' of social relations throughout his life.

Recognition of the crucial role of this original relationship, the mother–infant 'dyad' as the genetic psychologist Edward Simmel has called it,[1] for the development of all subsequent social relations has been relatively late in coming in the social sciences. Thus, although Freud mentioned its importance in 1895 in one of his earliest papers and often elaborated on the psychological reciprocity between mothers and infants, he came to appreciate its full significance in emotional development only towards the end of his life. By 1938, he described the mother's importance to the infant as 'unique, without parallel, established unalterably for a whole lifetime as the first and strongest love-object and as the prototype of all later love-relations—for both sexes'.[2] It is within this dyad that a person first learns to relate to the 'other' and begins to develop his capacity to love (in its widest sense); it is here that an individual originates as a social being. As adults, all of our affiliations and

*From *The Inner World: A Psychoanalytic Study of Childhood and Society in India,* Delhi and New York: Oxford University Press, 1978.

intimacies bear the stamp of our particular kind of infancy. Indeed, as anthropologists such as Kardiner, Benedict and Mead have shown, the specific emotional colouring of many of a society's cultural institutions can be directly attributed to the dominant quality or mode of the first relationship, not in the sense of simple causal connection, but in the complementarity and reciprocal influence between the mother–infant dyad and other institutionalized forms of social relations.

In spite of the general consensus on its significance, the mother–infant dyad remains intellectually elusive and relatively unexplored. In part, because of its archaic, wordless nature, it is but dimly reflected in the free associations of psychoanalytic patients and hence in clinical reconstructions. Hypotheses and speculations on the emotional development of the infant and on what actually transpires between him and his mother in the course of their repeated early encounters are thus derived from a variety of sources: direct observation of infants, experimental data in neonatal cognition, treatment of psychotic patients, and deductions from the conceptual framework of psychoanalysis. The following short summary of existing knowledge of the emotional state of infancy is highly condensed.[3] Such a description, however minimal, is a necessary background for the elaboration of the dominant mode of the mother–infant relationship in Hindu society and for an interpretation of its consequences for adult personality, its influence on the organization of social relations and its relevance to the elaboration of cultural ideals.

During the first few months of life, the infant lives in a psychological state which has variously been termed 'undifferentiated', 'non-differentiated', or 'unintegrated'. These terms are basically similar; all imply that at the beginning of life there is no clear and absolute distinction between conscious and unconscious, ego and id, psyche and *soma*, inside and outside, 'I' and what is 'not-I', nor even between the different parts of the body. Only gradually, through constant exchanges with the mothering person, does the infant begin to discriminate and differentiate these opposites which are initially merged, and thus to take his first steps on the road to selfhood. The emotional or affective quality of this process of differentiation and inner integration is determined by the vicissitudes of the infant's tie to his mother. Whether all that is 'not-I' will forever remain vaguely threatening, replete with forebodings of an undefined nature, a danger to be avoided, whether the infant will emerge from this phase feeling that the outside world is benevolently disposed and basically trustworthy, or whether a reassuring sense of inner continuity and wholeness will predominate over a sense of falling to pieces and life forever lived in disparate segments are some of the developmental questions which originate in infancy. Furthermore, there is no comparable period of life in so far as the adaptive learning that takes place, learning which is mediated almost solely through the mother's instrumentality, when the mother is the principal caretaker of infants as she is in most cultures.

It is the mother's face—which the baby's eyes begin to 'grasp' and follow from about the age of four weeks, even when nursing—which becomes crystallized as the first visual precept from a jumble of light blurs, the first meaningful image out of a chaos of 'things' without meaning. It is on the mother's body, on her breast and through her hands that tactile perception and orientation are learned and practised. It is her rhythms of movement and quiet, her body warmth and smell, which differentiate the baby's other sensitivities, his sense of equilibrium and movement and his sensuality, while her voice is the sound stimulus which is the prerequisite for his own development of speech. Thus, the mother's *sensory presence* is of vital importance for the infant's earliest developmental experiences and awakenings.[4]

This emphasis on the mother's significance and power does not mean that the infant is completely helpless or passive in his relationship with her. From the beginning, he, too, is actively involved—looking, listening and, with the development of manual coordination, touching, handling, grasping—in maintaining connection and communication with his mother. Ethnologists have designated this innate predisposition to activity—the five basic instinctive responses of sucking, clinging, following, crying, and smiling—as a 'species-specific behaviour pattern' designed to further the human infant's survival by keeping him near the mother. Whether the ethological hypothesis is appropriate remains a controversial issue;[5] and even given the infant's predisposition to this kind of activity and the innate equipment which makes it possible, 'the vital spark has to be conferred on the equipment through exchanges with another human being, with a partner, with the mother'.[6] She is the 'facilitating environment' for these earliest processes of development. Without her contact and facilitation, the infant's first experiences take place in a psychosocial void, and his development is likely to be severely disturbed.

The infant's development and the relationship with the mother which nurtures it are optimal only when that relationship becomes a kind of psychological counterpart to the biological connection of pregnancy. Psychologists have variously described this optimal condition as 'mutuality', 'dual unit', 'reciprocity', or 'dialogue'. All these terms seek to convey that what is good and right for one partner in the relationship is also good and right for the other. The reciprocity between the mother and infant is a circular process of action–reaction–action in which, ideally, the mother welcomes her infant's unfolding activities and expressions of love with her own delighted and loving responses, which in turn stimulate the baby to increase his efforts and to offer his mother further expressions of gratification and attachment. This mutuality is by far the most important factor in enabling an infant to create a coherent inner image of a basically reassuring world and to lay the foundation for a 'true self'; without it, he is likely to become a bundle of reactions which resignedly complies with, or is in constant struggle against, the outer world's infringements. It is the mother who helps her infant learn to deal with anxiety without feeling devastated, and to temper and manage the inevitable feelings of frustration and anger.

For many years, psychoanalytic psychologists were preoccupied with the infant's need for succour in its most literal form: the need to be fed. The manifest nature of this need, together perhaps with the symbolic nostalgia and charm evoked by the image of a nursing baby and his mother, led to an almost exclusive focus on the variability of feeding practices in the mother–infant relationship as the central dynamic factor in personality formation. Anthropological observations of feeding and weaning activities were relied upon in an almost ritualized manner, as a primary source for the explanation of dominant personality characteristics within a given culture. Without underestimating the effect of the nursing situation and the feeding moment on personality—the vicissitudes of orality, as psychoanalysts would call it—it is fair to note that the nutritional need and its satisfaction is only one element, albeit an important one, in the total configuration of the mother–infant dyad. For the crucial social interaction, through which an individual begins to separate himself out and become a person, the infant needs his mother as a whole human being, not merely as a satisfier of hunger and thirst; or, to state it plainly, what the infant requires is not a breast but a mother. Feeding must be viewed as a part of a total communication process in which not only the mother's breast but also the quality of her movement, voice and touch affects the quality of the infant's sensory and emotional lease on life. The breast can be viewed, then, as a symbol for the mother, while feeding and weaning are but symbols for the inevitable processes of attachment and separation in human development. That is, whether or not they are representative of the quality of mothering in any culture, they are the most tangible (and symbolically loaded) aspects of nurturing. What psychologists and anthropologists alike must observe more carefully is not the false controversy between breast and bottle feeding, or how conscientiously the mother carries out her nursing duties, or how and when she weans her child, but the total emotional climate, the gestalt, of mothering.

Psychosocial Matrix of Infancy: Feminine Identity in India

Whether her family is poor or wealthy, whatever her caste, class or region, whether she is a fresh young bride or exhausted by many pregnancies and infancies already, an Indian woman knows that motherhood confers upon her a purpose and identity that nothing else in her culture can. Each infant borne and nurtured by her safely into childhood, especially if the child is a son, is both a certification and a redemption.

At the same time, each individual woman approaches motherhood at her particular crossroads of *desa*, *kala*, *srama and gunas*, and with her unique constellation of values, expectations, fears and beliefs about the role and the experience of mothering. She meets her newborn infant with the emotional resources and limitations of her particular personality; these are the 'matrix' of her child's infancy.[7] Her identity as a Hindu woman has evolved out of the *particulars* of her life cycle and childhood, out of the dailiness of her relationships as daughter in her parents' family and as wife and daughter-in-law in her husband's family, and out of the universals of the traditional ideals of womanhood absorbed by her from childhood onwards. Whether a particular mother is reserved or responsive to a particular infant, and in what circumstances, depends on a wide range of variables, not the least of which is her ordinal position in her original family (whether she was a firstborn female or the fourth daughter in a row, or the first little girl after a line of sons ...) as well as the sex and ordinal position of the infant who now needs and claims her love and care. It is not the purpose of this study to explore the range of individual maternal receptivity. Rather, we will focus on the vivid ideals of womanhood and motherhood in India, the common themes which in a traditional society such as India pervade and circumscribe the identities of individual women.

First of all, where and when tradition governs, an Indian woman does not stand alone; her identity is wholly defined by her relationships to others. For, although in most societies a woman (more than a man) defines herself in relation and connection to other intimate people, this is singularly true of Indian women. The dominant psychosocial realities of her life can be condensed into three stages:

First, she is a daughter to her parents.

Second, she is a wife to her husband (and daughter-in-law to his parents).
Third, she is a mother to her sons (and daughters).

How, then, do daughters fare in 'mother India'? The frank answer is that it is difficult to know, at least as exhaustively and 'in depth' as I would like to. The reason for this lies in the fact that data, of all kinds, are uneven or unavailable. Anthropological accounts refer, implicitly or explicitly, to the development of boys, and skim the subject of female childhood or skip it altogether. Myths, too, are sparing of their bounty towards daughters, for in a patriarchal culture myths are inevitably man-made and man-oriented. Addressing as they do the unconscious wishes and fears of men, it is the parent–son rather than the parent–daughter relationship which becomes charged with symbolic significance.[8]

These limitations are real enough, but they need not be forbidding. On the contrary, they challenge the psychoanalytic researcher to mine the existing material thoroughly and to construct an interpretive bridge for future work. There are, for example, in anthropological accounts, both a consistent indication of the marked preference for sons all over India, and at the same time, somewhat paradoxically, abundant allusion to the warmth, intimacy and relaxed affection of the mother–daughter bond.[9] Statistics document the higher rate of female infant mortality, and call attention to the fact that whatever health care and schooling are available in India, daughters are the last to receive it.[10] In the realm of literature, although the mainstream mythology and classical texts of Hinduism have been the preserves of men, there are parts of the oral tradition—ballads, folk songs, and couplets sung by women in different parts of the country, and a few folktales—which give us clues to the psychological constellation of daughterhood in India. Leavened with clinical impressions, these various sources can be judiciously drawn together to sketch a portrait of Indian girlhood.

The preference for a son when a child is born is as old as Indian society itself. Vedic verses pray that sons will be followed by still more male offspring, never by females. A prayer in the *Atharvaveda* adds a touch of malice: 'The birth of a girl, grant it elsewhere, here grant a son.'[11] As MacDonell observes,

> Indeed daughters are conspicuous in the *Rigveda* by their absence. We meet in hymns with prayers for sons and grandsons, male offspring, male descendants and male issue and occasionally for wives but never daughters. Even forgiveness is asked for ourselves and grandsons, but no blessing is ever prayed for a

daughter. When *Agni* is born it is as if it were a male infant. They clap their hands and make sounds of rejoicing like the parents of a newborn son. There is no such rejoicing over the birth of a daughter.[12]

The ancient *Pumsavana* rite, still performed over pregnant women in traditional Hindu households, is designed to elicit the birth of a male infant and to magically change the sex of the unborn child if it be a female.

Contemporary anthropological studies from different parts of India and the available clinical evidence assure us that the traditional preference for sons is very much intact.[13] At the birth of a son drums are beaten in some parts of the country, conch shells blown in others and the midwife paid lavishly, while no such spontaneous rejoicing accompanies the birth of a daughter. Women's folk songs reveal the painful awareness of inferiority—of this discrepancy, at birth, between the celebration of sons and the mere tolerance of daughters. Thus, in a north Indian song the women complain:

Vidya said, *'Listen, O Sukhma, what a tradition has started!*
Drums are played upon the birth of a boy,
But at my birth only a brass plate was beaten.'[14]

And in Maharashtra, the girl, comparing herself to a white sweet scented jasmine (*jai*) and the boy to a big, strong smelling thorny leaf (*kevada*), plaintively asks: 'Did anyone notice the sweet fragrance of a *jai*? The hefty *kevada* however has filled the whole street with its strong scent.'[15]

Of course there are 'valid' ritual and economic reasons—we will come to the psychological ones later—for 'sexism' in Indian society. The presence of a son is absolutely necessary for the proper performance of many sacraments, especially those carried out upon the death of parents and imperative to the well-being of their souls. In addition to her negligible ritual significance, a daughter normally is an unmitigated expense, someone who will never contribute to the family income and who, upon marriage, will take away a considerable part of her family's fortune as her dowry. In the case of a poor family, the parents may even have to go deep in debt in order to provide for a daughter's marriage. The *Aitareya Brahmana* (like other older texts) probably refers as much as anything else to the economic facts of life when it states flatly that a daughter is a source of misery while a son is the saviour of the family.[16]

As in other patriarchal societies, one would expect the preference for sons, the cultural devaluation of girls, to be somehow reflected in the psychology of Indian women. Theoretically, one possible consequence of this kind of inequity would be a heightened female hostility and envy towards males, together with a generally pronounced antagonism between the sexes. I do not have sufficient evidence to be categorical; yet my impression is that these phenomena do not, in general, characterize the inner world of Indian women. The dominant myths, for example—unlike, say, *A Thousand and One Nights*—show little evidence of strain in relationships between the sexes. And, as I have shown elsewhere, aggression occurring between members of the same sex is significantly greater than between members of opposite sexes in India.[17]

It can be argued that male dominance and strong taboos against feminine aggression may inhibit the expression of female resentment against men and serve to redirect this hostility against male children. For if a woman perceives that the fundamental premise of the absolute status hierarchy between the sexes is merely gender, and if she is prevented from expressing her rage and resentment at this state of affairs, either because of cultural taboos, social inferiority or her dependence upon men, then her unconscious destructive impulses towards male children are liable to be particularly strong, this being her only possible revenge against a pervasive oppressive masculinity. Again, excepting certain communities, this does not appear to be characteristic of Indian women, given the evidence of songs, tales and other kinds of folklore.[18]

The third possibility is that girls and women in a dramatically patriarchal society will turn the aggression against themselves and transform the cultural devaluation into feelings of worthlessness and inferiority. There is scattered evidence that such a propensity indeed exists among many communities of Indian women, that hostility towards men and potential aggression against male infants are often turned inward, subsumed in a diffuse hostility against oneself, in a conversion of outrage into self-depreciation. At least among the upper-middle-class women who today seek psychotherapy, the buried feeling, 'I am a girl and thus worthless and "bad"', is often encountered below the surface of an active, emancipated femininity. One patient, for example, staunchly maintained that her parents' separation took place because of her father's disappointment that she was born a girl and not a boy, although in fact, as she herself was aware, the parents had separated shortly before her birth. Some of the traits connected with low self-esteem—depressive moodiness, extreme touchiness, and morbid sensitivity in interpersonal relations—come through in the testimony of modern, educated Indian girls in the non-clinical interviews reported by Margaret Cormack in *The Hindu Woman.*[19] Their less educated, rural sisters give vent to similar feelings through the medium of folk songs: 'God Rama, I fall at your feet and fold my hands and pray to you, never again give me the birth of a woman.'[20]

I have deliberately used the words 'possibility' and 'propensity' in the above discussion rather than ascribe to Indian women a widespread depressive pattern. In the first place, for the cultural devaluation of women to be translated into a pervasive psychological sense of worthlessness in individual women, parents' and other adults' behaviour and attitudes towards the infant girls in their midst—the actualities of family life—must be fully consistent with this female depreciation. Secondly, the internalization of low self-esteem also presupposes that girls and women have no sphere of their own, no independent livelihood and activity, no area of family and community responsibility and dominance, no living space apart from that of the men, within which to create and manifest those aspects of feminine identity that derive from intimacy and collaboration with other women. And, in fact, these two circumstances exist in India, to mitigate the discriminations and inequities of patriarchal institutions.

From anthropological accounts and other sources, we know of the lenient affection and often compassionate attention bestowed by mothers on their daughters throughout their lives.[21] 'I turn the stone flour mill with the swiftness of a running deer; that is because my arms are strong with the mother's milk I drank.'[22] This, and other couplets like it, sung by women all over India, bear witness to the daughter's memory of her mother's affection for her and to the self-esteem and strength of will this has generated in turn. Thus, in the earliest period of emotional development, Indian girls are assured of their worth by whom it really matters: by their mothers.

The special maternal affection reserved for daughters, contrary to expectations derived from social and cultural prescriptions, is partly to be explained by the fact that a mother's unconscious identification with her daughter is normally stronger than with her son.[23] In her daughter, the mother can re-experience herself as a cared-for girl. And, in Indian society, as we shall see later, a daughter is considered a 'guest' in her natal family, treated with the solicitous concern often accorded to a welcome outsider, who, all too soon, will marry and leave her mother for good. Mindful of her daughter's developmental fate, the mother re-experiences the emotional conflicts her own separation once aroused, and this in turn tends to increase her indulgence and solicitude towards her daughter.

In addition to her mother's empathic connection with her, as an Indian girl grows up, her relationships with others within the extended family further tend to dilute any resentment she may harbour for her brothers. Among the many adults who comprise a Hindu family, there is almost always someone in particular who gives a little girl the kind of admiration and sense of being singled out as special that a male child more often receives from many. In such a family system, every child, irrespective of sex, stands a good chance of being some adult's favourite, a circumstance which softens the curse of rivalry, envy, and possessiveness which often afflicts 'modern' nuclear families. And of course when a girl is the only daughter, such chances are increased immeasurably. Thus, in folktales, however many sons a couple may have, there is often one daughter in their midst who is the parents' favourite.

Finally, in traditional India, every female is born into a well-defined community of women within her particular family. Although by no means does it always resound with solidarity and goodwill, the existence of this exclusive sphere of femininity and domesticity gives women a tangible opportunity to be productive and lively, to experience autonomy and to exercise power. It also allows a special kind of inviolate feminine privacy and familiar intimacy. Getting along with other women in this sphere, learning the mandatory skills of householding, cooking, and childcare, establishing her place in this primary world … these relationships and these tasks constitute the dailiness of girlhood in India. Moreover, this experience of 'apprenticeship' and the activities that transpire in this feminine sphere are independent of the patriarchal values of the outside world. And when necessary, other women in the family—her mother, grandmother, aunts, sisters, and sisters-in-law—are not only an Indian girl's teachers and models but her allies against the discriminations and inequities of that world and its values. Often enough, in the 'underground' of female culture, as reflected in ballads, wedding songs, and jokes, women do indeed react against the discriminations of their culture by portraying men as vain, faithless, and infantile.[24] All these factors help to mitigate (if not to prevent) the damage to a girl's self-esteem when she discovers that in the eyes of the culture, she is considered inferior to a boy, a discovery which usually coincides with the awareness of gender identity in late childhood.

Late childhood marks the beginning of an Indian girl's deliberate training in how to be a *good woman*, and hence the conscious inculcation of culturally designated feminine roles. She learns that the 'virtues' of womanhood which will take her through life are submission and docility as well as skill and grace in the various household tasks. M.N. Srinivas, for example, reports on the training of young girls in Mysore:

It is the mother's duty to train her daughter up to be an absolute docile daughter-in-law. The *summum bonum* of a girl's life is to please her parents-in-law and her husband. If she does not 'get on' with her mother-in-law, she will be a disgrace to her family, and cast a blot on the fair name of her mother. The Kannada mother dins into her daughter's ears certain ideals which make for harmony (at the expense of her sacrificing her will) in her later life.[25]

In the *bratas*, the periodical days of fasting and prayer which unmarried girls keep all over India, the girl's wishes for herself are almost always in relation to others; she asks the boons of being a good daughter, good wife, good daughter-in-law, good mother, and so forth.[26] Thus, in addition to the 'virtues' of self-effacement and self-sacrifice, the feminine role in India also crystallizes a woman's connections to others, her embededness in a multitude of familial relationships.

If the self-esteem of Indian girls falters during the years of early puberty, this is intimately related to the fact that at precisely this developmental moment, a time of instinctual turbulence and emotional volatility, her training in service and self-denial in preparation for her imminent roles of daughter-in-law and wife is stepped up. In order to maintain her family's love and approval—the 'narcissistic supplies' necessary for firm self-esteem—the girl tends to conform, and even over-conform, to the prescriptions and expectations of those around her.

The adult personality of Indian women is not only moulded through this (unconscious) manipulation of her precarious feelings of worthiness as an adolescent, it is also distinctly influenced by the culturally sanctioned maternal indulgence of daughters. As we have noted above, daughterhood in India is not without its rewards, precisely because the conditions of womanhood are normally so forbidding. In contrast to the son's, a daughter's training at her mother's hands is normally leavened with a good deal of compassion, for which, as ever, there are traditional as well as psychological explanations. Manu expressly enjoins that kindness be shown to the daughter as she is 'physically more tender and her emotions are more delicate', and other ancient commentators forbid any harshness towards her, even in words.[27] The learned Medhatithi puts the whole matter into its 'proper', that is, its ritual, perspective:

By reason of the marriage having taken the place of *Upanayana* it follows that just as in the case of men all the ordinances of the *Srutis*, *Smritis* and custom become binding upon them after the *Upanayana*, before which they are free to do what they like and are unfit for any religious duties, so for women also there is freedom of action before marriage, after which they also become subject to the ordinances of the *Srutis* and *Smritis*.[28]

Little wonder that for an Indian girl, rebellion against the constraints of impinging womanhood with its circumscription of identity, becomes impossible. She internalizes the specific ideals of womanhood and monitors her behaviour carefully in order to guarantee her mother's love and approval, upon which she is more than ever dependent as she makes ready to leave home. For all the reasons described above, the irony of an Indian girl's coming of age is that to be a good woman and a felicitous bride she must be more than ever the perfect daughter.

Sita—The Ego Ideal

For both men and women in Hindu society, the ideal woman is personified by Sita, the quintessence of wifely devotion, the heroine of the epic *Ramayana.* Her unique standing in the minds of most Hindus, regardless of region, caste, social class, age, sex, education, or modernization, testifies to the power and pervasiveness of the traditional ideal of womanhood. Sita, of course, is not just another legendary figure, and the *Ramayana* is not just another epic poem. It is through the recitation, reading, listening to, or attending a dramatic performance of this revered text (above all others) that a Hindu reasserts his or her cultural identity as a Hindu, and obtains religious merit. The popular epic contains ideal models of familial bonds and social relations to which even a modernized Hindu pays lip service, however much he may privately question or reject them as irrelevant to the tasks of modern life.

Sita, like the other principal figures in the epic—Rama, Lakshman, Hanuman—is an incomparably more intimate and familiar heroine in the Hindu imagination than similar figures from Greek or Christian mythology are in the fantasies and deliberations of an average Westerner. This intimate familiarity does not mean historical knowledge, but rather a sense of the mythical figure as a benevolent presence, located in the individual's highly personal and always actual space–time. From earliest childhood, a Hindu has heard Sita's legend recounted on any number of sacral and secular occasions; seen the central episodes enacted in folk plays like the *Ram Lila*; heard her qualities extolled in devotional songs; and absorbed the ideal feminine identity she incorporates through the many everyday metaphors and similes that are associated with her name.

Thus, 'She is as pure as Sita' denotes chastity in a woman, and 'She is a second Sita', the appreciation of a woman's uncomplaining self-sacrifice. If, as Jerome Bruner remarks, 'In the mythologically instructed community there is a corpus of images and models that provide the pattern to which the individual may aspire, a range of metaphoric identity',[29] then this range, in the case of a Hindu woman, is condensed in one model. And she is Sita.

For Western readers unacquainted with the myth, the legend of Sita, in bare outline, goes like this: One day as King Janaka was ploughing, an infant sprang up from the ground whom he named Sita. The child grows up to be a beautiful girl whom the king promises to give in marriage to any man who can bend the wonderful bow in his possession. Many suitors—gods, princes, kings, demons—vie for Sita's hand but none is even able to lift the bow, until Rama, the reincarnation of Vishnu and the hero of the epic, comes to Janaka's country and gracefully snaps the bow in two. After their wedding, Sita and Rama return to Ayodhya, which is ruled by Rama's father, Dasharatha.

After some time Dasharatha wants to abdicate in favour of Rama who is his eldest son. But because of a promise given to the mother of one of his younger sons, he is forced to banish Rama to the forest for fourteen years. Rama tries to persuade Sita to let him proceed in his exile alone, pointing out the dangers, discomforts and deprivations of a homeless life in the forest. In a long, moving passage Sita emphasizes her determination to share her husband's fate, declaring that death would be preferable to separation. Her speech is an eloquent statement of the *dharma* of a Hindu wife:

> For a woman, it is not her father, her son, nor her mother, friends nor her own self, but the husband, who in this world and the next is ever her sole means of salvation. If thou dost enter the impenetrable forest today, O Descendant of Raghu, 1 shall precede thee on foot, treading down the spiky *Kusha* grass. In truth, whether it be in palaces, in chariots or in heaven, wherever the shadow of the feet of her consort falls, it must be followed.[30]

Both Rama and Sita, mourned by the citizens of Ayodhya who adore their prince and future king, proceed to the forest in the company of Rama's brother Lakshman. The *Ramayana* then recounts their adventures in the forest, most prominent and terrible among them being Sita's kidnapping by the powerful king of the demons, Ravana, and her abduction to Lanka. In Lanka, Ravana's kingdom, Sita is kept imprisoned in one of the demon-king's palaces where he tries to win her love.

Neither his seductive kindnesses nor his grisly threats are of any avail as Sita remains steadfast in her love and devotion to Rama.

Meanwhile, Rama raises an army from the *Vanar* (monkey) tribes in order to attack Lanka and bring back Sita. After a long and furious battle, he is victorious and Ravana is killed. Doubting Sita's fidelity through the long term of her captivity, Rama refuses, however, to accept her again as his wife until she proves her innocence and purity by the fire ordeal in which the fire-god Agni himself appears to testify to her virtue. The couple then return to Ayodhya where, amidst the citizens' happy celebrations, Rama is crowned king.

However, Sita's ordeal is not yet over. Hearing of rumours in the city which cast suspicion on the purity of his queen, Rama banishes her to the forest where she gives birth to twins, Lava and Kusha. She and her children live an ascetic life in a rustic hermitage, Sita's love for Rama unfaltering. When the twins grow up, she sends them back to their father. On seeing his sons, Rama repents and Sita is brought back to Ayodhya to be reinstated as queen. On her arrival, however, Rama again commands her to assert her purity before the assembled court. His abiding mistrust and this further demand prove too much for the gentle queen who calls on her mother, the earth, to open up and receive her back. The earth obliges and Sita disappears where she was born.

How are we to interpret the legend of Sita? Philip Slater has pointed out that a myth is an elaborately condensed product, that there is no one 'correct' version or interpretation, for no matter how many layers one peels off, there will remain much to be explained.[31] In the interpretation that follows, I will set aside such elements as social history, religious ritual, and artistic embellishment, although I am well aware of their importance to myth-making. Rather, my aim is to attend to the themes in the Sita legend from a psychoanalytic and psychosocial perspective. In this kind of interpretation, we must ask questions such as the following. How does the myth influence the crystallization of a Hindu woman's identity and character? What role does it play in helping to ward off or assuage feelings of guilt and anxiety? How does it influence her attitude towards and images of men? How does it contribute to the individual woman's task of 'adapting to reality' and to the society's task of maintaining community solidarity? And finally do the different mythological versions of a single underlying theme correspond to different 'defensive editions' of unconscious fantasy at different life stages of those to whom the myths speak?[32]

The ideal of womanhood incorporated by Sita is one of chastity, purity, gentle tenderness, and a singular faithfulness which cannot be destroyed or even disturbed by her husband's rejections, slights, or thoughtlessness. We should note in passing that the Sita legend also gives us a glimpse into the Hindu imagery of manliness. Rama may have all the traits of a godlike hero, yet he is also fragile, mistrustful and jealous, and very much of a conformist, both to his parents' wishes and to social opinion. These expectations, too, an Indian girl incorporates gradually into her inner word.

The legend of Nala and Damayanti provides a variation on the ideal of the good wife; Damayanti cheerfully accompanies Nala, her husband, into the forest after he has gambled away everything they own, including his clothes. And when he leaves her sleeping in the forest at night, taking away half of the only garment she possesses to clothe his own nakedness, Damayanti does not utter a single word of reproach as she wanders through the forest, looking for her husband. The 'moral' is the familiar one: 'Whether treated well or ill a wife should never indulge in ire.'

In another popular myth, Savitri, in spite of the knowledge that her chosen husband is fated to die within a year, insists on marrying him and renouncing the luxuries of her palace to join him in his poverty. When at the end of the year, Yama, the god of death, takes away her husband, Savitri follows them both. Although Yama assures her that she has loved her husband faithfully, that she need not sacrifice her own life but should return, Savitri replies that wherever her husband goes she must follow for that is the eternal custom: 'Deprived of my husband, I am as one dead!'[33]

In the Savitri myth, the ideal of fidelity to one man takes on an added dimension and categorical refinement: exclusive devotion to one's husband becomes the prerequisite for the all-important motherhood of sons. Thus, as Savitri follows Yama to his country, the land in which all wishes come true, she refuses to accept his assurance that with her husband's death all her wifely obligations have expired. Only through her demonstration of wifely devotion, even after her husband's death, can she finally persuade Yama to revive him and grant her the boon of offspring: 'Of Satyavan's loins and mine, begotten by both of us, let there be a century of sons possessed of strength and prowess and capable of perpetuating our race.'[34]

To be a good wife is, by definition, to be a good woman. Thus, Markandeya discourses to Yudhishthira of 'wives restraining all their senses and keeping their hearts under complete control. [They] regard their husbands as veritable gods. For women, neither sacrifice, nor *sraddhas* (penances), nor fasts are of any efficiency. By serving their husbands only can they win heaven.'[35] This is the ideal, purveyed over and over again, in numberless myths and legends, through which the Hindu community has tried to mould the character and personality of its female members. Moreover, a woman is enjoined that her devotion to her husband should extend also to his family members, especially to his parents. A married woman's duties have been nowhere more fully described than in Draupadi's advice to Satyabhama, Lord Krishna's wife:

> Keeping aside vanity, and controlling desire and wrath, I always serve with devotion the sons of Pandu with their wives. Restraining jealousy, with deep devotion of heart, without a sense of degradation at the services I perform, I wait upon my husbands … Celestial, or man, or Gandharva, young or decked with ornaments, wealthy or comely of person, none else my heart liketh. I never bathe or eat or sleep till he that is my husband hath bathed or eaten or slept. … When my husband leaveth home for the sake of any relative, then renouncing flowers and fragrant paste of every kind, I begin to undergo penances. Whatever my husband enjoyeth not, I even renounce … Those duties that my mother-in-law had told me in respect of relatives, as also the duties of alms-giving, of offering worship to the gods … and service to those that deserve our regards, and all else that is known to me, I always discharge day and night, without idleness of any kind.[36]

I have quoted from the ancient texts in detail in order to emphasize the formidable consensus on the ideal of womanhood which, in spite of many changes in individual circumstances in the course of modernization, urbanization, and education, still governs the inner imagery of individual men and women as well as the social relations between them in both the traditional and modern sectors of the Indian community.

Together with this function as a more or less conscious ideal which leaves indelible traces in the identity formation of every Hindu woman, the Sita myth also plays an unconscious role as a defence against the anxiety aroused by a young girl's sexual impulses, whose expression would almost seem to be invited by the nature of family life in traditional India. Freud has clarified for us the universal themes of infantile psychosexual development in terms of the vicissitudes of the libido. He left it primarily to others to differentiate among the social influences and cultural variations. Thus, sexual development in Hindu daughters is *socially* influenced by the communal living pattern, the close quarters of the extended family and the indulgent adult attitudes towards infant sexuality. In this intimate daily setting where constant close contact with many members of the family of both sexes and several generations is part of a little girl's early bodily experience, where the infant girl is frequently caressed and fondled by the many adults around her, and where playful exploratory activities of an explicitly sexual nature among the many cousins living in the same house or nearby in the neighbourhood are a common early developmental experience, often indulgently tolerated by the more or less 'permissive' adults, a promiscuous sexual excitation, as well as the fear of being overwhelmed by it, looms large in the unconscious fantasies of an Indian girl. Later, as she leaves childhood behind, the identification with Sita helps in the necessary renunciation of these childhood fantasies, in the concentration of erotic feeling exclusively on one man, and in the avoidance of all occasions for sexual temptation and transgression. Sita sets the compelling example: although Rama's emissary, the monkey-god Hanuman, offers to rescue Sita from her ordeal of imprisonment in Lanka by carrying her on his shoulders and transporting her through the air to her waiting husband, she must refuse the offer since it means touching Hanuman's body, and of her own free will she may, on no account, permit herself to touch any man except her husband. This enigmatic tension between the memory of intense and pleasurable childhood sexuality and the later womanly ideal which demands restraint and renunciation, between an earlier indiscriminate 'availability' and the later unapproachability, may account for that special erotic presence in Indian women which has fascinated the imagination of many writers and artists.

Perhaps the most striking mythological elaboration of the connection between the young girl's sexuality, in particular, her fantasized erotic wishes towards her father, and her later repudiation of these wishes by transforming them into their opposite, aloofness and chastity, is the myth of Arundhati, who, next to Sita, is the most famous chaste wife in Hindu mythology. I have reproduced the myth in detail not only to illustrate this aspect of feminine identity in India but also because of its special relevance for psychoanalytic theory, for it explicitly acknowledges the existence of infantile sexuality:

Brahma (the Creator) had displayed desire for his daughter, Sandhya (Twilight), as soon as she was born, and she had desired him. As a result of this, Brahma cursed Kama (Eros), who had caused the trouble, to be burnt by Siva. When everyone had departed, Sandhya resolved to purify herself and to establish for all time a moral law: that new-born creatures would be free of desire. To do this, she prepared to offer herself as an oblation in the fire. Knowing of her intention, Brahma sent the sage Vasistha to instruct her in the proper manner of performing *tapas*. Vasistha disguised himself as a *brahmacarin* with matted locks and taught her how to meditate upon Siva. Siva then appeared to her and offered her a boon. She said, 'Let all new-born creatures be free of desire, and let me be reborn as the wife of a man to whom I can just be a close friend. And if anyone but my husband gazes upon me with desire, let his virility be destroyed and let him become an impotent eunuch.' Siva said, 'Your sin has been burnt to ashes, purified by your *tapas*. I grant what you ask; henceforth, creatures will only become subject to desire when they reach youth, and any man but your husband who looks upon you with desire will become impotent.' Then Sandhya, meditating upon the chaste Brahmin for her husband, entered the sacrificial fire. Her body became the oblation, and she arose from the fire as an infant girl, named Arundhati. She grew up in a sage's hermitage and married Vasistha.[37]

Another version of the myth offers a diametrically opposite resolution of the conflict. Here the 'plot' works to lift the repression of childhood memories and to remove defences against erotic impulses and guilt feelings, and, according to the principle of the identity of opposites, the daughter of Brahma is reborn not as the most chaste of women, but as Rati, the incarnation of sexuality and the goddess of sexual pleasure. The unconscious fantasy elaborated in this version belongs of course to adolescence rather than to the Oedipal years of childhood.

On still another level, the identification with Sita contributes to the Hindu woman's adaptation to married life in her husband's extended family and to the maintenance of this family as a functioning unit. Such a family, composed as it is of other men besides her husband, affords the Hindu wife temptations and opportunities for sexual transgression, the indulgence of which would destroy the necessary interdependence and cooperation of the Indian family. At some level of consciousness, every Hindu couple is aware, for instance, of Sita's exemplary behaviour towards Rama's brother Lakshman during the fourteen years of their exile together. There exist, of course, elaborate codes and rituals of social behaviour and discretion between the male and female members of an extended family, such as the injunction that the elder brother never directly address his younger brother's wife (nor enter her room when she is alone). Like most taboos, these are broken in fantasy. In a Bengali folk song; for example, a woman expresses her desire for amorous relations with the elder brother of her husband, regretting that he is not the younger brother so that her desire might be gratified.[38] These taboos are designed to preclude intolerable jealous passions and disruptive rivalries; the reigning presence of Sita in the Indian inner world, in all her serene forbearance, is an important psychological reinforcement of these special codes.

The short description of daughterhood and the elaboration of the Sita ideal of womanhood cannot fully account for an Indian woman's emotional preparation for motherhood. Her chronological and developmental stage of life at marriage, her experiences and relationships within her husband's family, and the meaning of childbirth in her particular personal and social setting: these factors too are paramount. Taken together, they are the 'psychosocial matrix of infancy' in India.

Life Stage at Marriage

An Indian girl is usually married during early adolescence, between the ages of twelve and eighteen; the average age of a Hindu bride is fifteen to sixteen.[39] In urban areas, or among higher castes, where daughters are more likely to receive some kind of formal education, the age may be somewhat higher. The traditional ideal holds that a girl should be married soon after her first menstrual period, for it is feared that 'if she remains long a maiden, she gives herself to whom she will'. The custom of early marriage, it seems, recognizes and is designed to guard against the promiscuous resurgence in adolescence of a girl's playful childhood sexuality and the threat this would pose to Hindu social organization. To marry one's daughters off propitiously is considered one of the primary religious duties of Hindu parents. Indeed, 'Reprehensible is the father who gives not his daughter at the proper time.' If married at eleven or twelve, the girl may remain in her parents' home for another three to four years before moving away to live with her husband. In any case, when she joins her husband's family, she is still a young adolescent and vulnerable to the universal psychological problems of this age.

First of all, before her departure for her husband's family and household, a very special relationship tends to develop between an Indian girl and her mother,[40] who becomes at this time her daughter's confidante and counselor in the bewildering turmoil of adolescence and the newness of the prospect of marriage. Although the relationship between daughter and mother is surely characterized by the tension between the conflicting modalities of 'getting away' and 'coming nearer', the daughter none the less seeks to recreate the emotional closeness to the protective mother of her childhood. She has also formed intimate attachments to girl friends of her age in the village or neighbourhood among whom the secret fears and delights concerning the physical changes of puberty are shared, and fantasies about men and marriage are collectively evoked as each girl tries to envision and secure a clear sense of herself as a woman. These processes—the renunciation of dependency on the 'pre-Oedipal' mother, the integration of what she was as a girl with the woman she is now suddenly becoming, and the acceptance of her inevitable marriage to a stranger—all these require time, her mother's support and love, the reassuring exchange of confidences with peers, and the 'trying out' of new, as yet unexperienced identities in fantasy. This whole process of feminine adolescent development is normally incomplete at the time an Indian girl gets married and is transplanted from her home into the unfamiliar, initially forbidding environment of her in-laws.

The alien, often threatening and sometimes humiliating nature of the setting in which an Indian girl's struggle for identity and adult status takes place cannot be stressed enough. In much of northern India, for example, the exogamous rule, that the bride comes from a village which does not border on the groom's village, strictly applies. In some other parts of the country, marriage customs are governed by a further rule which stipulates that a man who lives in a *gotra* village—that is, a village which is predominantly composed of a related caste group—is unacceptable as a potential bridegroom for any daughter of the village. In his study of social life in a village in Delhi, Oscar Lewis found that the 266 married women of the village came from 200 different villages, a pattern repeated by those who married outside this, their native village.[41] Consequently, this small village of 150 households was linked with over 400 other villages in its region; at the same time, no woman in the village could call for company or, in a moment of crisis or loneliness, on a friend or neighbour or relative known to her from childhood.

Whatever the contribution of these marriage rules to the integration of Indian society, and it is considerable, this integration is ultimately based on the insistence that women not only renounce their erotic impulses and primary loyalties to their parents—a universal developmental requirement—but also sever their attachments, in fact and in fantasy, to all the other boys and men they have known during their early lives who inevitably belong to one of the forbidden extended kinship or village groups. Instead, upon marriage, an Indian woman must direct her erotic tenderness exclusively towards a man who is a complete stranger to her until their wedding night, and she must resolve the critical issues of feminine identity in unfamiliar surroundings without the love and support of precisely those persons whom she needs most. Little wonder that the themes of the young girl pining for her parental home, her grief at separation from her mother, constantly recur in popular folk songs and ballads.[42] The staunch presence of ideal feminine figures like Sita and Savitri is crucial to making the traumatic transition which an Indian girl undergoes at precisely the most sensitive and vulnerable period of her development.

Status Within her Husband's Family—Not Wife but Daughter-in-law

An Indian girl's entry into the married state and the new world of social relations within her husband's family thus does not take place under auspicious psychological conditions. In spite of her inner ideals and conscious resolutions to be a good wife and an exemplary daughter-in-law, a bride comes into her husband's family with a tremendous burden of anxiety and nostalgia, with a sense of antagonism towards her mother-in-law who has, after all, usurped the place of her own sorely missed and needed mother, with a mixture of shy anticipation and resentment towards her husband's sisters and other young female relatives who have presumed to replace the sisters and cousins and friends at home, and with ambivalent feelings of tenderness and hostility towards the unknown person who is now her husband and claims her intimacy.[43] And if her husband turns out to be unworthy, she knows that there is no recourse for her. Manu enjoins: 'Though destitute of virtue or seeking pleasure elsewhere, or devoid of good qualities, yet a husband must be constantly worshipped as a god by a faithful wife.'[44] And: 'By violating her duty towards her husband, a wife is disgraced in this world, [after death] she enters the womb of a jackal and is tormented by the punishment of her sin.'[45] These precepts, in spirit if not in these precise words, have been instilled into Hindu girls from the age of earliest understanding. For, as mentioned above, although treated with indulgence and demonstrative affection in the years immediately before her marriage, an Indian girl is so indulged partly because of her status as a guest in her own house. Her 'real' family is her husband's family. Whatever her future fortunes, when she marries, an Indian girl knows that, in a psychological sense, she can never go home again.

In the social hierarchy of her new family, the bride usually occupies one of the lowest rungs. Obedience and compliance with the wishes of the elder women of the family, especially those of her mother-in-law, are expected as a matter of course. Communication with the older men is minimal (if it exists at all) since they, as mentioned earlier, are traditionally expected to maintain a posture of formal restraint in the presence of the newcomer. Unflinchingly and without complaint, the new daughter-in-law is required to perform some of the heaviest household chores, which may mean getting up well before dawn and working till late at night. Any mistakes or omissions on her part are liable to incur sarcastic references to her abilities, her looks, or her upbringing in her mother's home. For it must be noted once again that the new bride constitutes a very real threat to the unity of the extended family. She represents a potentially pernicious influence which, given family priorities, calls for drastic measures of exorcism. The nature of the 'danger' she personifies can perhaps best be suggested by such questions as the following. Will the young wife cause her husband to neglect his duties as a son? As a brother? A nephew? An uncle? Will social tradition and family pressure be sufficient to keep the husband–wife bond from developing to a point where it threatens the interests of other family members? Will 'sexual passion' inspire such a close relationship in the bridal couple that the new girl becomes primarily a wife rather than a daughter-in-law and her husband transfers his loyalty and affection to her rather than remaining truly a son of the house?

These are, of course, not either/or choices; however, custom, tradition and the interests of the extended family demand that in the realignment of roles and relationships initiated by marriage, the roles of the husband and wife, at least in the beginning, be relegated to relative inconsequence and inconspicuousness. Any signs of a developing attachment and tenderness within the couple are discouraged by the elder family members by either belittling or forbidding the open expression of these feelings. Every effort is made to hinder the development of an intimacy within the couple which might exclude other members of the family, especially the parents. Oblique hints about 'youthful infatuations', or outright shaming virtually guarantee that the young husband and wife do not publicly express any interest in (let alone affection for) each other; and they are effectively alone together only for very brief periods during the night. If women's folk songs are any indication, even these brief meetings are furtive affairs; there is hardly a song which does not complain of the ever-wakeful *sas* (mother-in-law) and *nanad* (sister-in-law) preventing the bride from going to her husband at night. Madhav Gore's study of a sample of Indian men of the Agarwal community further confirms that these constraints, masterminded by the older women, usually succeed in their aims: 56 per cent of the men described themselves as being closer to their mothers than to their wives, while only 20 per cent felt they were closer to their wives.[46]

I do not intend to imply that marriage in India lacks intimacy—that mutual enhancement of experience within culturally determined patterns of love and care which is the commonly held criterion of a 'good marriage' in the West. Rather, in India, this intimacy develops later in married life, as both partners slowly mature into adult 'householders'. Ideally, parenthood and the shared responsibility for offspring provide the basis for intimacy, rather than the other way around as in the West. This postponement of intimacy is encouraged by the family, for in the years of middle age the husband–wife bond no longer seems to threaten the exclusion of other family members, but incorporates or rather evolves out of the responsibility to take care of the next generation. Thus, it is not antithetical to communal and family solidarity but, in its proper time, a guarantor of it.

Has the newly-married girl's situation in her husband's family no redeeming, or even relieving, features? I have neglected to point out that an Indian girl prepares for the harsh transition of marriage for some time before her actual departure for her husband's household. Stories, proverbs, songs, information gleaned from conversations with newly-married friends who come back home on visits, all more or less 'prepare' her for her role as an obedient daughter-in-law. Moreover, as in many other parts of the world, puberty rites such as seclusion during her menstrual period, or fasting on certain days, are designed to separate the young girl, both physically and symbolically, from her parents and to enable her to tolerate 'oral deprivation', for in her husband's household, at any meal, she will be the last one to eat.

These and other procedures bring the Indian girl to the end of childhood and introduce her, in a measured, ritual way, to the realities of womanhood. If married *very* young, the bride's initiation into her new life and family is gradual, interspersed with long visits to her parents' home where much of the accumulated loneliness and resentment can be relieved by the indulgent love showered on her by everyone, and particularly by her own mother's constant presence as a sympathetic listener and a gentle mentor. The young wife's isolation in her husband's home, moreover, is not necessarily as extreme as I have implied. She often develops relationships of informal familiarity and friendly consolation with certain younger members of her husband's family; and it usually happens that one or another of the many children in the family forms a strong attachment to her. Above all, it should be emphasized that the suspicion and hostility towards her rarely degenerate into deliberate oppression. This reflects a cultural tradition of restraint and prudence, which manifests itself in the Hindu conscience. Respect for and protection of the female members of society are a prime moral duty, the neglect of which arouses anxiety and a sense of being judged and punished. Manu the law-giver, a misogynist by modern standards, leaves no doubt about the virtuous treatment of the female members of the family:

Where women are honoured, there gods are pleased; but where they are not honoured, no sacred rite yields rewards ... Where the female relations live in grief, the family soon wholly perishes; but that family where they are not unhappy ever prospers. ... The houses on which female relations, not being duly honoured, pronounce a curse, perish completely, as if destroyed by magic.[47]

Thus, the head of the family, or other elder males who feel themselves entrusted with the family's welfare, gently but firmly seek to mitigate the excesses of the mother-in-law and the elder women. On balance, however, the conclusion is unavoidable that the identity struggle of the adolescent Indian girl is confounded by the coincidence of marriage, the abrupt and total severance of the attachments of childhood, and her removal from all that is familiar to a state of lonely dependency upon a household of strangers.

Pregnancy and the Anticipation of Motherhood

The young Indian wife's situation, in terms of family acceptance and emotional well-being, changes dramatically once she becomes pregnant. The prospect of motherhood holds out a composite solution for many of her difficulties. The psychological implications of her low social status as a bride and a newcomer; the tense, often humiliating relationships with others in her husband's family, her homesickness and sense of isolation, her identity confusion, the awkwardness of marital intimacy, and thus, often, the unfulfilled yearnings of her sexual self ... these are tangled up in a developmental knot, as it were. With the anticipation of motherhood, this knot begins to be unraveled.

The improvement in an Indian wife's *social* status, once she is pregnant, has been universally noted by cultural anthropologists.[48] Elder family members, particularly the women, become solicitous of her welfare, seeing to it that she eats well and rests often. Many irksome tasks, erstwhile obligations and restrictions are removed, and gestures of pride and affection towards her as a daughter-in-law of the house increase markedly.

The growing feeling of personal well-being throughout the course of pregnancy is also reinforced by social customs. Thus, in many parts of India, the expectant mother goes back to stay at her own mother's house a few months before the delivery. This stay helps her to strengthen her identification with her mother, a prerequisite for her own capacity for motherhood. The anticipation of the birth itself, in spite of the primitive medical facilities available, does not seem to provoke strong anxiety or fears of dying since she knows her own parents, the all-powerful protectors, will be constantly at her side during labour. Once having given birth, the new mother can bask in her delight in her child and also in her satisfaction with herself, all of this taking place in a circle of greatly pleased and highly approving close kin.

This unambiguous reversal in an Indian woman's status is not lost on her; moreover, the belief that pregnancy is a woman's ultimate good fortune, a belief that amounts to a cultural reverence for the pregnant woman, is abundantly broadcast in the favourite folktales and familiar myths of Hindu tradition. Thus, this passage from a Bengali tale: 'Suddenly it seemed that God had taken notice of the prayer. The youngest queen, Sulata, was expecting. The king was overjoyed at the happy news. His affection for Sulata grew even more. He was always looking after her comforts and attending to her wishes.'[49]

The roots of this solicitous respect for the pregnant woman lie deep in a religious and historical tradition which equates 'woman' with 'mother', and views the birth of a male child as an essential step in the parents' and the family's salvation. 'To be mothers women were created, and to be fathers men,' Manu states categorically.[50] Further on in the *Laws*, appraising the status of motherhood, he adds, 'The teacher is ten times more venerable than the sub-teacher, the father a hundred times more than the teacher, but the mother is a thousand times more than the father.'[51] 'She is a true wife who hath borne a son,' Shakuntala tells Dushyanta as she reminds him of his forgotten marriage vows, for wives who produce children are 'the root of religion and of salvation. They are fathers on occasions of religious acts, mothers in sickness and woe.'[52] And the goddess Parvati, with divine disdain for convention, remarks: 'Among all the pleasures of women, the greatest pleasure is to unite with a good man in private, and the misery that arises from its interruption is not equalled by any other. The second greatest misery is the falling of the seed in vain, and the third is my childlessness, the greatest sorrow of all.'[53]

Numerous passages in legends and epics vividly describe the sufferings of the souls of departed ancestors if a couple remain childless and thus unable to guarantee the performance of the rituals prescribed for salvation. 'Because a son delivers his father from the hell called *put*,'

Manu says, 'he was therefore called *put-tra* [a deliverer from *put*] by the self-existent himself.'[54] Hindu society is of course not unique in revering motherhood as a moral, religious, or even artistic ideal,[55] but the absolute and all-encompassing social importance of motherhood, the ubiquitous variety of motherhood myths, and the function of offspring in ritual and religious (not to mention economic) life all give to motherhood in Indian culture a particularly incontrovertible legitimacy.

Subjectively, in the world of feminine psychological experience, pregnancy is a deliverance from the insecurity, doubt and shame of infertility: 'Better be mud than a barren woman', goes one proverb. Moreover, until very recently, in Hindu society, as among the Jews, Muslims and certain West African tribes, a childless wife could be repudiated (even if not divorced) by her husband who was permitted then to take another wife. On the positive side, pregnancy marks the beginning of the psychological process which firmly establishes a Hindu woman's adult identity. The predominant element in this identity, the ideal core around which it is organized, is what Helene Deutsch has called 'motherliness'.[56] Its central emotional expressions are those of *tenderness*, *nurturing* and *protectiveness*, directed towards the unborn child. Many of the other psychic tendencies generally associated with the young woman's life-stage now become subordinate. The need for emotional closeness with her 'pre-Oedipal' mother and the wish to be loved can be transformed into the wish to love; hostility, especially towards her new surroundings, can be directed towards the protection of her child from the environment; the longing of her reawakened sensuality can be temporarily sublimated, given over to physical ministrations to her child.

To be sure, the development of motherliness as the dominant mode in a Hindu woman's identity and its harmony with other personality traits vary among individual women. Nonetheless, a Hindu woman's 'motherliness' (including manifestations of maternal excess) is a relatively more inclusive element of her identity formation than it is among Western women. Given her early training and the ideals of femininity held up to her, motherhood does not have connotations of cultural imposition or of confinement in an isolating role.

For an Indian woman, imminent motherhood is not only the personal fulfilment of an old wish and the biological consummation of a lifelong promise, but an event in which the culture confirms her status as a renewer of the race, and extends to her a respect and consideration which were not accorded to her as a mere wife. It is not surprising that this dramatic improvement in her social relations and status within the family, the resolution of her emotional conflicts and the discovery of a way of organizing her future life around the core of motherliness tend to be experienced unconsciously as a gift from the child growing within her. The unborn child is perceived as her saviour, instrumental in winning for its mother the love and acceptance of those around her, a theme which recurs in many legends and tales. Thus, Rama repents and is ready to take Sita back from her exile in the forest after he sees his sons for the first time; Dushyanta remembers and accepts Shakuntala as his legitimate wife after he comes face to face with his infant son; while in the two Bengali folktales of Sulata and Kiranmala, it is through their children's instrumentality that the injustice done to the mothers is redressed and they assume their rightful places as queens. In the case of a Hindu woman, at least in the imagery of the culture, maternal feelings of tenderness and nurturance occur in combination with a profound gratitude and the readiness for a poignantly high emotional investment in the child.

The 'Good Mother'

Although in the usage of paediatrics and medicine, 'infant' refers to a child who cannot yet walk, the actualities of childhood and identity development in India suggest that the psychosocial *quality* of infancy extends through the first four or five years of life, the entire span of time in which feeding, toileting, and rudimentary self care, as well as walking, talking, and the initial capacity for reasoning, become matters of course. This extension of the definition is not arbitrary. As we shall see, in India, the first developmental stage of childhood, characterized by a decisive, deep attachment to the nurturing mother, by dependence upon her for the necessities and the pleasures of succour and comfort, and by the 'crisis' of trust in the benign intentions of others towards oneself, is prolonged in such a way that the second and third developmental stages seem not to take place sequentially but are compressed into one. Thus, it is not until between the ages of three and five that an Indian child moves away (in a psychological sense) from the first all-important 'other' in his life, his mother. And it is at this time that he[57] confronts simultaneously the developmental tasks of separation and individuation, of autonomy and initiative, of wilful self definition and Oedipal rivalry, and moves as it were from 'infancy' to 'childhood' all at once.

During this period of prolonged infancy, the Indian child is intensely and intimately attached to his mother. This attachment is an exclusive one, not in the sense of being without older and younger siblings close in age who claim, and compete for, the mother's love and care, but in that the Indian child up to the age of four or five exclusively directs his demands and affections towards his mother, in spite of the customary presence in the extended family of many other potential caretakers and 'substitute mothers'.[58] Nor does the father play a significant caretaking role at this time.

This attachment is manifested in (and symbolized by) the *physical closeness* of the infant and his mother. Well up to the fifth year, if not longer, it is customary for Indian children to sleep by their mother's side at night. During the day she carries the youngest, or the one most needing attention, astride her hip, the others within arm's reach, as she goes about on visits to neighbours, to the market, to the fields and on other errands. At home, if not suckling or nestling in his mother's lap, the infant is playing on the floor or resting in a cot nearby. Constantly held, cuddled, crooned, and talked to, the Indian infant's experience of his mother is a heady one, his contact with her is of an intensity and duration that differentiate it markedly from the experience of infancy in Western worlds. At the slightest whimper or sign of distress the infant is picked up and rocked, or given the breast and comforted. Usually it is the infant's own mother who swiftly moves to pacify him, although in her occasional absence on household matters it may be a sister or an aunt or a grandmother who takes him up to feed or clean or just to soothe with familiar physical contact. It is by no means uncommon to see an old grandmother pick up a crying child and give him her dried-up breast to suck as she sits there, rocking on her heels and crooning over him. The intensity of the infantile anxiety aroused by inevitable brief separations from the mother is greatly reduced by the ready availability of the other female members of the extended family. Hindu cultural tradition enjoins women not to let their infants cry, and maternal practice in India anticipates the findings of contemporary empirical research on infancy which attributes infant distress, when a baby is not hungry, cold or in pain, to separation from the mother (or her substitute).

From the moment of birth, then, the Indian infant is greeted and surrounded by direct, sensual body contact, by relentless physical ministrations. The emotional quality of nurturing in traditional Indian families serves to amplify the effects of physical gratification. An Indian mother is inclined towards a total indulgence of her infant's wishes and demands, whether these be related to feeding, cleaning, sleeping, or being kept company. Moreover, she tends to extend this kind of mothering well beyond the time when the 'infant' is ready for independent functioning in many areas. Thus, for example, feeding is frequent, at all times of the day and night, and 'on demand'. And although breast feeding is supplemented with other kinds of food after the first year, the mother continues to give her breast to her child for as long as possible, often up to two or three years: in fact, suckling comes to a gradual end only when there is a strong reason to stop nursing, such as a second pregnancy. Even then, weaning is not a once-and-for-all affair, for an older child may also occasionally suckle at his mother's breast. It is not uncommon to see a five- or six-year-old peremptorily lift up his mother's blouse for a drink as she sits gossiping with her friends, an event which is accepted as a matter of course by all concerned.

Similarly, without any push from his mother or other members of the family, the Indian toddler takes his own time learning to control his bowels, and proceeds at his own pace to master other skills such as walking, talking and dressing himself. As far as the mother's and the family's means permit, a young child's wishes are fully gratified and his unfolding capacities and activities accepted, if not always with manifest delight, at least with affectionate tolerance.

The predisposition of an Indian mother to follow rather than lead in dealing with her child's inclinations and with his tempo of development does not spring from some universal component of maternal pride. In part, it reflects the cultural conception of and respect for the specific 'inborn' individuality of every child. In part, it has been influenced by the facts of life in traditional India; given the infant mortality rate which used to range above twenty per cent, a surviving child was accorded by his mother the most deferential care, for he would become the parents' source of economic support in later life, and through his participation in the rituals of death and mourning, their guarantee of *religious* merit and of righteous passage into the next life. Above all, this quality of deference and indulgence in Indian motherhood has *psychological* origins in the identity development of Indian women. As I have described above, in daughterhood, an Indian girl is a sojourner in her own family, and with marriage, she becomes less a wife than a daughter-in-law. It is only with motherhood that she comes into her own as a woman, and can make a place for herself in the family, in the community and in the life cycle. This accounts for her unique sense of maternal obligation and her readiness for practically unlimited emotional investment in her children. These are the cultural, social, religious, and developmental threads which are woven together in the formation of conscious attitudes and unconscious images in the mother which, in turn, give Indian infancy its special aura and developmental impact.

Given the experience of his mother's immediacy and utter responsiveness, an Indian generally emerges from infancy into childhood believing that the world is benign and that others can be counted on to act in his behalf. The young child has come to experience his core self as lovable: 'I am lovable, for I am loved.' Infancy has provided him with a secure base from which to explore his environment with confidence. This confidence in the support and protection of others, together with the memory traces of maternal ministrations, provide the basic modality for his social relations throughout the life cycle. In other words, Indians are apt to approach others with an unconscious sense of their own lovability and the expectation and demand that trustworthy benefactors will always turn up in times of difficulty. Suspicion and reserve are rare. Many character traits ascribed to Indians are a part of the legacy of this particular pattern of infancy: trusting friendliness with a quick readiness to form attachments, and intense, if short-lived, disappointment if friendly overtures are not reciprocated; willingness to reveal the most intimate confidences about one's life at the slightest acquaintance and the expectation of a reciprocal familiarity in others; and the assumption that it is 'natural both to take care of others … *and* to expect to be cared for'.[59] Considering the oppressive economic environment in which most Indians live, I find no other explanation than the emotional capital built up during infancy for the warmth that is abundantly and unreservedly given and received in the most casual encounters, for the bouts of spontaneous laughter (and crying), and for the glow of intimacy and vitality that characterizes social relations.

Setting aside our consideration of the unconscious for a moment, we can observe that an Indian child tends to experience his mother almost totally as a 'good mother'. The proportion of Indian men who express or experience an active dislike, fear, or contempt for their mothers at a conscious level is infinitesimally small. This is strikingly apparent in clinical work; in initial interviews and in the early stages of psychotherapy, patient after patient invariably portrays his mother as highly supportive and extremely loving. In studies of family relations, sociologists and anthropologists confirm the existence of a very close mother–son relationship of the 'good mother' variety in different regions and social classes throughout India.[60]

Literary evidence further corroborates her sentimental prevalence. Thus, short stories and novels by Indian writers such as Sarat Chandra and Premchand tend to portray the mother in her benign and nurturing aspect, with a nostalgia uncomplicated by the slightest trace of hostility or guilt. Nor do autobiographical accounts deviate from this psychological stance of conscious devotion to the 'good mother'. Nehru, recalling his mother, writes, 'I had no fear of her, for I knew that she would condone everything I did, and because of her excessive and undiscriminating love for me, I tried to dominate over her a little.'[61] And Yogananda recollects, 'Father ... was kind, grave, at times stern. Loving him dearly, we children yet observed a certain reverential distance. But mother was queen of hearts, and taught us only through love.'[62]

It needs to be noted here that this idealized image of the 'good mother' is largely a male construction. Women do not sentimentalize their mothers in this way. For daughters, the mother is not an adoring figure on a pedestal: she is a more earthy presence, not always benign but always *there.*

I have so far described the core of Indian personality in terms of confidence in the safeguarding supportiveness of others and trust in the fundamental benevolence of the environment. Mythological and religious representations of the 'good mother' as she is personified in the widely worshipped goddesses, Lakshmi, Sarasvati, Parvati, or Gauri, allow us to elaborate on the Indian experience of this 'basic trust'. In Hindu mythology we find that the specifically oral aspect of maternal nurturing is represented by very minor deities such as Annapurna, portrayed as a fair woman standing on a lotus holding a rice bowl, or by the heavenly cow Surabhi who gives an eternal fountain of milk. But the central feature of the 'good mother', incorporated by every major goddess in the Hindu pantheon and dramatized either in her origins or in her function, is not her capacity to feed but to provide life-giving reassurance through her *pervasive presence.* Thus Lakshmi, the goddess of prosperity and good fortune, comes to *dwell* with men, while those in adversity are spoken of as being *forsaken* by her. Sarasvati, the goddess of learning, is identified as *vak* (speech)—the mother soothing, consoling, talking to her infant. And Parvati, according to one of the Puranic accounts, came into existence to protect the gods against the distress caused by the demon Andhaka (born of Darkness), the representation of one of the elemental fears of childhood. The reassurance provided by the goddesses Sarasvati and Parvati against the terrific estrangements of infancy reminds me of Freud's account of the child who called out of a dark room, 'Auntie, speak to me! I'm frightened because it's so dark!' His aunt answered him, 'What good would that do? You can't see me.' 'That does not matter,' replied the child, 'if anyone speaks, it gets light.'[63]

This emphasis on a nurturing, fear-dispelling presence as the fundamental quality of the 'good mother' is unmistakable in the descriptions of the appearance of these goddesses: They *shine* 'with pearl and golden sheen', *glow* 'with splendour, bright as burnished gold' and *gaze* with faint smiles upon the worshippers.[64] Erikson has called this the 'numinous element, the sense of hallowed presence'.[65] This is the 'good mother', in earthly mothers and in maternal divinities, smiling down on the dependent infant, or on the devoted believer, who, each in his own way, yearns to be at one with that gracious presence. Shiva's lament at the loss of Parvati evokes the sense of intactness the mother's presence gives, as well as the dread of separation or abandonment:

> With thee I am almighty, the framer of all things, and the giver of all bliss; but without thee, my energy, I am like a corpse, powerless and incapable of action: how then, my beloved, canst thou forsake me? With smiles and glances of thine eyes, say something sweet as *amrita*, and with the rain of gentle words sprinkle my heart which is scorched with grief ... O mother of the Universe! arise.[66]

The theme of isolation and its transcendence constitutes the core of the *moksha* ideal. This theme has its ontogenetic source in the specific form and quality of the interactions between mothers and infants in Indian society; and it is vividly elaborated in Hindu mythology as the persistent nostalgic wish for the benevolent presence of the 'good mother' as she was experienced in infancy.

The preoccupation with the themes of loneliness and separation together with the strong unconscious desire for the confirming presence of the 'good (M)other', stays with the individual in India throughout the course of his life. This is in striking contrast to most Western cultures in which the yearning for a loved one and distress caused by her or his absence are often held to be 'childish' and 'regressive'. However, as Bowlby, marshalling impressive evidence from clinical, empirical, and ethological research, has demonstrated, the tendency to react with fear to the threat of being left alone is a natural one which has developed out of a genetically determined bias in man and has the character of an instinctive response.[67]

Yet, in Western culture on the whole, and especially in psychotherapy, '... little weight is given to the component of "being alone"'. Indeed, in our culture, for someone to confess himself afraid when alone is regarded as shameful or merely silly. Hence there exists a pervasive bias to overlook the very component of fear-arousing situations that a study of anxious patients suggests is most important![68] When a patient's suffering stems from certain phobias, or even when it involves free-floating anxiety, clinicians resort all too readily to complex explanations hinging on 'internal dangers'; no other anxiety-provoking situation is overlooked or camouflaged, either by the patient or by the clinician, as is the common fear of isolation and separation. In India, on the other hand, patients openly allude to, and even insist upon, the fear of being cut off from 'attachment figures' and the consequent threat of loneliness. This fear is acknowledged by family and society in India (however negligible it is to the clinician trained in the West); it has a cultural legitimacy which reinforces its vicissitudes in the course of an individual neurosis and hence merits serious consideration by clinicians. Indeed in India, the fear of isolation is projected on to the Creator himself: In one of the Hindu myths we are told that Creation began because Purusha, the soul of the universe, was alone and 'hence did not enjoy happiness'.[69]

The yearning for the confirming presence of the loved person in its positive as well as negative manifestation—the distress aroused by her or his unavailability or unresponsiveness in time of need—is the dominant modality of social relations in India, especially within the extended family. This 'modality' is expressed variously but consistently, as in a person's feeling of helplessness when family members are absent or his difficulty in making decisions alone. In short, Indians characteristically rely on the support of others to go through life and to deal with the exigencies imposed by the outside world. Some Western as well as Indian social scientists have chosen to interpret this as a 'weakness' in the Indian personality, the price to be paid for the indulgence enjoyed in infancy and early childhood. Statements like, 'Training in self-reliance and achievement are conspicuous by their absence. Children are not encouraged to be independent. They, like adults, are expected to seek aid in difficulty',[70] or, 'Family life tends to develop an acute sense of dependence with a strong sense of security, and a clear sense of responsibility without an accompanying sense of personal initiative or decision',[71] are the rule in studies which touch on the developmental aspects of Indian character. And this invariably carries with it the general value implication that independence and initiative are 'better' than mutual dependence and community. Nevertheless, it depends, of course, on the culture's vision of a 'good society' and 'individual merit', whether a person's behaviour in relationships approaches the isolation pole of the fusion–isolation continuum, as postulated by the dominant cultural tradition in the West today, or the fusion pole as maintained in traditional Indian culture. To borrow from Schopenhauer's imagery, the basic problem of human relations resembles that of hedgehogs on a cold night. They creep closer to each other for warmth, are pricked by quills and move away, but then get cold and again try to come nearer. This movement to and fro is repeated until an optimum position is reached in which the body temperature is above the freezing point and yet the pain inflicted by the quills (the nearness of the other) is still bearable. In Indian society the optimum position entails the acceptance of more pain in order to get greater warmth.

The Indian resolution of the tension between the coldness of distance and the price (in dependency) of nearness is not 'deviant', nor are the consequences in patterns of social behaviour 'regressive'. Even in the West, as Bowlby points out, a consensus is emerging among clinicians of many theoretical persuasions that emotional maturity includes the capacity to rely trustingly on others, and that true self-reliance is not only compatible with the capacity for mutual dependence but grows out of it and is complementary to it.[72] The capacity to be truly alone is greatest when the 'other', originally equated with the accepting, giving 'good mother', has become a constant and indestructible presence in the individual's unconscious mind and is fused with it in the form of self-acceptance. We have seen in an earlier chapter that this paradox also underlines the Indian guru's meditation, his striving towards the attainment of *moksha*, wherein he attempts to reach the *sine qua non* of autonomy through the total introjection of the 'other', the not-self. And, as ever, the imagery of Hinduism is uncompromising: Shiva, arch-ascetic and the epitome of lonely self-sufficiency, is often portrayed in such close embrace with Shakti, the 'mother of the universe', that they are one, inseparable for the duration of a world–age.

The 'Bad Mother'

I have suggested above that much of the so-called dependent behaviour observed in individuals and in social relations in India is a manifestation of the universal wish to avoid isolation and the need to share the responsibility for one's life with others. The apparent ubiquity of these needs in India, and their open, undisguised expression, reflect not so much a regressive striving or an 'oral fixation' as the cultural acceptance and even encouragement of such needs and behaviour, an acceptance that is itself rooted in an ideal model of human relationships which diverges sharply from the corresponding ideal in the West. Yet even if we can transfer the larger part of 'dependent' behaviour from the domain of the 'infantile' to that of the 'normal', the fact remains that anxiety around the theme of separation is much more common and intense in India than in Western cultures. However, it is inappropriate to attribute the neurotic warp of an otherwise normative element in Indian identity to a prolonged infancy characterized by affectionate care. This theory of 'spoiling', which often crops up in discussions of personality development and psychopathology in India, rests on an uncritical acceptance of Freud's contention that an excess of parental love serves to magnify for the child the danger of losing this love, and renders him in later life incapable of either temporarily doing without love or accepting smaller amounts of it.[73] In spite of the widespread popularity of this hypothesis and its dogged influence on studies of character formation, there is little evidence to support it. In fact, all the available data[74] point in the opposite direction, namely, that a child becomes anxious and clinging if parental affection is insufficient or unreliable.

In India, the anxiety that may fester around the theme of separation stems at least partly from that moment in later infancy when the mother may suddenly withdraw her attention and her presence from her child. And indeed, retrospective accounts of adults as well as anthropological observations of child rearing practices suggest that this is a widely used method of disciplining young children in India. 'I don't remember my mother ever scolding me or hitting me. If I became too much for her she would become sad and start crying and would refuse to speak to me.' Or: 'She often told me that she would go away and leave me. If I was especially bothersome, she would say that the ghost living in the mango tree outside our courtyard would take me. I still cannot pass that mango tree without shivering a little inside.' These are typical recollections of patients in a culture where frightening a child with ghosts or goblins, or locking him up alone in a dark room—in short, threats of abandonment and isolation—are deemed the most effective methods of socialization. These are the apprehensions that make an Indian child 'be good'; yet if these punishments are threatened or carried out in a context of reliable mothering and family affection they do not immobilize development, but recede into the depths of the psyche, a flickering trace of the dark side of the Indian inner world.

If there is disease in the mother–infant relationship (with its probable consequences in the formation of the Hindu psyche) it stems not so much from styles of maternal reprimand and punishment, and not from the duration or the intensity of the connection between mother and infant, but rather from the danger of inversion of emotional roles—a danger which all too frequently becomes a reality particularly in the case of the male child. By inversion of emotional roles I mean this: an Indian mother, as we have shown, preconsciously experiences her newborn infant, especially a son, as the means by which her 'motherly' identity is crystallized, her role and status in family and society established. She tends to perceive a son as a kind of saviour and to nurture him with gratitude and even reverence as well as with affection and care. For a range of reasons, the balance of nurturing may be so affected that the mother unconsciously demands that the child serve as an object of her own unfulfilled desires and wishes, however antithetical they may be to his own. The child feels compelled then to *act* as her saviour. Faced with her unconscious intimations and demands, he may feel confused, helpless and inadequate, frightened by his mother's overwhelming nearness, and yet unable (and partly unwilling) to get away. In his fantasy, her presence acquires the ominous visage of the 'bad mother'.

Before I elaborate on the specific form the 'bad mother' theme takes in Hindu psyche and culture, it is necessary to emphasize that the 'bad' aspect of the mother is not unique to India. The 'bad mother' lives at the opposite pole from the 'good mother' in the fantasies of all of us. As Erich Neumann has shown in an analysis of the myths of ancient cultures, and as clinical reports have demonstrated in contemporary society, a generative, nurturing and compassionate femininity has always had its counterpoint in the demanding, destroying, and devouring maternal image.[75] And, in unconscious fantasy, the vagina as the passage between being and non-being is not only perceived as a source of life and equated with emergence into light, but also shunned as the forbidding dark hole, the entrance into the depths of a death womb which takes life back into itself. At this most fundamental level of the psyche, no one is entirely free from ambivalent feelings towards the mother. The theme of the 'bad mother' merits particular attention in the Indian context not just because it exists, but because it is characterized by a singular intensity and pervasiveness. Considered from this angle, the idealization of the 'good mother' doubtless betrays the intensity of emotion aroused by her during infancy and suggests a secondary repression of the anxious and hostile elements of these feelings.

Images of the 'bad mother' are culturally specific. To a large extent, they are a function of the relationship between the sexes in any society. In patriarchal societies, moreover, they reflect the nature of the mother's own unconscious ambivalence towards the male child. Thus, for example, aggressive, destructive impulses towards the male child are a distinct probability in societies which blatantly derogate and discriminate against women. Traditional psychoanalytic theory compresses the abundant variety of affect and fantasy deriving from the basic duality of the sexes into the concept of penis envy, claims for it a stubborn prominence in the feminine unconscious, and concludes that this prevents women from finding the satisfaction of emotional and psychosexual needs in marriage, and predisposes them to seek this satisfaction from their infant sons. The invariability of these propositions in individual lives is questionable; however, it is more than likely that erotic feelings towards the child will be more intense and closer to consciousness in a society such as India where a woman is expected and encouraged to find emotional fulfilment primarily in her relationship with her children.

In all societies the image of the 'bad mother' combines both the aggressively destroying and the sexually demanding themes. The question as to which of the two aspects, in any society, casts a longer shadow over the infant's earliest experience and thus contributes to the formation of a culturally specific image of the 'bad mother' depends upon the position and status of women within the society and also upon the means and circumstances of socially sanctioned feminine expression of aggressive and erotic impulses. It goes without saying that in this analysis I am speaking of the imagery that informs a collective fantasy of the 'bad mother', and necessarily setting aside individual variations, attributable to the life-historical fates of individual mothers within a given culture.

In Indian society as a whole, for reasons suggested earlier, the aggressive dimension of maternal feeling towards the male child is comparatively weak. Rather, it is in the sphere of unsatisfied erotic needs, a seductive restlessness that the possibility of disturbance lies. By this I do not mean to imply that Indian women are without feelings of envy and hostility for the males among them; the castration fantasy of turning all men into eunuchs in the Arundhati myth, however much a patriarchal projection, is but one illustration of the ambivalence that governs relations between the sexes. Given the overwhelming preference in Indian society for the birth of male offspring, it would indeed give the psychoanalytic interpreter pause if such envy were non-existent or totally repressed. However, for the purposes of elaborating the imagery of the 'bad mother' in Indian personality development, we must shift our attention from the 'aggressive' sphere of rivalry and rage to the 'erotic' sphere of love and longing. We must attend to the outcome of female psychosexual development in traditional Indian society.

The fate of an Indian girl's sexuality is a socially enforced progressive renunciation. The birth of a child does not change this prescription; in fact, maternity often demands an even greater repudiation of a woman's erotic impulses. The familial and social expectation that she now devote herself exclusively to her child's welfare, the long periods of post-partum taboo on sexual intercourse in many communities, her increasing confinement to female quarters—these are a few of the social factors which dispose a young mother to turn the full force of her eroticism towards an infant son.

Here, it must be remembered that a mother's inner discontents are conveyed to her infant, wordlessly, in the daily intimacy of her contact with him, and that the relief of his mother's tension may become as important to the child as the satisfaction of his own needs. And indeed, clinical experience has consistently and convincingly demonstrated that the displacement of a woman's sexual longings from her husband to her son poses one of the most difficult problems for a boy to handle. At a certain point, the mother's touch and stimulation, whether or not her ministrations are deliberately seductive or overtly sexual, together with the unconscious erotic wishes that infuse her caretaking, arouse an intensity of feeling in the male child with which his still weak and unstructured ego cannot cope. The surge of unbidden and uncontrollable affect seems to threaten to engulf him while at the same time it arouses acute anxiety. The son's predicament is extreme: although he unconditionally needs the physical tending and emotional sustenance that at first only his mother provides, he is profoundly wary of the intensity of his feelings for her (and of hers for him) and unconsciously afraid of being overwhelmed and 'devoured' by her. As the infant boy grows—cognitively, psychosexually, and socially—as he develops the capacity to 'put it all together', he senses that he cannot do without his mother nor remove himself from her presence, but, at the same time, he is incapable of giving her what she unconsciously desires. 'Realizing' his inadequacy in this regard, he also begins to fear his mother's anger and the separation which her disappointment in him seems to forebode. In his fantasy, the mother's body and specially her genitals may assume an ominous aspect. As Philip Slater in his interpretation of child-rearing in ancient Greece has expressed: 'In so far as the child receives a healthy, non-devouring love from the mother he will regard the female genitalia as the source of life. However, in so far as he fails to receive such love, or receive it at the price of living solely for the satisfaction of maternal needs, he will regard the female genitalia as threatening to his very existence.'[76]

In the child's fantasy, the menace implicit in the female genitalia may become concrete, magnified in horrific imagery—a chamber full of poison, causing death in the sexual act, or jaws lined with sharp teeth, the so-called *vagina dentata.* This ferocious motif, which occurs frequently in Indian legends and myths, is vividly illustrated in the following myth from the *Kalika Purana*:

> During a battle between the gods and the demons, Sukra, the guru of the demons, was able to revive all the demons who were slain. Siva knew that Sukra could not be killed because he was a Brahmin, and so he resolved to throw Sukra into the vagina of a woman. From Siva's third eye there appeared a horrible woman with flowing hair, a great belly, pendulous breasts, thighs like plantain tree trunks, and a mouth like a great cavern. There were teeth and eyes in her womb. Siva said to her, "Keep the evil guru of the demons in your womb while I kill Jalandhara [the chief of the demon army], and then release him!" She ran after Sukra and grabbed him, stripped him of his clothes and embraced him. She held him fast in her womb, laughed and vanished with him.[77]

Whereas the Sukra myth is a symbolic dramatization of the child's helplessness in the face of the dreadful mother, another Siva myth from the *Matsya Purana* manages to incorporate the child's own sexual excitement and his fantasized revenge through the complementary motif of *penis aculeatus*—the sharp phallus. Siva once teased Parvati about her dark skin, so she resolved to perform *tapas* to obtain a golden skin. As Parvati departed, she said to her son Viraka, 'My son, I am going to do *tapas* [ascetic practices], but Siva is a great woman-chaser, and so I want you to guard the door constantly while I am gone, so that no other woman may come to Siva!' Meanwhile, Adi, the son of the demon Andhaka, who had resolved to kill all the gods to revenge his father's death, learned that Parvati had gone to do tapas. Adi did tapas and won from Brahma the boon that he would only die when he had transformed himself twice. Then he came to Siva's door and seeing Viraka there, he changed himself into a serpent to delude him, forgetting the stipulation about the manner of his death. Once inside the house, he took the form of Parvati in order to deceive Siva, and he placed teeth as sharp as thunderbolts inside her vagina, for he was determined to kill Siva. When Siva saw him he embraced him, thinking him to be Parvati, and

Adi said, 'I went to do *tapas* in order to be dear to you and lovely, but I found no pleasure there so I have returned to you.' When Siva heard this he became suspicious, for he knew that Parvati would not have returned without completing tapas, and so he looked closely for signs by which to recognize her. When he saw that the illusory Parvati did not have the mark of the lotus on the left side of her body, as the true Parvati did, he recognized the magic form of the demon, and he placed a thunderbolt in his own phallus and wounded the demon with it, killing him.[78]

The figure of the mother is indeed omnipresent in the psyche of Indian men. Yet, what these typical myth fragments make clear is the ambivalence with which she is regarded in fantasy: she is both nurturing benefactress and threatening seductress. The image of the 'bad mother' as a woman who inflicts her male offspring with her unfulfilled, ominous sexuality is not just a clinical postulate, supported by mythological evidence; it is indirectly confirmed by the staunch taboos surrounding menstrual blood and childbirth throughout traditional India.[79] A menstruating woman may not prepare food, nor make offerings, nor participate in family feasts. She is forbidden to go into the temple, into the kitchen, into the granary, or to the well. Men have a mortal horror of being near a woman during the time of menstruation. As with many other customs in India, the menstruation taboos have a hoary tradition. Manu is customarily blunt on the subject: 'The wisdom, the energy, the strength, the might and the vitality of a man who approaches a woman covered with menstrual excretions utterly perish.'[80]

Thus, underlying the conscious ideal of womanly purity, innocence, and fidelity, and interwoven with the unconscious belief in a safeguarding maternal beneficence is a secret conviction among many Hindu men that the feminine principle is really the opposite—treacherous, lustful, and rampant with an insatiable, contaminating sexuality. This dark imagery breaks through in such proverbs as, 'Fire is never satisfied with fuel, the ocean is never filled by the rivers, death is never satisfied by living beings and women are never satisfied with men.' In mythology, when Shiva destroys Kama, the god of sexual desire, Kama's essence enters the limbs of Devi, the great mother–goddess and archetypal woman. Or, the women in the Pine Forest, in their efforts to seduce Shiva, quote from a text which appears in several Upanishads and Brahmanas: 'The Vedas say, "Fire is the woman, the fuel is her lap; when she entices, that is the smoke, and the flames are her vulva. What is done within is the coals, and the pleasure is the sparks. In this Vaisvanara fire, the gods always offer seed as oblation." Therefore have pity. Hers is the sacrificial altar.'[81]

The anxiety aroused by the prospect of encountering female sexuality is also evident in the mildly phobic attitude towards sexually mature women in many parts of India. Dube's observations in a Hyderabad village—'Young people have a special fascination for adolescent girls "whose youth is just beginning to blossom." Young men who succeed in fondling "the unripe, half-developed breasts" of a girl and in having intercourse with one "whose pubic hair is just beginning to grow" easily win the admiration of their age-group. ... Success—real or imaginary—with an adolescent girl is vividly described'[82]—illustrate the widespread preference for immature girls and the concomitant fear of mature female sexuality. The fantasy world of Hindu men is replete with the figures of older women whose appetites debilitate a man's sexuality, whose erotic practices include, for example, vaginal suction, 'milking the penis'. These fantastic women recall the Hindu son's primitive dread of the maternal sexuality that drains, devours and sucks dry. Here we may note that the common term of abuse, 'Your mother's penis', whose meaning puzzles Dube, stems from precisely this dark side of the Hindu male's emotional imagery of maternity; as Karen Horney has shown, the attempt in male fantasy to endow the woman with a penis is an attempt to deny the sinister female genitals—in India, those of the mother.[83]

The latent sexual dread of the mature female is also the main *psychological* reason for the unusual disparity in age between men and women at the time of marriage in India, although this difference in age rarely approaches the number contemplated by Manu as right and proper: namely, sixteen to eighteen years! Yet, even a girl bride gets older, of course. She becomes an adult woman who, especially after childbirth, moves dangerously close to the sexually intimidating mother of infancy in her husband's unconscious fantasy. 'The most direct expression of this (generally unconscious) association in the male psyche is the myth of Skanda, the son of Shiva and Parvati:

When Skanda killed Taraka [a demon who had been terrorizing the gods], his mother, Parvati, wished to reward him, so she told him to amuse himself as he pleased. Skanda made love to the wives of the gods, and the gods could not prevent it. They complained to Parvati, and so she decided she would take the form of whatever woman Skanda was about to seduce. Skanda summoned the wife of Indra [the king of gods], and then the wife of Varuna [the wind-god], but when he looked at each one he saw his mother's form, and so he would let her go and summon another. She too became the image of his mother, and then Skanda was ashamed and thought, "the universe is filled with my mother", and he became passionless.[84]

On the other side of the coin, the counterphobic attitude, the conscious seeking out of what is unconsciously feared, is expressed in the following passage from the *Yogatattva Upanishad*: 'That breast from which one sucked before he now presses and obtains pleasures. He enjoys the same genital organs from which he was born before. She who was once his mother, will now be his wife and she who is now wife, mother. He who is now father will be again son, and he who is now son will be again father.'[85]

One of the likely psychosexual consequences of this anxiety-provoking process of association in unconscious fantasy is a heightened fear, or the actual occurrence, of impotence. And indeed this is a phenomenon to whose ubiquity Indian psychiatrists as well as their traditional counterparts—the *vaids* and *hakims* to whom a majority of Indians turn with psychosomatic complaints—can bear witness. This anxiety is plainly in evidence in the advertisements for patent medicines plastered or painted on the walls enclosing the railway tracks in any of the larger Indian towns. Together with cures for barrenness, the major worry of Indian women, these remedies hold out the promise of sexual rejuvenation for men. Psychosexual development and problems of intimacy between Indian men and women suggest the vicious circle that spirals inward in the Indian unconscious: mature women are sexually threatening to men, which contributes to 'avoidance behaviour' in sexual relations, which in turn causes the women to extend a provocative sexual presence towards their sons, which eventually produces adult men who fear the sexuality of mature women.

Given the concurrence of these phenomena, we must conclude that the sexual presence of the 'bad mother' looms large in the unconscious experience of male children in India and is therefore critical to an understanding of the Hindu psyche. And indeed, as I attempt to show below, the mine of collective fantasy around this theme is unusually rich. Certainly all societies call upon witches, vampires, ghosts and other spectres to symbolize the forbidding, negative aspect of a real mother; these phantoms, along with other mother surrogates such as a stepmother and evil goddesses, are infused with meanings derived from archaic early childhood fears of the mother's emotional needs and fantasized threats. These are familiar figures in individual and collective fantasy across cultures, and the *dayans, jinns,* and *bhoots* who people the Indian night and the Hindu imagination in such profusion are unexceptional. Female vampires who suck the blood from the toe of a sleeping man suggest (even without an analysis of the obvious sexual symbolism) the fantasized rapacious mother as graphically as Ghitachi, Menaka, Rambha, Urvasi, Chitralekha and all the other *apsaras*, or 'heavenly damsels', who lure men from their practice of 'rigid austerities' and deprive them of their 'spiritual' life substance.

A vivid illustration of the collective male fantasy of the child's encounter with the sexual mother is the mythical meeting of Arjuna, a hero of the epic Mahabharata, with the *apsara* Urvasi, which is one of the most popular and frequently enacted subjects in Indian dance drama. As described in the Mahabharata, the episode has a dreamlike quality. It begins with the child's pleasurable feeling of wonderment at his mother's beauty and his desire for her presence, a tender expectancy which gradually changes into its opposite—anxiety about his inadequacy to fulfil her sexual needs. The conflict is resolved through a self-castration which appeases the mother. In fantasy, the mother takes the initiative and approaches the child:

And when the twilight had deepened and the moon was up, that *Apsara* of high hips set out for the mansions of Arjuna. And in that mood, her imagination wholly taken up by thoughts of Arjuna, she mentally sported with him on a wide and excellent bed laid over with celestial sheets, and with her crisp, soft and long braids decked with bunches of flowers, she looked extremely beautiful. With her beauty and grace, and the charm of the motions of her eyebrows and of her soft accents, and her own moonlike face, she seemed to tread, challenging the moon himself. And as she proceeded, her deep, finely tapering bosoms, decked with a chain of gold and adorned with celestial unguents and smeared with fragrant sandal paste, began to tremble. And in consequence of the weight of her bosom, she was forced to bend slightly forward at every step, bending her waist exceedingly beautiful with three folds. And her loins of faultless shape, the elegant abode of the god of love, furnished with fair and high and round hips, and wide at their lower part as a hill, and decked with chains of gold and capable of shaking the saintship of anchorites, being decked with this attire, appeared highly graceful. And her feet with fair suppressed ankles, and possessing flat soles and straight toes of the colour of burnished copper and high and curved like a tortoise back and marked by the wearing of ornaments furnished with rows of little bells, looked exceedingly handsome. And exhilarated with a little liquor which she had taken and excited by desire, and moving in diverse attitudes and expressing a sensation of delight, she looked more handsome than usual.

Urvasi enters Arjuna's palace. 'Upon beholding her at night in his mansion, Arjuna, with a fear-stricken heart, stepped up to receive her, but from modesty, closed his eyes. And Arjuna said, "O thou foremost of the Apsaras, I reverence thee by bending my head down. O lady, let me know thy commands. I wait upon thee as thy servant."' Without the circumlocution and hyperbole so dear to the Hindu, Urvasi expresses her sexual desire for Arjuna frankly and directly. However,

Hearing her speak in this strain, Arjuna was overcome with bashfulness. And shutting his ears with his hands, he said, 'O blessed lady, fie on my sense of hearing, when thou speakest thus to me. For, O thou of beautiful face, thou art certainly equal in my estimation unto the wife of a superior. Even as Kunti [his mother] of high fortune or Sachi the queen of Indra [King of gods] art thou to me, O auspicious one ... O blessed Apsara, it behoveth thee not to entertain other feelings towards me, for thou art superior to my superiors, being the parent of my race.'

Urvasi, however, insists, and Arjuna expresses the increasing helplessness of the child who desires the mother's comfort and care but instead is confronted with her sexuality: '"Return, O thou of the fairest complexion: I bend my head unto thee, and prostrate myself at thy feet. Thou deservest my worship as my own mother and it behoveth thee to protect me as a son."' The conflict now crescendos, for thus addressed, 'Urvasi was deprived of her sense by wrath. Trembling with rage, and contracting her brows, she cursed Arjuna saying that since he disregarded a woman who is pierced by shafts of Kama, the god of love, "... Thou shalt have to pass thy time among females unregarded, and as a dancer and destitute of manhood and scorned as a eunuch."'

As in all Hindu myths and legends, there is a benevolent power in the background who comes forward to mitigate the extreme consequences of the curse. In striking contrast to ancient Greek mythology with its blood-thirsty homicides, mutilations, and castrations, in Indian fantasy the murderous impulses of parents towards children or of children towards their parents do not result in permanent injury or death. Even in the rare instance when an actor goes beyond the attempt to actual fulfilment, there is always a good figure, a god or goddess or ancestral spirit, who helps to undo the act that has been committed. Thus, Arjuna must live only one year in the castrated state as eunuch, a solution with which he 'experienced great delight and ceased to think of the curse'.[86]

The renunciation of masculine potency and prowess, mythically depicted in Arjuna's transient fate, is one of the principal unconscious defences of the male child against the threat posed by the mother's sexuality. This 'typical' defence is cartooned in yet another, less well-known myth:

The demon Ruru with his army attacked the gods, who sought refuge with Devi. She laughed and an army of goddesses emerged from her mouth. They killed Ruru and his army, but then they were hungry and asked for food. Devi summoned Rudra Pasupati (Siva by another name) and said, 'You have the form of a goat and you smell like a goat. These ladies will eat your flesh or else they will eat everything, even me.' Siva said, 'When I pierced the fleeing sacrifice of Daksa, which had taken the form of a goat, I obtained the smell of a goat. But let the goddesses eat that which pregnant women have defiled with their touch, and newborn children and women who cry all the time.' Devi refused this disgusting food, and finally Siva said, 'I will give you something never tasted by anyone else: the two balls resembling fruits below my navel. Eat the testicles that hang there and be satisfied.' Delighted by this gift, the goddess praised Siva.[87]

Here, in spite of commendable efforts to dilute the elements of disgust and dread at the heart of the fantasy by adding such details as the multitude of goddesses, the goat, and so on, that maternal threat and the defence of self castration are unmistakable, although perceived and couched in the rapacious oral imagery of earliest infancy.

The fantasized renunciation of masculinity is but one resolution which the male child may resort to in his helplessness in this dilemma. Hindu mythology gives dramatic play to others—such as the unsexing of the 'bad mother'. Consider the myth of Surpanakha, sister of the demon-king Ravana. The giantess, 'grim of eye and foul of face', tells Rama that he should

This poor misshapen Sita leave
And me, thy worthier bride, receive.
Look on my beauty, and prefer
A spouse more like me than one like her;
I'll eat that ill-formed woman there,
Thy brother, too, her fate shall share.
But come, beloved, thou shalt roam
Through our woodland home.[88]

Rama staunchly refuses her advances. Thinking Sita to be the chief obstacle to her union with him, Surpanakha is about to kill her, but is forcibly prevented from doing so when Rama's brother cuts off Surpanakha's nose. In accordance with the well-known unconscious device of the upward displacement of the genitals, this becomes a fantasized clitoridectomy, designed to root out the cause and symbol of Surpanakha's lust.

Another 'defence' in the mythological repertoire against the sexually threatening 'bad mother' is matricide followed by resurrection and deification. Philip Spratt, summarizing the legends of twenty-nine popular goddesses locally worshipped in the villages of southern India, points out that nineteen of the women who were eventually deified had met first with a violent death; moreover, in fourteen of these legends the woman's forbidden sexual activity is the central theme.[89] Thus: 'Podilamma was suspected of sexual misconduct. Her brothers, who were farmers, threw her under the feet of their oxen. She vanished, and all they could find was a stone. Her spirit demanded that they [the villagers] worship the stone.' Or: 'A widow named Ramama had immoral relations with her servant. Her brother murdered them both. Cattle-plague broke out, and the villagers attributed it to her wrath and instituted rites to pacify her spirit.'[90] On the one hand, the fantasy underlying these legends aims to accomplish and gratify the sexual wishes of the mother, while on the other, the child revenges himself upon her for putting him, with his own unsettling 'wishes', his inexperience and his woeful lack of mature genital equipment, in this hopeless predicament. By the 'murder' of the sexual mother, however, the child's source of affirmation, protection, and motherly love is also eliminated, thus arousing an unbearable sense of longing and guilt. To reclaim the filial relationship, to restore the forfeited mutuality, the mother must be resurrected as no less than a goddess.

Yet another defence in the male child's struggle against the 'bad mother' is the fantasy of having been born of a man, in which case one's existence has nothing whatsoever to do with the mother and is thus unquestionably masculine. This fantasy is expressed in one version of the birth of Ganesha, one of the most popular deities in the Hindu pantheon. Ganesha is usually portrayed as a short, corpulent god with an elephant's head and a large belly. His image, whether carved in stone or drawn up in a coloured print, may be found in almost any Hindu home or shop. Important matters of householding, whether in the sphere of the family or of business, whether the task at hand is the construction of a house or embarking on a journey or even writing a letter, are not undertaken without an invocation to Ganesha. In the particular version of his birth I have in mind here from the *Varaha Purana*, it is related that gods and holy sages, realizing that men are as liable to commit bad acts as good ones, came to Shiva and asked him to find a way of placing obstacles in the path of wrongdoing. While meditating on this request, Shiva produced a beautiful youth with whom all the heavenly damsels fell in love and who was charged by his father with the task of hindering evil. However, Shiva's wife, the great mother–goddess Uma (also known as Durga, Parvati or Gauri), became extremely jealous of the youth's immaculate conception and incomparable beauty, and so she cursed him with a large belly and the head of an elephant.

Other accounts in Hindu mythology of the origin of Ganesha's incongruous physiognomy reflect the strikingly different sequential 'editions' of unconscious fantasy that inform infantile psychosexual development. Thus, in the version of the *Brahmavaivarta Purana*, it is narrated that Parvati who was very desirous of having a child is finally granted her wish after a long period of penance and prayer. All the gods come to Shiva's house to congratulate the couple and to admire the newborn. However, Sani, the ill-omened Saturn, refuses to look at the baby, and keeps his gaze firmly fixed on the ground. When asked the reason for this discourtesy, Sani replies that he is cursed and that any child he looks upon will lose its head. Parvati, however, forces Sani to look at the infant, whereupon Ganesha's head is severed from his body and flies off. Parvati's pitiful lamentations over her son's decapitation attract the sympathy of Vishnu who intercedes and finds an elephant's head which he joins to the infant's trunk. Thus Ganesha is resurrected.

In the sequence of developmental time within the individual psyche, these two versions of the Ganesha myth exist in close proximity. Without elaborating on the unconscious equation of genitals and head so prominent in Hindu fantasy, it is clear that each version of Ganesha's genesis threatens the son, symbolically, with the loss of his penis at the behest of the 'bad mother'. Moreover, when Ganesha's head is restored, we witness one of the psyche's marvellous compensations, for the replacement is not an ordinary human head, but the head of an elephant, with a trunk for good measure!

In the third version of the Ganesha story, which is from the *Shiva Purana*, the variation of the fantasy is more advanced; it condenses and reflects the dominant themes of a later, Oedipal stage of development. A new conflict arises out of the intrusive presence of the father, his claims on both mother and child, and the threat this poses to their earlier symbiosis. In this version of the myth, Siva has nothing to do with Ganesha's birth. Rather, the infant is said to have been fashioned solely by Parvati from the impurities of her own body and brought to life by being sprinkled with 'maternal water' from the holy river Ganges. Charged by Parvati to stand at the door and guard her from intruders while she is bathing, Ganesha refuses to let his father enter. In his anger at being kept from his wife, Shiva cuts off Ganesha's head. However, when Parvati tells Shiva that her son was only carrying out her orders and when she proves inconsolable at the loss of her son, Shiva restores Ganesha to life by taking the head of a passing elephant and fitting it to the child's headless body.

The Oedipal struggle in this version of the myth and the way the son resolves it, through castration by the father, is not my main concern here. I merely want to indicate, and stress, the various sequential transformations of fantasy from stage to stage in psychological development and their coexistence in the unconscious. Moreover, this may occur in relation to a *single* mythological figure who, thus, comes to represent a plurality of psychic propensities. The enormous popularity enjoyed by Ganesha throughout India, a phenomenon of considerable puzzlement to Indologists, can thus be partially explained if we recognize Ganesha as a god for all psychic seasons, who embodies certain 'typical' resolutions of developmental conflicts in traditional Hindu society.

These, then, are the legendary elaborations of the Indian boy's encounters with the 'bad mother'. The evidence of popular myths, religious customs, and anthropological observations converges to suggest that the modal resolution of the conflict is a lasting identification with the mother.[91] This process of identification contrasts with the earlier grateful incorporation of the 'good mother' into the infant's budding ego in that it contains an element of hostility, for the source of anxiety, the mother, is only eliminated by being taken inside oneself.

In psychosexual terms, to identify with one's mother means to sacrifice one's masculinity to her in order to escape sexual excitation and the threat it poses to the boy's fragile ego. In effect, the boy expresses his conviction that the only way he can propitiate the mother's demands and once again make her nurturing and protective is to repudiate the cause of the disturbance in their mutuality: his maleness. In myths, we witnessed this process in Arjuna's encounter with Urvasi, in Shiva's offer of his testicles, in Ganesha's losing his head because of Parvati's jealousy.[92] In the ancient and medieval tales collected, for example, in *Hitopadesha*, *Vikramaditya*'s *Adventures,* and *Kathasaritsagar*, the cutting off of one's own head (symbolic of self-castration) as an act of sacrificial worship to the mother–goddess occurs frequently. Western readers may recollect Thomas Mann's treatment of the Indian tale, in *The Transposed Heads*, in which two friends caught in a sexually tempting and dangerous situation repair to the goddess Bhavani's temple and cut off their heads.

In its purely sexual sense, the puerile identification with the mother is even more explicit in the story of King Bhangaswana in the Mahabharata, who, after being transformed into a woman by Indra, wished to remain in that state. Refusing Indra's offer to restore his masculinity, the king contended that a woman's pleasure in intercourse was much greater than a man's.[93] Philip Spratt's painstaking collection of anthropological evidence—traditional village ceremonies in which men dress as women, the transvestite customs of low-caste beggars in Bellary, the possession of men of the Dhed community in Gujarat by the spirit of the goddess Durga, the simulated menstrual period among certain followers of Vallabhacharya—need not be further catalogued.[94] And although we may be tempted to view these phenomena as aberrant, as extreme manifestations of marginal behaviour, we must nevertheless acknowledge the possibility that, just as the 'sick' member may act out the unconscious conflict of the whole family, thereby permitting other family members to remain 'normal', so these marginal groups disclose the governing emotional constellations within Hindu society as a whole. Nor is this to deny that transvestism, like any aspect of behavioural style, is 'overdetermined'. As a re-enactment of a powerful infantile conflict, rituals such as these represent not only the boy's attempt to identify with his mother but also the man's effort to free himself from her domination. By trying to be like women—wearing their clothes, acquiring their organs, giving birth—these men are also saying that they do not need women (mothers) any longer. The counterpart of such extreme 'femininity' rituals among men are those rites, common in many parts of the world, in which men behave in a rigid, symbolic masculine way. Both extremes suggest a family structure in which the mother is perceived by the male child as a dangerous, seductive female presence during his early years. However compelling the sexual idiosyncrasies spawned by this childhood identification with the mother may be, our main concern is the broader question of its consequences on the evolution of Indian identity.

Infancy and Ego—Origins of Identity in a Patriarchal Culture

We have seen that minimal demands are placed on the Indian infant to master the world around him and to learn to function independently of his mother. The main emphasis in the early years of Indian childhood is avoidance of frustration and the enhancement of the pleasurable mutuality of mother and infant, not encouragement of the child's individuation and autonomy. By and large, an Indian child is neither pressed into active engagement with the external world, nor is he coerced or cajoled to master the inner world represented, temporarily at least, by his bodily processes. Thus, with respect to elimination, the toddler in India is exempt from anxious pressure to learn to control his bowel movements according to a rigid schedule of time and place. Soiling of clothes or floor is accepted in a matter-of-fact way and cleaned up afterwards by the mother or other older girls or women in the family without shame or disgust.

This does not of course mean that no attempts of any kind are made at training toddlers in cleanliness. A child may indeed be taken outside in the morning, seated on a hollow made by his mother's feet and coaxed to relieve himself. What is relevant here is that such attempts are not a matter of systematic instruction or *a priori* rules; therefore they rarely become occasions for a battle of wills in which the mother suddenly reveals an authoritarian doggedness that says her nurturing love is, after all, conditional. More often than not, an Indian child gradually learns to control his bowels by imitating older children and adults in the family as he follows them out into the fields for their morning ablutions. This relaxed form of toilet training, as Muensterberger (among others) has observed,[95] can contribute to the formation of specific personality traits such as a relative feeling of timelessness, a relaxed conscience about swings of mood and a certain low-key tolerance of contradictory impulses and feelings not only in oneself but in others as well. Indians do tend to accept ambiguity in emotions, ideas and relationships, with little apparent need (let alone compulsion) to compartmentalize experience into good/evil, sacred/profane—or inner/outer, for that matter.

In India the process of ego development takes place according to a model which differs sharply from that of Western psychologists. Indian mothers consistently emphasize the 'good object' in their behaviour. They tend to accede to their children's wishes and inclinations, rather than to try to mould or control them. Hindu children do not have a gradual, step-by-step experience of the many small frustrations and disappointments which would allow them to recognize a mother's limitations harmlessly, over some time. Rather her original perfection remains untarnished by reality, a part of the iconography of the Hindu inner world. Thus, the detachment from the mother by degrees that is considered essential to the development of a strong, independent ego, since it allows a child almost imperceptibly to take over his mother's functions in relation to himself, is simply not a feature of early childhood in India. The child's differentiation of himself from his mother (and consequently of the ego from the id) is structurally weaker and comes chronologically later than in the West with this outcome: the mental processes characteristic of the symbiosis of infancy play a relatively greater role in the personality of the adult Indian.

In these, the so-called primary mental processes, thinking is representational and affective; it relies on visual and sensual images rather than the abstract and conceptual secondary process thinking that we express in the language of words. Primary-process perception takes place through sensory means—posture, vibration, rhythm, tempo, resonance, and other non-verbal expressions—not through semantic signals that underlie secondary-process thought and communication.[96] Although every individual's thinking and perception are governed by his idiosyncratic mixture of primary and secondary processes, generally speaking, primary-process organization looms larger in the Indian than the Western psyche.[97] The relative absence of social pressure on the Indian child to give up non-logical modes of thinking and communication, and the lack of interest or effort on the part of the mother and the family to make the child understand that objects and events have their own meaning and consequences independent of his feelings or wishes, contribute to the protracted survival of primary-process modes well into the childhood years.

Compared with Western children, an Indian child is encouraged to continue to live in a mythical, magical world for a long time. In this world, objects, events and other persons do not have an existence of their own, but are intimately related to the self and its mysterious moods. Thus, objective, everyday realities loom or disappear, are good or bad, threatening or rewarding, helpful or cruel, depending upon the child's affective state; for it is his own feelings at any given moment that are projected onto the external world and give it form and meaning. Animistic and magical thinking persists, somewhat diluted, among many Indians well into adulthood. The projection of one's own emotions onto others, the tendency to see natural and human 'objects' predominantly as extensions of oneself, the belief in spirits animating the world outside and the shuttling back and forth between secondary and primary process modes are common features of daily intercourse.

The emphasis on primary thought processes finds cultural expression in innumerable Hindu folktales in which trees speak and birds and animals are all too human, in the widespread Hindu belief in astrology and planetary influence on individual lives, and in the attribution of benign or baleful emanations to certain precious and semi-precious stones. The Indian sensitivity to the non-verbal nuances of communication—all that is perceived with the 'sixth sense' and the 'inner eye'—has been noted not only by Western psychiatrists but also by Western writers such as Hesse, Kipling, and Forster with fascination or horror or both.

Traditionally, moreover, Indians have sought to convey abstract concepts through vivid concrete imagery. Whether we consider the instruction in political science by means of the animal fables of *Panchatantra*, or the abundance of parables in Upanishadic metaphysics, a good case can be made that symbolic imagery rather than abstract concepts, and teleology rather than causality, have historically played a prominent role in Indian culture. Causal thinking has never enjoyed the pre-eminence in Indian tradition that it has in Western philosophy.

Clinically, the persistence of primary processes in an individual's thinking and perception has been asociated with psychopathology, in the sense that it suggests the persistence in adult life of an 'infantile' mode of behaviour. As Pinchas Noy has pointed out, however, in many kinds of normal regression (such as reveries and daydreams), artistic activity and creative endeavour, primary processes govern in the sphere of thought without signs of regression in other aspects of the individual's life.[98] And though the supremacy of primary processes in an individual's mental life may indeed lead to distorted perceptions of outside reality or to an impaired ability to grasp the 'real meaning' of external events and relationships, these processes serve a fundamental human purpose, namely, preserving the continuity of the self in the flux of outer events and maintaining one's identity by assimilating new experiences into the self. Throughout our lives, we must deal not only with an outer world but also an inner one, and whereas the secondary processes of logical thought and reasoning govern our mastery of the outside world, the primary processes of condensation, displacement and symbolization—the language of children, dreams and poetry—contribute to the unfolding and enrichment of the inner world.

The Western cultivation of secondary processes, by and large at the expense of primary processes, contributes (almost inevitably) to a sense of disorientation among Westerners who confront Indian culture for the first time. This confusion has often resulted in a foreclosure of experience and explicit or implicit negative value judgements of the Indian mode of experiencing the world, rather than in a questioning of the basic cultural assumption. As Noy remarks:

The ability to represent a full experience, including all the feelings and ideas involved, is a higher achievement than merely operating with abstract concepts and words, and the ability to transcend time limits and organize past experiences with the present ones is a higher ability than being confined to the limitations of time and space … The schizophrenic, for example, tries to deal with reality by his primary processes, and accordingly tries to organize reality in terms of his own self. The obsessive-compulsive does the opposite—he tries to assimilate and work through his experience with the aid of secondary processes. He tries to 'understand' and analyse his feelings in terms of logic and reality. Both fail because you cannot deal with reality by self-centred processes nor can you deal with your self by reality-oriented processes.[99]

The different emphases placed by Western and Indian cultures on one or the other of the two basic modes thus reflect two diametrically opposed stances to the inner and outer worlds.

We can now appreciate that certain elements of the Hindu world image are strikingly consistent and reciprocal with the ego configuration generated in the developmental experience of Indian childhood. The widespread (conscious and pre-conscious) conviction that knowledge gained through ordering, categorizing, logical reasoning, is *avidya*, the not-knowledge, and real knowledge is only attainable through direct, primary-process thinking and perception; the imperative that inspires the yogi's meditation and the artist's *sadhana* namely, that to reach their avowed goals they must enlarge the inner world rather than act on the outer one; the injunction inherent in the *karma* doctrine to accept and use outer reality for inner development rather than to strive to alter worldly realities; the indifferent respect given to eminent scientists and professionals, compared with the unequivocal reverence for Sai Baba, Anandamai, Tat Baba, Mehr Baba, and the innumerable shamanic gurus who act as spiritual preceptors to Hindu families: these are a few of the indicators of the emphasis in Hindu culture on the primary processes of mental life.

Unless the social organization makes some special provision for it, however, no group can survive for long if its members are brought up to neglect the development of those secondary processes through which we mediate and connect outer and inner experience. An 'underdeveloped' ego in relation to the outer world is a risky luxury except under the most bountiful and Utopian of natural conditions. Indian social organization traditionally 'took care' of the individual's adaptation to the outer world. That is, traditionally, in the early years, the mother serves as the child's ego, mediating his most elementary experiences well into the years of childhood proper, until around the age of four. The ego's responsibility for monitoring and integrating reality is then transferred from the mother to the family-at-large and other social institutions. Thus, when making decisions based on reasoning through the pros and cons of a situation, the individual functions as a member of a group rather than on his own. With the help of traditional precedents and consensual (as opposed to adversary) modes of decision-making, based on the assumption that no two people have identical limits on their rationality, Indians cope effectively with their environment (if it does not change too fast). Similarly, as far as the environment of relationships is concerned, the myriad, detailed rules and regulations governing social interaction and conduct define the individual Hindu's interpersonal world in most conceivable situations and spell out appropriate behaviours. By making social interactions very predictable, these norms make it unnecessary (and usually imprudent) for each individual to assess the exigencies of a particular encounter or circumstance on his own, and encourage him to respond according to a tried-and-true traditional pattern.

The highly structured and elaborated social organization that seems oppressive to many Westerners is functional in the sense that it strengthens and supplements the individual's basic ego fabric in which the world of magic and animistic projection looms large. In Indian society, this complementary 'fit' between ego and social organization remains functional only so long as the process of environmental change is a slow one, as it has been in the past, affording enough time for gradual, barely perceptible evolution of cultural ideals, social institutions, and generational relationships. Difficulties arise when the pace of change quickens. Today, the outer world impinges on the Indian inner world in an unprecedented way. Harsh economic circumstances have resulted in higher social and geographical mobility, which has meant, in turn, that dealings with the outer world are more and more on an individual, rather than a social, footing. Under these 'modern' conditions, an individual ego structure, weak in secondary and reality-oriented processes and unsupported by an adequate social organization, may fail to be adaptive.

I have discussed the influence of the protracted intimacy between mother and infant in India—subsuming childhood, as it does—on the entrenchment of primary mental processes in the Hindu inner world. These processes, as we have seen, are supported by the structures of Hindu social organization and traditional cultural mores. The second lifelong theme in the Indian inner world (more actual for men by far than for women) that derives from the special psychosocial features of Indian motherhood is the simultaneous, often unintegrated presence in fantasy of images of the 'good' and the 'bad' mother.

These contradictory aspects of the maternal presence can coexist in the very young child's psyche without disturbing each other, for it is a feature of primary mental processes characteristic of infancy that contradictions do not cause urgent conflicts pressing for resolution. It is only later, when the ego gains strength and attempts to synthesize and integrate experience, that conflicts erupt and ambivalence comes into its own, and that the negative, threatening aspects of earliest experience may be forcibly repressed or projected onto the external world.

Taken into the child's ego, the 'good mother's' maternal tolerance, emotional vitality, protectiveness, and nurturing become the core of every Indian's positive identity. Alongside this positive identity, however, and normally repressed, is its counterpart: the negative identity that originates in experiences with the demanding, sometimes stifling, all too present mother. Whatever the contours of the negative identity, they reflect certain defences against the 'bad mother' who may have been most undesirable or threatening, yet who was also most real at a critical stage of development.[100] In conditions of psychological stress and emotional turmoil, the negative identity fragments tend to coalesce in a liability to a kind of psychological self-castration, in a predisposition to identify with rather than resist a tormentor, and in a longing for a state of perfect passivity.

Although the inner world of Indian men is decisively influenced by both the 'good' and the 'bad' versions of the maternal–feminine, the adult identity consolidation of men is of course not to be cast exclusively in these terms. For identity is constituted not only out of early feminine identifications but also from later masculine ones, all of them rearranged in a new configuration in youth. Normally, the biological rock-bottom of maleness limits the extent to which a boy can or will identify with his mother as he grows up. The view advanced here, namely, that the length, intensity and nature of the mother–infant relationship in India, together with the sexualized nature of the threat posed by the mother to the male child in fantasy, contribute to the Hindu male's strong identification with his mother and a 'maternal–feminine' stance towards the external world, only make's sense in the light of these self-evident reservations. The expression of the maternal–feminine in a man's positive identity is, however, neither deviant nor pathological, but that which makes a man more human. Its presence precludes that strenuous phallicism which condemns a man to live out his life as half a person, and it enhances the possibility of mutuality and empathic understanding between the sexes. Of course, in its defensive aspect, the maternal–feminine identification of men may serve to keep the sexes apart and may even contribute to discrimination against women. A precarious sense of masculine identity can lead to a rigid, all-or-nothing demarcation of sex roles; this kind of rigid differentiation is a means of building outer bulwarks against feared inner proclivities.

The seeds of a viable identity, if they are not to mutate into plants of a 'false self', require the supportive soil of a compatible family structure and a corresponding set of cultural values and beliefs. In India, the child learns early that emotional strength resides primarily in his mother, that she is 'where the action is'. The cultural parallel to the principal actuality of infancy is the conviction that mother–goddesses are reservoirs of both constructive and destructive energy. The very word for energy, Shakti, is the name of the supreme mother–goddess. And although the spirit of the godhead is one, its active expression, worshipped in innumerable forms ranging from particular local village goddesses to the more or less universal manifestations of Mahadevi ('great goddess'), is decisively female. The male gods of the Hindu pantheon, Shiva, Vishnu, Brahma, may be more dignified beings, but the village deities, earthy, mundane, attuned to the uncertainties and troubles, the desires and prayers of daily life, are generally female. In South India, as Whitehead has shown, village deities are almost exclusively feminine; and the exceptional male gods, such as Potu-Razu in Andhra Pradesh, are not worshipped in their own right, but in conjunction (as brother or husband) with the local village goddess, the position of the male gods being often subordinate if not outright servile.[101]

Hindu cosmology is feminine to an extent rarely found in other major civilizations. In its extremity (for example) in Tantric beliefs, god and creation are unconditionally feminine; in *Mahanirvana Tantra*, even the normally male gods Vishnu and Brahma are portrayed as maidens with rising breasts. The essence of this deepest layer of Hindu religiosity is conveyed in the following prayer to the goddess Durga:

> O thou foremost of all deities, extend to me thy grace, show me thy mercy, and be thou the source of blessings to me. Capable of going everywhere at will, and bestowing boons on thy devotees, thou art ever followed in thy journeys by Brahma and the other gods. By them that call upon thee at daybreak, there is nothing that cannot be attained in respect either of offspring or wealth. O great goddess, thou art fame, thou art prosperity, thou art steadiness, thou

art success; thou art the wife, thou art man's offspring, thou art knowledge, thou art intellect. Thou art the two twilights, the night sleep, light, beauty, forgiveness, mercy and every other thing. And as I bow to thee with bended head, O supreme goddess, grant me protection. O Durga, kind as thou art unto all that seek thy protection, and affectionate unto all thy devotees, grant me protection![102]

The most striking illustration of the cultural acceptance and outright encouragement of the passive feminine aspects of identity in Indian men is the *bhakti* cult associated with Lord Krishna. Its appeal is dramatically simple. Renouncing the austere practices of yoga, the classical Hindu means of attaining *moksha*, the Krishna cult emphasizes instead the emotional current in religious devotion. Personal devotion to Lord Krishna absorbs a devotee's whole self and requires all his energies. Depending on individual temperament and inclination, this devotional emotion—-*bhava*—may express itself in a variety of modes: *santa*, awe, humility, a sense of one's own insignificances; *dasya*, respect, subservience, and pious obedience; *vatsalya*, nurturing, protective (maternal) feelings of care; and so on.

The most intensely and commonly desirable feeling towards the godhead, a rudimentary prerequisite for the state of pure bliss, is held to be *madhurya bhava*, the longing of a woman for her lover, of the legendary *gopis* for their Lord. In an interview with Milton Singer, a Krishna devotee in the city of Madras articulates the systematic cultivation of this feminine-receptive stancc and its transformation into a religious ideal:

The love of a woman for her husband or for her lover is very much more intense than any other sort of love in the world, and I mentioned the gopis, Radha, Rukmini, Satyabhama, and so forth, as instances in point. Their love was indeed transcendent. Even when the husband or lover is a man the woman's love for him is of a very high order and when the Lord Supreme is the husband or lover of a woman, you can find no other love excelling or surpassing this love. The ladies mentioned above can therefore be said to be the most blessed in the world. If we concede this, we can ourselves aspire for this kind of supreme love for God. We can imagine ourselves to be those women on at any rate ordinary women, imagine that the Lord is our husband or lover and bestow the maximum love on Him ... Think constantly that you are a woman and that God is your husband or lover, and you will be a woman and God will be your husband or lover ... You know the philosophy here that all men and women in the world are spiritually women, and the Lord alone is male—the Purusa. The love of the gopis, Radha, Rukmini, and Satyabhama explains the principle of the human soul being drawn to the Supreme Soul and getting merged in it.[103]

Fragments from the life history of the widely revered nineteenth century Bengali saint, Sri Ramakrishna, further highlight the respect and reverence Indian society pays to the ontogenetically motivated, religiously sublimated femininity in a man. As a child, it is related, Ramakrishna often put on girl's clothing and sought to mimic the village women as they went about their daily chores. In adolescence, he would imagine that he was a forsaken wife or child–widow and would sing songs of longing for Krishna. In his quest for union with the god-head, he systematically practised madhurya bhava. For six months during his youth, he wore women's clothes and ornaments, adopted women's gestures, movements and expressions, and 'became so much absorbed in the constant thought of himself as a woman that he could not look upon himself as one of the other sex even in a dream'.[104]

If interpreted solely from an individual developmental viewpoint, Sri Ramakrishna's behaviour would seem deviant, the eruption of negative elements latent in Indian masculine identity. Yet the meaning of any thematic event or behaviour cannot be grasped in one dimension only. What appears to be an episode in Ramakrishna's life of 'psychopathological acting out' is, when viewed culturally and historically, an accepted, representative phenomenon in the tradition of Krishna worship. It is profoundly consistent with the basic 'mood' of all schools of Hindu miniature painting and of the *bhajan*, *kirtan,* and even *dadra* forms of vocal music. Finally, the feminine stance is consistent with the life style of certain specialized religious groups, and its aim dramatizes a cultural ideal of the whole society, namely, a receptive absorption rather than an active alteration and opposition.

To conclude, the primary themes of Indian identity, emerging from the infant's relationship with his mother, are inextricably intertwined with the predominant cultural concerns of Hindu India. These concerns, both individual and social, govern, inform and guide the Indian inner world in such a way that they reverberate throughout the identity struggles of a lifetime.

Notes and References

1 I am adopting Simmel's term 'dyad' for the mother–infant relationship, since no other word conveys so well the feeling of complementarity and interdependence of two independent entities.

2 Freud, Sigmund, 1940, *An Outline of Psychoanalysis*, Standard Edition, vol. 23, p. 188. For a comprehensive historical account of Freud's writings on the

mother–infant relationship, see Bowlby, John, 1958, 'The Nature of the Child's Tie to his Mother', *International Journal of Psychoanalysis*, 39, pp. 350–73.

3 The literature on the earliest human relationship has grown rapidly during the last few years; a complete bibliography of sources would cover many pages. The most important psychoanalytic writings upon which this summary is based are Spitz, René A., 1965, *The First Year of Life*, New York: International Universities Press; Winnicott, D.W., 1952, *The Family and Individual Development*, London: Tavistock Publications; Erikson, Erik H., 1950, *Childhood and Society*, New York: W.W. Norton; Jacobson, Edith, 1964, *The Self and the Object World*, New York: International Universities Press, especially Part 1; Mahler, Margaret S., 1969, *On Human Symbiosis and the Vicissitudes of Individuation*, New York: International Universities Press; Murphy, L.B., 1964, 'Some Aspects of the First Relationship', *International Journal of Psychoanalysis*, 45, pp. 31–43; and Bowlby, J., 1969, *Attachment*, New York: Basic Books. And of course no psychoanalytic study of motherhood (however liable to cultural specialization) can be complete without reference to Deutsch, Helene, 1945, *The Psychology of Women*, vol. 2 (*Motherhood*), New York: Grune and Stratum.

4 Spitz, *First Year of Life*, p. 96.

5 For an elaboration of this view, see Bowlby, *Attachment*, pp. 265–96.

6 Spitz, *First Year of Life*, p. 95.

7 For a psychoanalytic consideration of some of these issues, see, for example, Bibring, Grete L. *et al.*, 1961, 'A Study of the Psychological Processes in Pregnancy and of the Earliest Mother-Child Relationship', *The Psychoanalytic Study of the Child*, vol. 16, New York: International Universities Press, pp. 9–72, and Moss, H.A.,1967, 'Sex, Age and State as Determinants of Mother-Infant Interaction', *Merrill Palmer Quarterly*, 13, pp. 19–36.

8 Although the patrilineal and patrilocal family type is dominant all over India, there are some castes and communities, especially in South India, which are matrilineal and in which women enjoy relatively greater freedom. For the similarities and contrasts in kinship organization of different regions in India, see Karve, Irawati, 1968, *Kinship Organization in India*, 3rd edn., Bombay: Asia Publishing House.

My remarks are intended to apply only to the dominant patriarchal culture where by unconscious necessity it is the *mater* who is of primary symbolic significance, or, as the Jungians would put it, the mother is the primary constituent of a man's *anima*. The problem of feminine figures in the myths of a patriarchal society is compounded by the fact that these *animas* are not solely male projections but also represent some aspects of feminine psychology in these cultures. The reason for this intertwining of *anima* images and feminine psychology is that very early in childhood, girls learn to accurately perceive and conform to the patriarchal images of femininity entertained by the men around them in the household. In this connection, see von Franz, Marie-Louise, 1972, *The Feminine in Fairy Tales*, Zurich: Spring Publications.

9 The anthropological accounts which have a bearing on this section are Madan, T.N., 1965, *Family and Kinship: A Study of the Pandits of Rural Kashmir*, Bombay: Asia Publishing House; Minturn, Leigh and John T. Hitchcock, 1963, 'The Rajputs of Khalapur, India' in B.B. Whiting (ed.), *Six Cultures: Studies of Child-rearing*, New York:

John Wiley and Sons, pp. 301–61; Minturn, L. and W.W. Lambert, 1964, *Mothers of Six Cultures*, New York: John Wiley; Lewis, Oscar, 1958, *Village Life in Northern India*, New York: Vintage Books; Dube, S.C., 1967, *Indian Village*, New York: Harper and Row; Srinivas, M.N., 1942, *Marriage and Family in Mysore*, Bombay: New Book Co.; Harper, Edward B., 'Spirit Possession and Social Structure', in B. Ratnam (ed.), *Anthropology on the March*, Madras: The Book Centre, pp. 165–97; and Ross, Aileen D., 1961, *The Hindu Family in its Urban Setting*, Toronto: University of Toronto Press. Two other useful studies, essentially descriptive, based on intensive interviewing with women who represent the progressive, well-educated parts of Indian society are Cormack, Margaret, 1961, *The Hindu Woman*, Bombay: Asia Publishing House, and Kapur, Promilla, 1973, *Love, Marriage and Sex*, Delhi: Vikas Publishing House. For older, impressionistic yet sensitive studies of Indian women, see Billington, Mary F., 1973, *Woman in India* (18—?), New Delhi: Amarko Book Agency, and Das, Frieda M., 1932, *Purdah, the Status of Indian Women*, New York: The Vanguard Press.

10 The infant mortality rate in 1969 for females was 148.1 as compared to 132.3 for males; the life expectancy between 1961–71 was 45.6 for females, 47.1 for males, while the number of girls enrolled in the educational system in 1970–1 was 18.4 per cent as compared to 39.3 per cent for boys. See the relevant statistical tables in Indian Council of Social Science Research, 1975, *Status of Women in India: A Synopsis of the Report of the National Committee on the Status of Women* (1971–4), New Delhi: Allied Publishers, pp. 140–75.

11 *Atharvaveda*, VI. 2. 3, quoted in Das, R.M., 1962, *Women in Manu and his Seven Commentators*, Varanasi: Kanchana Publications, p. 43. See also *Atharvaveda*, VIII. 6. 25, VI. 9. 10, III. 23. 3, for prayers in a similar vein.

12 MacDonell, A.A., *Vedic Religion*, p. 165, quoted in R.M. Das, *Women in Manu*, p. 43.

13 See, for example, Mintum and Hitchcock, 'Rajputs of Khalapur', pp. 307–8; Madan, *Family and Kinship*, p. 77; Dube, *Indian Village*, pp. 148–9; Cormack, *Hindu Woman*, p. 11. See also, Goode, William J., 1963, *World Revolution and Family Patterns,* New York: The Free Press, pp. 235–6; and Mandelbaum, D.G., 1970, *Society in India*, vol. 1, Berkeley: University of California Press, p. 120. Cases of *post-partum* depression, for example, are much more commonly reported among mothers who give birth to a daughter than among those who have a son. See Gaitonde, M.R., 1958, 'Cross-Cultural Study of the Psychiatric Syndromes in Out-Patient Clinics in Bombay, India, and Topeka, Kansas', *International Journal of Social Psychiatry*, 4, p. 103.

14 Lewis, *Village Life*, p. 195.

15 Karve, *Kinship Organization*, p. 206.

16 See Das, *Purdah*, p. 44. A contemporary Bengali proverb expresses this thought more bluntly, 'Even the piss of a son brings money; let the daughter go to hell.'

17 Kakar, Sudhir, 1974, 'Aggression in Indian Society: An Analysis of Folk Tales', *Indian Journal of Psychology*, 49 (2), p. 124.

18 Ibid., pp. 125–6.

19 Cormack, *Hindu Woman*, pp. 75–8.

20 Karve, *Kinship Organization*, p. 210.

21 See Ross, *Hindu Family*, pp. 150–1; Dube, *Indian Village*, pp. 148–9; Srinivas, *Marriage and Family*, p. 173; Whiting, *Six Cultures*, p. 303; Harper, 'Spirit Possession', pp. 171–2; Madan, *Family and Kinship*, p. 77; and Cormack, *Hindu Woman*, p. 9. Folk songs from all over India also bear witness to this close mother–daughter tie. See, for example, songs no. 4, 5, 6, 7, 8, and 9 in Karve, *Kinship Organization*, p. 205.

22 Karve, *Kinship Organization*, p. 205.

23 As Helene Deutsch expresses it, 'In her relation to her own child, woman repeats her own mother-child history.' See *The Psychology of Women*, vol. 1, p. 205. See also Chodorow, Nancy, 1975, 'Family Structure and Feminine Personality', in M. Rosaldo and L. Lamphere (eds), *Woman, Culture and Society*, Stanford : Stanford University Press, pp. 52–3.

24 Thus in many ballads whereas the women are depicted as tolerant, self-sacrificing, and faithful, the men are weak, timid, and faithless. See Sen Gupta, Sankar, 1970, *A Study of Women of Bengal*, Calcutta: Indian Publications, p. 107.

25 Srinivas, *Marriage and Family*, p. 195.

26 For example, in the *Dasa Puttal Brata* of Bengali girls it is wished that 'I shall have a husband like Rama, I shall be *sati* like Sita, I shall have a *devara* (younger brother-in-law) like Lakshman; I shall have a father-in-law like Dasharatha; I shall have a mother-in-law like Kousalya; I shall have sons as Kunti had; I shall be a cook like Draupadi; I shall acquire power like Durga; I shall bear the burden like earth; I shall be like Sasthi whose offspring know no death.' See Akshay Kumar Kayal, 'Women in Folk Sayings of West Bengal', in Sen Gupta, *Study of Women of Bengal*, p. xxii.

27 Das, *Purdah*, p. 49.

28 Ibid., p. 72.

29 Bruner, Jerome S., Spring 1959, 'Myths and Identity', *Daedalus*, p. 357. In a study carried out in the North Indian province of Uttar Pradesh 500 boys and 360 girls between the ages of 9 and 22 years were asked to select the ideal woman from a list of 24 names of gods, goddesses, and heroes and heroines of history. Sita was seen as the ideal woman by an overwhelming number of respondents: there were no age or sex differences. See Pratap, P., 1960, 'The Development of Ego Ideal in Indian Children', unpublished Ph.D. thesis, Banaras Hindu University.

30 *Ramayana of Valmiki*, translated by H.P. Shastri, 1962, vol. 1 (Ayodhyakanda), London: Shantisadan, p. 233.

31 Slater, Philip, 1966, *The Glory of Hera*, Boston: Beacon Press, p. xi.

32 In this connection, see also Arlow, J.A., 1961, 'Ego Psychology and the Study of Mythology', *Journal of American Psychoanalytic Association*, 9, p. 375.

33 *Mahabharata*, translated by P.C. Roy, Calcutta: Oriental Publishing Co., n.d., vol. 3 (Vanaparva), p. 634.

34 Ibid., p. 633. The Savitri myth is also a striking demonstration of Ernest Jones's thesis that the conscious fantasy of dying together possesses the unconscious significance of the wish to have children. See Jones, E., 1951, 'On "Dying Together" with Special Reference to Heinrich von Kleist's Suicide' and 'An Unusual Case of Dying Together', *Essays on Applied Psychoanalysis*, London: Hogarth Press, pp. 9–21.

35 Ibid., p. 488.

36 Ibid., pp. 506–7.

37 *Siva Purana*, 2. 2. 5. pp. 1–68, 6. pp. 1–62. The translation is from Wendy O'Flaherty, 1973, *Asceticism and Eroticism in the Mythology of Siva*, London: Oxford University Press, p. 64–5. A perusal of Hindu law texts reveals that our ancient law-givers—Manu, Kautilya, Kullika, Medhatithi—were obsessed with the chastity of young, unmarried girls. The punishments for all conceivable kinds of chastity-violation, depending on the castes of the actors, their sex (whether the violator is a man or a woman), the degree of consent, and so on, are elaborately detailed. Thus, for example, if a man forcibly 'pollutes' a maiden with his fingers, the fingers shall be amputated and he shall pay a fine of 500 *panas*. If the man is of equal caste, the fine is reduced. If the fingers have been inserted with the consent of the maiden, the fingers are not amputated and the fine is reduced to 200 *panas*. If the initiative is taken by the girl, the punishment is lighter or non-existent; instead, her guardians are to be punished in so much as they presumably did not keep a proper watch on her. There are similar fines in the case of an older woman seducing a young girl, depending on their castes and the 'violation'. See Das, *Purdah*, pp. 63–70.

38 *Rangila Bhasur go tumi keno deyor haila na.*
Tumi jodi haita re deyor khaita batar pan
(aar) ranga rasa kaitam katha juraito paran.
Sen Gupta, *Study of Women in Bengal*, p. 94.

39 The mean age according to the 1961 census was 15.8 years. For a discussion of the subject, see Singh, K.P., 1974, 'Women's Age at Marriage', *Sociological Bulletin*, 23 (2), pp. 236–44. See also Goode, *World Revolution*, pp. 232–6.

40 See Ross, *Hindu Family*, p. 151.

41 Lewis, *Village Life*, p. 161; see also Karve, *Kinship Organization*, p. 137 for evidence on the widespread existence of this custom.

42 Here is an example from Bengal (freely translated):
O, Kaffu [a bird], you are from my mother's side.
Speak, O speak in the courtyard of my parents.
My mother will hear you; She will send my brother to fetch me.
O what sorrowful days have come!
I wish to get out of this,
I wish to reach my father's house.
Sen Gupta, *Study of Women of Bengal*, p. 149.

43 Folklore especially singles out the sas (mother-in-law) and the nanad (sister-in-law) as the natural enemies of the young bride. See Karve, *Kinship Organization*, p. 130. Here are lines from some of the songs in Bengal depicting the bride's plight (and her anger) in these two relationships. 'My husband's sister is nothing but a poisonous thorn, her poisonous stings give me much pain'; 'My mother-in-law expired in the morning, if I find time in the afternoon after eating lunch, I will weep for her.' In North India the bride sings:
O my friend! My in-laws' house is a wretched place.
My mother-in-law is a very hard woman
She always struts about full of anger,

and so forth. There are also many songs which complain of the husband's indifference. For example, see songs no. 39, 40, 41, in Karve, *Kinship Organization*, pp. 209–10. The presence of hidden hostility towards the new husband can also be inferred from the results of a Thematic Apperception Test administered to forty school girls in the South who were shown a picture of a death scene, with a covered unidentifiable body in the centre of the room and a doctor nearby consoling a young woman. In the stories written by the girls, by far the largest number (45 per cent) 'saw' the covered figure as the body of a dead husband. See Narain, D., 1964, 'Growing up in India', *Family Process*, 3, pp. 132–3.

44 *The Laws of Manu*, translated by G. Buhler, 1886, in M. Muller (ed.), *Sacred Books of the East*, vol. 25, Oxford: Clarendon Press, p. 196.

45 Ibid., p. 197.

46 Gore, Madhav S., 1961, 'The Husband-Wife and Mother-Son Relationship', *Sociological Bulletin*, 11, pp. 91–102. See also Ross, *Hindu Family*, p. 147, for evidence of a similar relationship existing in urbanized families.

47 *The Laws of Manu*, p. 85. Similar sentiments are expressed in the Mahabharata.

48 See, for example, Mandelbaum, *Society in India*, p. 88, and Lewis, *Village Life*, p. 195.

49 Majumdar, Geeta, 1911, *Folk Tales of Bengal*, New Delhi: Sterling Publishers, p. 17.

50 *The Laws of Manu*, p. 344.

51 Ibid., p. 56.

52 *Mahabharata*, translated by P.C. Roy, vol. 1 (*Adi-parva*), pp. 177–8.

53 *Brahmavaivarta*, 3. 2. pp. 19–24, in O'Flaherty, *Asceticism and Eroticism*, p. 225.

54 *The Laws of Manu*, p. 354. Although it is primarily the son who is responsible for the performance of these rites, in case a couple has no son the rites may be performed by the daughter's son.

55 The Hindu attitude is similar to Malinowski's characterization of the Melanesians: 'The woman shows invariably a passionate craving for her child and the surrounding society seconds her feelings, fosters her inclinations, and idealizes them by custom and usage.' See Malinowski, B., 1927, *Sex and Repression in Savage Society*, New York: Harcourt, p. 21.

56 Deutsch, Helene, 1945, *The Psychology of Women*, vol. 2, Ch. II.

57 Unless specifically mentioned, the following sections deal with the male infant only, the pattern being somewhat different in the case of daughters.

58 For anthropological accounts which confirm the widespread existence of this pattern of attachment all over India, see Carstairs, G.M., 1957, *The Twice Born*, London: Hogarth Press, pp. 63–4; Dube, *Indian Village*, pp. 148–9; Narain, Dhirendra N., 1964, 'Growing up in India', *Family Process*, 3, pp. 134–7; Elder, John W., 1959, 'Industrialization in Hindu Society; A Case Study in Social Change', unpublished Ph.D. thesis, Harvard University, p. 242.

59 Murphy, Gardner, 1953, *In the Minds of Men*, New York: Basic Books, p. 56.

60 See Mayer, Adrian C., 1970, *Caste and Kinship in Central India*, London: Routledge and Kegan Paul; Ross, *Hindu Family*; Gore, 'Husband–Wife and Mother–Son Relationship'; and Narain, D., 'Interpersonal Relationships in the Hindu Family', in R. Hill and R. Konig (eds), *Families in East and West*, Paris: Mouton, pp. 454–80.

61 Nehru, Jawaharlal, 1961, *Toward Freedom*, Boston: Beacon Press, p. 22.

62 Yogananda, Paramhansa, 1972, *Autobiography of a Yogi*, Los Angeles: Self Realization Fellowship, p. 4.

63 Freud, Sigmund, 1916, *Introductory Lectures on Psychoanalysis*, Standard Edition, vol. 16, p. 407.

64 Wilkins, W.J., 1882, *Hindu Mythology*, Delhi: Delhi Book Store, 1972, pp. 107–12 and 238–47.

65 Erikson, Erik H., 1966, 'Ontogeny of Ritualization', in R.M. Loewenstein *et al.* (eds), *Psychoanalysis—A General Psychology: Essays in Honor of Heinz Hartmann*, New York: International Universities Press, p. 604.

66 *Vaivarta Purana*, quoted in Wilkins, *Hindu Mythology*, p. 244.

67 Bowlby, J., 1973, *Separation: Anxiety and Anger*, London: Hogarth Press.

68 Ibid., p. 314.

69 *Satapatha Brahmana*, quoted in Wilkins, *Hindu Mythology*, p. 286.

70 Hitchcock, J., 'Pregnancy and Childbirth', quoted in Narain, 'Growing up in India', p. 139.

71 Taylor, William S., 1948, 'Basic Personality in Orthodox Hindu Culture Patterns', *Journal of Abnormal Psychology*, 43, p. 11. See also Spratt, P., 1966, *Hindu Culture and Personality*, Bombay: Manaktalas, pp. 181–6.

72 See Bowlby, *Separation*, p. 359, and Winnicott, D.W, 1958, 'The Capacity to be Alone', *International Journal of Psychoanalysis*, 39, pp. 416–20. A similar position has also been adopted by the intellectual spokesmen of what has come to be known as the 'counter-culture' in the United States. Thus Philip Slater suggests that the present American social order deeply frustrates three fundamental human needs: 'The desire for *community*—the wish to live in trust and fraternal cooperation with one's fellows. The desire for *engagement*—the wish to come directly to grips with social and interpersonal problems. The desire for *dependence*—the wish to share the responsibility for the control of one's impulses and the direction of one's life.' See Slater, Philip, 1970, *The Pursuit of Loneliness: American Culture at the Breaking Point*, Boston: Beacon Press, p. 5.

73 Freud, Sigmund, 1916, *Introductory Lectures on Psychoanalysis*, Standard Edition, vol. 16, p. 408 and 1926, *Inhibitions, Symptoms, and Anxiety*, Standard Edition, vol. 20, p. 167.

74 See Bowlby, *Attachment*.

75 Neutmann, Erich, 1963, *The Great Mother: An Analysis of the Archetype* (2nd edn), Princeton: Princeton University Press, pp. 147–203.

76 Slater, *The Glory of Hera*, p. 68. Slater's brilliant discussion of the mother-son constellation in ancient Greece shows some parallels, though not a complete identity, with the corresponding situation in modern India and has been a rich source of comparative material.

77 *Kalika Purana*, 47. pp. 114–119, paraphrased from O'Flaherty, *Asceticism and Eroticism*, p. 190.

78 *Matsya Purana*, 155, pp. 1–34.

79 William N. Stephens, in a cross-cultural study of the family, has demonstrated these taboos to be positively correlated with indicators of sexual arousal. See Stephens, 1963, *The Family in Cross-Cultural Perspective*, New York: Holt, pp. 80 ff.

80 *The Laws of Manu*, p. 135.

81 *Aitareya Brahmana*, 1. 6. pp. 1–6; see O'Flaherty, *Asceticism and Eroticism*, p. 275.

82 Dube, *Indian Village*, pp. 190–7.

83 Horney, Karen, 1932, 'The Dread of Woman', *International Journal of Psychoanalysis*, 13, pp. 349–53.

84 *Brahma Purana*, 81. pp. 1–5; paraphrased from O'Flaherty, *Asceticism and Eroticism*, p. 204.

85 *Thirty Minor Upanishads*, translated by K.N. Aiyar, quoted in Spratt, *Hindu Culture*, p. 118.

86 *Mahabharata*, vol. 2 (*Vanaparva*), pp. 102–5.

87 *Padma Purana*, 5. 26. pp. 91–125; O'Flaherty, *Asceticism and Eroticism*, p. 280.

88 *Ramayana of Valmiki*, vol. 1 (*Aranyakanda*), 18: pp. 15–16. In psychoanalytic literature, it was Wilhelm Stekel who pointed to the relationship between the nose and feminine genitalia, basing some of his conclusions on the earlier work of Fliess Wilhelm, 1897, *Die Beziehungen zwischen Nase und weiblichen Geschlechtsorganen in ihrer biologisches Bedeutungen*; see Stekel, 1923, *Conditions of Nervous Anxiety and their Treatment*, London: Paul Trench and Trubner, p. 49.

89 Spratt, *Hindu Culture*, p. 254.

90 Ibid., pp. 252–7.

91 I suspect this will be corroborated convincingly by clinical evidence, once this evidence becomes available in sufficient quantity and depth. Meanwhile, we cannot dismiss the common game of 'playing the wife' among boys of a certain age. The case history of a young boy who used to tie a piece of string around his prepuce and draw his penis so tightly into the scrotum that it was covered by the folds of the scrotum, thereby giving the genitalia a remarkable female resemblance is one aberrant manifestation of this identification. See Bose, G., 1949, 'The Genesis and Adjustment of the Oedipal Wish', *Samiksa*, 3, p. 231. This behaviour is reminiscent of the commonly accepted (and admired) ability of Hatha-Yogis to draw the penis and the testes back into the pubic arch so that the whole body takes on the appearance of a woman.

92 The second version of the Ganesha myth, in which Sani first avoids and then looks at the infant Ganesha (thus depriving him of his head) is reminiscent of cases of scotophilic women whose compulsive avoidance of, and looking at, men's genitals is a distorted expression of their castration wish.

93 *Mahabharata*, vol. 10 (*Anusasnaparva*), pp. 35–8.

94 Spratt, *Hindu Culture*, p. 193, and p. 237.

95 Muensterberger, Warner, 1969, 'Psyche and Environment', *Psychoanalytic Quarterly*, 38, p. 204.

96 For Freud's distinction between the primary and the secondary processes, see 1911, *Formulations on the Two Principles of Mental Functioning*, Standard Edition, vol. 12.

97 This is of course an impressionistic generalization based on personal and professional experience in Indian and western societies. Empirical studies comparing Indian and western children are rare. For an older study lending support to the impression that primary thought processes persist well beyond infancy in Indian childhood, see Hoyland, J.C., 1921, *An Investigation Regarding the Psychology of Indian Adolescence*, Jubbulpore: Christian Mission Press. In a study based on student responses to Rorschach cards, Asthana concludes that fantasy and imagination characterize the entire sample with some subjects given to intense and vivid imagery. See Asthana, Hari S., 1956, 'Some Aspects of Personality Structuring in Indian (Hindu) Social Organization', *Journal of Social Psychology*, 44, pp. 155–63.

98 Noy, Pinchas, 1969, 'A Revision of the Psychoanalytic Theory of the Primary Process', *International Journal of Psychoanalysis*, 50, pp. 155–78.

99 Ibid., pp. 176–7.

100 See Erikson, *Identity: Youth and Crisis*, p. 174, for a discussion of the concept of negative identity.

101 Whitehead, Henry, 1921, *The Village Gods of South India*, Calcutta: Association Press, p. 18.

102 *Mahabharata*, vol. 4 (Virataparva), p. 12.

103 Singer, Milton, 1966, 'The Radha-Krishna Bhajans of Madras City', in M. Singer (ed.), *Krishna: Myths, Rites, and Attitudes*, Honolulu: East-West Center Press, p. 130.

104 Swami Saradananda, n.d., *Sri Ramakrishna, The Great Master*, Madras: Ramakrishna Math, p. 238.

The Hierarchical Man*

IN AN ARTICLE TITLED 'Where Rank Alone Matters', the well-known Indian journalist, Sunanda K. Datta-Ray, writes that the gratification of 300 million middle-class consumers, the 'new Brahmins', does not lie in their being consumers in a global market place but in their being 'somebody' in a profoundly hierarchical society.[1.] Retired judges, ex-ambassadors, and other sundry officials of the Indian state, who are no longer in service, are never caught without calling cards prominently displaying who they once were. India is not a country for the anonymous, he concludes. You must be somebody to survive with dignity since rank is the only substitute for money. He could have added that India provides, by far, the largest number of aspirants for the Guiness Book of Records. The Indian ingenuity in finding ever new fields for setting up records (and we are not talking about the well known ones for the longest fingernails or the largest moustache) is remarkable, amusing ... and oddly touching. Commercially astute British and American publishers of biographical dictionaries and compendia of 'Who's Who'—a lucrative branch of vanity publishing—have discovered that India provides the biggest market for people wanting to be included in such publications which are then prominently displayed in the living room of their homes.

The need to be noticed, to stand out from an anonymous mass, is, of course, not uniquely Indian but a part of the narcissistic heritage of all

*From *The Indians: Potrait of a People*, Delhi: Viking-Penguin, 2007.

human beings that fuels our self-esteem as also excesses of self-regard. What makes this phenomenon particularly ubiquitous (and poignant) in India is that a person's self worth is almost exclusively determined by the rank he (alone or as part of a family) occupies in the profoundly hierarchical nature of Indian society. If the perception—conscious or below the surface of consciousness—of another person has first to do with gender ('Is this individual male or female?'), followed by age ('Is he/she young or old?') and by other markers of identity, then in India the determination of relative rank ('Is the person superior or inferior to me?') remains very near the top of subconscious questions evoked in an interpersonal encounter.

The deeply internalized hierarchical principle, the lens through which men and women in India view their social world, has its origins in the earliest years of a child's life in the family. Indeed, a grasp of the psychological dynamics of family life is vital for understanding Indian behaviour not only towards authority but also in a wide variety of other social situations.

Web of Family Life

The Indian family: large and noisy, with parents and children, uncles, aunts, and cousins, presided over by benevolent grandparents, all of them living together under a single roof. There are intrigues and secret liaisons, fierce loving and jealous rages. Its members often squabble among themselves but are intensely loyal to each other and always present a united front to the outside world. The Indian family is animated with such a powerful sense of life that a separation from it leaves one with a perpetual sense of exile.

This is the 'joint' family of Bollywood movies which, social scientists tell us, has never been a universal norm. It is also untrue that the large joint family is more often found in villages than in cities; studies tell us that the joint family is more common in urban areas as also among the upper landholding castes than in the lower castes of rural India. Economic reasons, especially the high cost of urban living space, are certainly factors contributing to the joint family staying together and not splitting into nuclear cells. The contemporary nostalgia at the supposed withering away of the large Indian family with the increasing pace of modernization may be misplaced; the prevalence of joint families may be increasing rather than declining.[2] It is important to note that irrespective of demographic changes and the desire of many modern middle-class couples to escape the tensions of joint family life and live on their own in a nuclear family, the joint family continues to remain the most desirable form of family organization and has a *psychic reality* independent of its actual occurrence.[3]

What is this 'joint' family that is so much a feature of an Indian's inner landscape even in places and social strata where it is not the dominant form of family organization in contemporary India?[4] As an ideal type, a joint family is one in which brothers remain together after marriage and bring their wives into the parental household. It is governed by the ideals of fraternal loyalty and filial obedience which stipulate common residence and common economic, social, and ritual activities. In addition to this core group, there may be others who are either permanent or temporary residents in the household: widowed or abandoned sisters and aunts, or distant male relatives, euphemistically called 'uncles', who have no other family to turn to. In practice, of course, brothers and their families may not share a common kitchen or may live in adjacent houses rather than in a single residence, or a brother may have migrated to the city in search for economic opportunity. Yet, even in cases of many families that appear 'nuclear' in the sense that they are composed of parents and their unmarried children, a social and psychological (as distinguished from a residential) 'jointness' continues to operate. When a brother from the village family moves to the city, his wife and children frequently continue to live with the village family while he himself remits his share to the family income; or if he takes his family with him, they return 'home' as often as they can. Even in the upper- and upper-middle classes, it is the psychic reality of the joint family which makes them take it for granted that they can visit and live for weeks, if not months, with their adult married children who are working in distant parts of the country or even outside India.

The point we wish to make here is that most Indians spend the formative years of their life in family settings that approximate to the joint rather than the nuclear type. Even grown children who normally live in a nuclear family make long and frequent visits to members of the joint family. Families not only get together to celebrate festivals but people also prefer to go on vacations or on religious pilgrimage in the company of other family members. The ideals of fraternal solidarity and filial devotion incorporated by the joint family are so strong that a constant effort is made to preserve the characteristic 'jointness', at the very least, in its social sense. Anyone who has been surprised at the amount of traffic in an Indian city on a late Sunday morning, only needs to remember that many of the men, women, and children, dressed in their best clothes and precariously perched on scooters, or crammed into buses and small Maruti cars, are on their way to visit family members living in other parts of the city.

In part, the demography of childhood in India reflects Indian marriage patterns. Leaving aside the urban middle and upper classes where the marriageable age has been increasing, most couples marry in adolescence and have neither the economic nor psychological resources to set up an independent household. Separation from the joint family, if and when it does takes place, comes later when the children are well into the middle years of childhood. Thus, it is not surprising that uncles, aunts, and cousins, not to mention grandparents, figure prominently in the childhood recollections of most Indians. They occupy a much greater space in the inner world of Indians than is the case with Europeans and Americans growing up in nuclear families where it is only the mother and the father (and perhaps also the siblings) who cast such a long shadow on their emotional lives.

More than the recent high rate of economic growth, the improvement in the status of previously oppressed sections of society, and even more than the continuing strength of religious belief, it is the *family* and the role family obligations play in the life of an Indian which is the glue that holds Indian society together. Of course, the other side of the coin is—and there is always another side—that a focus on the family as the exclusive source of satisfaction of *all* needs, also reflects a continuing lack of faith in other institutions of Indian society.

Economically, in a country without large government programmes of social security, unemployment compensation and old age benefits, it is the family, if anyone, which must provide temporary relief when a man loses work, a young mother is ill, or the monsoon floods destroy the harvest. If one excludes the rising middle-class and small upper-class elite, it is the family that provides the only life insurance most Indians have.

In the imagination of most Indians, a man's worth and, indeed, recognition of his identity are inextricable from the reputation of his family. How a man lives and what he does are rarely seen as a product of individual effort or aspiration, but are interpreted in the light of his family's circumstances and reputation in the wider society. Individual success or failure makes sense only in a family context. 'How can a son of family X behave like this!' is as much an expression of contempt as 'How could he not turn out well! After all he is the son of family Y!' is a sign of approval.

Psychologically, an individual derives much of his self-esteem from family myths that ascribe to his family some kind of distinction or prominence in the past, or exaggerate its importance in the present. His closest ties, including friendships will be not outside but within the family. As a Hindi proverb puts it: 'A mustard seed of relationships is worth a cartload of friendship.' These special relationships within the family are a major source of support needed to go through life and for the recurrent affirmation of one's identity.

It is not as if family interactions and obligations have been static and unchanging. The alarm expressed in Hindu nationalist writings and in women's magazines about the Indian family being under attack by forces of Western modernization certainly points in this direction. Many of the changes have to do with the rise of individualism and the role of women in urban areas to which we will come back later. Family obligations, too, are changing. Thirty years ago, it was taken for granted that a man would look after a cousin or a nephew if he came and stayed with him for many years of schooling which was not available in his hometown or village. Some middle-class families will now hesitate to put themselves out to the same extent. The contraction of family obligations is taking place but they are not disappearing; one may not feel as obliged to look after a distant aunt but there is no question of not looking after the emotional, social, and financial needs of an aged parent. All in all, though, the Indian family remains distinctive (and distinctly conservative) in its views on marriage, parenthood, and the web of mutual responsibilities and obligations within wider ties of kinship.[5]

An unshakeable solidarity between the brothers as one of the highest ideals of family life can lead to some consequences that may be appear odd to a 'modern sensibility' which looks upon the husband–wife couple as the fulcrum of family life. Thus, a man often tolerates the adulterous relations of his wife with his brother, in the upper classes mostly by feigning ignorance although the poorer sections of society even dispense with this fig leaf. Thus the cook from the hill state of Uttaranchal once came to his employer asking for leave to go to his village since his wife had just given birth to a son.

'But how can your wife bear a son when you have not been to your village in the last one year?' asked the employer.

'How does that matter?" replied the man. "My brother is there.'

For a time in Indian social history, the erotic importance of the husband's younger brother—in the sense that he would or could have sexual relations with his elder brother's widow—was officially recognized in the custom of *niyoga*. The custom goes back thousands of years to the sacred book of the *Rig Veda* where a man, identified by the commentators as the brother-in-law, is described as extending his hand in promised marriage to a widow inclined to share her husband's funeral pyre.

Though the custom gradually fell into disuse, especially with the prohibition of widow remarriage (it still survives in some communities), the psychological core of niyoga, namely the mutual awareness of a married woman and her younger brother-in-law as potential or actual sexual partner, is very much alive even today. In psychotherapy practice, middle-class women, who are on terms of sexual intimacy with a brother-in-law, rarely express any feelings of guilt. Their distress is occasioned more by his leaving home or his impending marriage, which the women perceive as an end to their sensual and emotional life.

Authority in Family and Society

An Indian's sense of his relative familial and social position is so internalized that he qualifies, in Louis Dumont's phrase, as the original *homo hierarchicus*.[6] The internalization of hierarchy coincides with the acquisition of language. There are six basic nursery sounds, a universal baby language used by infants all over the world with only slight variation from one society to another.[7]. These 'words' are repeated combinations of the vowel 'ah' preceded by different consonants—'dada', 'mama', 'baba', 'nana', 'papa', and 'tata'. Infants repeat these or other closely related sounds over and over, in response to their own babbling and to their parents' modified imitations of their baby sounds. In most Western countries, only a few of these repetitive sounds, for example, 'mama', 'dada', or 'papa' are recognized and repeated by the parents and thus reinforced in the infant. In India, on the contrary, just about *all* of these closely related sounds are repeated and reinforced since each one is a name for various elder kin in the family which a child must learn to identify with the position he or she occupies in the family hierarchy. Thus, for example, in Punjabi, *ma* is mother, *mama* is mother's brother, *dada* is father's father, *nana* is mother's father, *chacha* is father's younger brother, *taya* is father's elder brother, *masi* for mother's sister and so on.

This transformation of basic baby language into names for kinship relations within the extended family is characteristic of all Indian languages. It not only symbolizes the child's manifold relationships with a range of potentially nurturing figures in the older generation but also emphasizes the importance of the child's familiarity with the hierarchy of the family organization. Indians must learn to adapt to the personality and moods of many authority figures, besides their parents, early in life. Whether a highly developed antenna that makes an Indian almost anticipate the wishes of a superior and adjust his behaviour accordingly is called 'flexibility' or 'a lack of a firm sense of self', is a cultural value judgment we are unwilling to make. The fact remains that early experiences in an extended family, the child's learning when to retreat, when to cajole, and when to be stubborn in order to get what he wants, also makes an Indian a formidable negotiator in later business dealings.

Regardless of personal talents or achievements, or of changes in the circumstances of his own or others' lives, an Indian's relative position in the hierarchy of the family, his obligations to those 'above' him, and his expectations of those 'below' him are immutable, lifelong. Already, in childhood, he begins to learn that he must look after the welfare of those subordinate to him in the family hierarchy so that they do not suffer either through their own misjudgment or at the hands of outsiders, and that he is reciprocally entitled to the obedience and respectful compliance of his wishes.

Since young people in Indian families generally receive a good deal of attention and nurturance from the older generation and maintenance of family integrity is valued higher than an unfolding of individual capacities, a young Indian neither seeks a radical demarcation from the generation of parents nor feels compelled to overthrow their authority in order to 'live my life on my own terms.' This is in stark contrast to the West where 'generational conflict' is not only expected but considered necessary for the renewal of a society's institutions and, moreover, is considered (we believe, erroneously) to be a universally valid psychological category. In India, it is not the rupture but the *stretching* of traditional values that becomes a means for the young person to realize his dreams for life. It is telling that, in spite of their fascination with the lives of sport and cinema stars and the omnipresence of these celebrities in advertising on billboards, in print, and in the electronic media, the primary role models for a large majority of Indian youth continue to hail from the family … most often a parent.

In spite of rapid social changes in the last decades, then, an Indian continues to be a part of a hierarchically ordered and, above all, stable network of relationships throughout the course of life. This complex relationship based on a pattern of behavior also manifests itself in work situations. Although intellectually the Indian professional or bureaucrat may agree with his Western counterpart that, for instance, the criterion for appointment or promotion to a particular job must be objective, a decision based solely on the demands of the task and 'merits of the case', emotionally he must still struggle against the cultural conviction that his relationship to the individual under consideration (if there is one) is the single most important factor in his decision. And among the vast majority of traditional-minded countrymen—whether it be a trader bending the law to facilitate the business transaction of a fellow caste member, or an industrialist employing an insufficiently qualified but distantly related job applicant as a manager, or the clerk in the municipal office accepting bribes in order to put an orphaned niece through school—dishonesty, nepotism, and corruption are merely abstract concepts. These negative constructions are irrelevant to the Indian experience, which, from childhood onwards, nurtures one standard of responsible adult conduct, and one only, namely, an individual's lifelong obligation to his kith and kin. Guilt and its attendant anxiety are aroused only when individual actions go against the principle of primacy of relationships, not when foreign, different ethical standards of honesty, equity, and justice are breached.

Although family relationships are hierarchical in structure, the mode of relationship is characterized by an almost maternal behaviour on the part of the superior, by filial respect and compliance on part of the subordinate, and by a mutual sense of highly personal attachment. We meet this kind of a superior—king, father, guru—in school textbooks where, in stories depicting authority situations, the ideal leader acts in a nurturing way so that his followers either anticipate his wishes or accept them without questioning.[8] He receives compliance by taking care of his people's needs, by providing the emotional rewards of approval, praise, and affection … or by arousing guilt. High-handed attempts to regulate behaviour through threat or punishment, rejection or humiliation, lead less to open defiance than to devious evasion on the part of the subordinate.

Another legacy of Indian childhood in superior-subordinate, leader-follower relations is the idealization of the former. The need to bestow *mana* on our superiors and leaders in order to partake of this magical power ourselves is an unconscious attempt to restore the narcissistic perfection of infancy, 'You are perfect and I am a part of you.' This is, of course, a universal tendency. In India, the automatic reverence for superiors is a widespread psychological fact. Leaders at every level of society, but particularly the patriarchal elders of the extended family and caste groups, as also religious and spiritual leaders, take on an emotional importance independent of any realistic evaluation of their performance, let alone an acknowledgment of their all too human weaknesses. Charisma, then, plays an unusually significant role among Indians and is a vital constituent of effective leadership in institutions.[9] In contrast to most people in the West, Indians are generally more prone to revere than admire.

It is not as if Indians are not sceptical of authority figures. Indeed, their cynicism towards leaders of many hues and especially political leadership is often extreme. It is only that when an Indian *grants* authority to a leader that his critical faculties disappear in the waves of credulity that wash over him. The granting of authority during childhood is involuntary in the case of family and caste leadership. It may be voluntary—to gurus of various hues, for instance—in situations of acute personal crisis or distress, the reason why, for example, healers of the most varied kinds flourish in the country. The effectiveness of these healers may be less because of their particular healing regimens and more due to the unconscious vital forces the healer's mana mobilizes and harnesses in the patient in service of a cure.

Do these patterns of family life, especially those connected with the hierarchical ordering of relationships, extend beyond their home base in the family to other institutions in Indian life, from university departments to corporate business life, from hospitals to political parties, from the traditional guru–disciple relationship to the institutions of state bureaucracy? The evidence suggests that they do—that authority relations in the Indian family provide a template for the functioning of most modern business, educational, political, and scientific organizations. Let us elaborate.

First, there is a strong preference for an authoritative, even autocratic (but not authoritarian) leader who is strict, demanding but also caring and nurturing—very much like the *karta*, the paternalistic head of the extended family. The organizational psychologist, Jai Sinha, has called this type of leader the 'nurturant-task' leader who is strict in getting the task accomplished and tries to dominate the activities of his subordinates.[10.] He is, however, not authoritarian but nurturing in the sense of being a benevolent guide to the subordinates and someone who takes a personal interest in their well-being and growth.

Among the subordinates, on the other hand, there is a complementary tendency to idealize the leader and look upon him as a repository of all virtues, an almost superhuman figure deserving of their faith and respect. Even in the upper echelons of modern business organizations, in senior managers with exposure to Western business education and practices, the influence of Indian culture on their perception of top leadership has not disappeared. The CEO of a modern company is the recipient of far greater idealization than is usually the case in the West.[11] The Indian idealization of the leader (and this is a potential strength of Indian organizations) has many advantages such as a greater *esprit de corps* in senior management and in a higher degree of loyalty, satisfaction and commitment to the organization of the managerial team. In case of the individual, it can lead to a work ethic and performance that is much more than what a leader might reasonably expect in most European and North American organizations. Yet, idealization, that great construct of human imagination which is capable of conceiving with the conviction of a known fact a more perfect and valuable reality, while ensuring that what is idealized is inevitably admired and held in awe, can also distort the perception of leadership. The Indian leader is thus often deprived of that critical feedback from the senior people of his organization which would help him eliminate his dysfunctional behaviours while helping him develop more effective leadership practices.

Since Indian institutions are markedly hierarchical, collaborative teamwork across levels of status and power often proves to be difficult. Decisions tend to be pushed upwards and the top leadership must often intervene in organizational processes. More than in most Western cultures, the legacy of Indian family and childhood ensures that the quality of leadership becomes pivotal for the success or failure of an institution.

The difficulty in working in teams is compounded by the cultural obstacles to giving or receiving negative feedback. With the preservation of relationships as the primary principle governing their actions in interpersonal situations, Indians find it difficult to say a frank 'No' to requests they are unable or unwilling to grant. The refusal has then to be interpreted from the words in which the rejection is couched ('Let's see' or 'It's difficult but I will try' and so on), from the tentative tone of voice and the cautious bodily language. One has to exercise the same kind of judgment when asking for directions on an Indian street. The man who might not have an idea of the right directions but nonetheless proceeds to guide you to your destination not only saves face by not admitting to his ignorance but also hesitates to introduce any negative vibes in the fleeting relationship that has just come into being.

The absence of a democratic mode of functioning in Indian institutions is not resented as long as those in leadership positions develop a close personal relationship with the led. In fact, effective leaders in

India, both in work and in the political arena, place great emphasis on the building and cultivating of relationships. This, as we have seen above, is consistent with an Indian's experience from his earliest years where he has learnt that the core of any social relationship—in family, caste, school, or at work—is caring and mutual involvement. What he should be sensitive to (and concerned with) are not only the goals of work that are external to the relationship, but the relationship itself, the unfolding of emotional affinity.

As in the extended family, where favouritism has to be avoided (for example, in the ideology of a joint family a father should not be seen as favoring his own son above the sons of his brothers) to maintain harmony, people in Indian organizations develop almost paranoid abilities in detecting signs of a leader's favouritism towards selected subordinates—not that they are particularly troubled by nepotism. As long as *they* are the intended beneficiaries, most accept that people in authority will make a distinction between their 'own people' and those who are not in the same privileged position. They have a sneaking sympathy for a senior politician's incredulous reaction to a journalist who questions the appointment of the politician's son to a high post within his party: 'Who else will I appoint? *Your* son?' If there is one 'ism' that governs Indian society and its institutions, then it is family-ism.

Given the strong need to be near the superior, to be considered 'his man', what is galling for an Indian is to feel that he has been excluded from a charmed circle that enjoys marks of the superior's favour. Not to be included in the group of the leader's 'own people' produces a good deal of hidden anger and passive-aggressive behaviour. Effective leaders in Indian institutions are thus constantly on their guard that they do not appear to show marks of favour to certain individuals which can be interpreted as favouritism and, in turn, may cause serious damage to the morale of the institution.

Indian Culture and Leadership

Some of the above values that govern Indian institutional and work life have been empirically demonstrated by the GLOBE (Global Leadership and Organizational Behaviour Effectiveness) research project, surveying over 17,000 middle managers in various industries in 62 societies, as characterizing Indian culture more than any of the other world cultures.[12] In this project, the 62 countries were grouped into ten cultural clusters: Latin Europe, Germanic Europe, Anglo Europe, Nordic

Europe, Eastern Europe, Latin America, Confucian Asia, Anglo (outside Europe), Sub-Saharan Africa, Southern Asia, and Middle East.

If one looks at South Asia, where India is by far the largest country, this cultural cluster stands out prominently in three of the nine dimensions of the study. South Asia has the greatest *power distance*, that is, the degree to which the culture's people are separated by power, authority, and prestige.[13] In other words, the difference in status between the chief executive and the office peon, *raja*, and *runk*, is at its maximum in India (the least is Nordic Europe, that is, Scandinavia). Irrespective of his educational status—a middle manager will tend to be a middle class, college educated individual—and more than in any other culture in the world, an Indian is a homo hierarchicus, even when the modern Indian manager wishes that this was not so and, as we shall see below, consciously aspires to a reduction in the power distance.

The second dimension on which South Asia stands out in international comparison is *humane orientation*, that is, the degree to which people are caring, altruistic, generous, and kind (the lowest here is Germanic Europe. Closely related to the humane orientation, although as its opposite, is assertiveness, the degree to which the culture's people are assertive, confrontational, and aggressive. Here, next only to Scandinavia, South Asia is the least assertive culture—Germanic Europe, followed by Eastern Europe, are the most aggressive and confrontational.)

Combining humane orientation with a high power distance produces the kind of Indian leader we have discussed earlier: authoritative but not autocratic, perhaps sometimes despotic, but generally benevolent.

South Asia also scores the highest on *in-group collectivism*, that is, the degree to which people feel loyalty towards small groups such as their family or circle of friends (Scandinavia, followed by Germanic Europe and North America scores least). We have seen that the habit of solidarity with the family group and later with members of one's caste which is inculcated in early childhood is regarded as one of the highest values guiding individual lives. This solidarity has the many economic advantages of informal networks that are based on trust rather than contractual obligations. We have already talked of the high *esprit de corps* when people working in an organization regard themselves as a 'band of brothers' and idealize the leader–father. The danger, of course, is of in-groupism which makes collaboration with other, out-groups in large organizations difficult, if not impossible.

This snapshot of Indian leadership practices says little about the changes taking place in modern urban families which will invariably have an impact on Indian institutions. The GLOBE study confirms that what Indian younger managers most dearly wish is a reduction in the power distance between the leader and the led.[14] We believe that leadership on this dimension is indeed in a state of transition. It is not a coincidence that the desired reduction in psychological distance between the leader and the led is congruent with the changes taking place in the father–son relationship in the middle-class family. Let us elaborate.

In traditional India, the father enters his son's life in a big way only in the later years of a boy's childhood. In the early and middle years, the relationship between the two was (and in large parts of the country continues to be) marked by formality and perfunctory daily social contact.[15] In older autobiographical accounts, fathers, whether strict or indulgent, cold or affectionate, are invariably portrayed as distant; the father's guiding voice is a prime element in a man's sense of identity, diffused among the voices of many older male family members, his individual paternity muffled.

The reasons for a traditional father not taking a demonstratively active role in the upbringing of his son are not difficult to fathom. A traditional father operates under the logic of the joint family. This demands that in order to prevent the building up of nuclear cells within the family that destroy its cohesion, a father be restrained in the presence of his own child and divide his interest and support equally among his own and his brothers' children. Moreover, as we shall see later in the chapter on sexuality, many a young father was embarrassed to hold his infant child in front of older family members since this fruit of his loins was clear evidence of activity in that particular region.

The second ideology impinging on traditional fathers in India (and in common with other patriarchal societies) is of a gender-based dichotomy in parenting roles and obligations. That is, decided notions of things that men do in household and childcare, and others that they don't. Playing with or taking care of their infant and small sons is not what fathers do, their major role lying in the disciplining of the child. As a north Indian proverb, addressed to men, pithily put it: 'Treat a son like a king for the first five years, like a slave for the next ten, and like a friend thereafter.'

Of course, behind the requisite façade of aloofness and impartiality, a traditional Indian father may be struggling to express his love for his son. Fatherly love is no less strong in India than in other societies. Even in ancient religious and literary texts, a son is not only instrumental in the fulfilment of a sacred duty but has often been portrayed as a source of intense emotional gratification.[16] Older autobiographical accounts often depict the Indian father as a sensitive man and charged with feelings for his son which he does not openly reveal. Thus, in *Autobiography of a Yogi*, Yogananda describes meeting his father after a long separation, 'Father embraced me warmly as I entered our Gurupur home. "You have come," he said tenderly. Two large tears dropped from his eyes. Outwardly undemonstrative, he had never before shown me these external signs of affection. Outwardly the grave father, inwardly he possessed the melting heart of a mother.'[17]

One of the more striking changes, associated with modernity and the rise of an urban middle class, is the active involvement of fathers in bringing up their infant and small children.[18] Given the intensity and ambivalence of the mother–son connection in the Indian setting, the need for the father's physical touch and guiding voice, his sponsorship for the son's separation from his mother, has always been pressing. Modern, generally urban and educated, fathers have begun to provide this early emotional access to the son, not only attenuating the overheated quality of the mother–son bond, but laying the foundations for a less hierarchical and closer father–son relationship. The early experience of fathers who are no longer distant and forbidding figures, who are available to both sons and daughters, often as playmates, cannot but help in moulding modern Indian notions of the desirable power distance in institutions and the expectations young Indians will increasingly have from their leaders.

Notes and References

1 Datta-Ray, S.K., 2005, 'Where Rank Alone Matters', *The Times of India*, July.

2 The various studies have been summarized by Patricia Uberoi in P. Uberoi (ed.), 1993, *Family, Kinship and Marriage in India*, Delhi: Oxford University Press, p. 387.

3 In a recent survey of young people from the ages of 18 to 35 in 14 Indian cities (*India Today*, 26 February 2006, p. 44), 68 per cent of the respondents preferred to live in joint families, the percentage being slightly higher in males than females.

4 Much of the following is based on Kakar, Sudhir, 1978, *The Inner World: A Psychoanalytical Study of Childhood and Society in India*, Delhi and New York: Oxford University Press, ch. 3.

5 See also Béteille, André, 1993, 'The Family and the Reproduction of Inequality', in P. Uberoi (ed.), *Family, Kinship and Marriage in India*, pp. 435–51.

6 Dumont, L., 1970, *Homo Hierarchicus: The Caste System and its Implications*, translated by M. Sainsbury, Chicago: University of Chicago Press.

7 Lewis, M., 1964, *Language, Thought and Personality in Infancy and Childhood*, New York: Basic Books, p. 33.

8 Kakar, Sudhir, 1971, 'The Theme of Authority in Social Relations in India', *Journal of Social Psychology*, 84, pp. 93–101. The authority relations in the family are elaborated in Kakar, *Inner World*, pp. 119–20.

9 See also Singh, P. and A. Bhandarker, 1990, *Corporate Success and Transformational Leadership*, New Delhi: Wiley Eastern.

10 Sinha, J.B.P., 1979, *The Nurturant Task Leader*, New Delhi: Concept.

11 Kakar, Sudhir, *et al.*, 2002, 'Leadership in Indian Organizations from a Comparative Perspective', *International Journal of Cross Cultural Management*, 2(2), pp. 239–50.

12 House, R.J., *et al.*, 2004, *Leadership, Culture, and Organizations: The GLOBE Study of 62 Societies*, Thousand Oaks, CA: Sage.

13 Javidan, M., *et al.*, 2005, 'Cross-border Transfer of Knowledge: Cultural Lessons from Project Globe', *Academy of Management Executive*, 19(2), pp. 59–76. The other comparisons are also taken from this article. For an earlier international study confirming the high power distance in Indian organizations, see Hofstede, G., 1980, *Culture's Consequences*, London: Sage.

14 Javidan, 'Cross-border Transfer of Knowledge', p. 63.

15 Older anthropological writings attest to this pattern being central to father–son relationship; see Mandelbaum, D.G., 1970, *Society in India*, Berkeley: University of California Press, vol.1, p. 60; Mayer, A.C., 1970, *Caste and Kinship in Central India*, London: Routledge, Kegan and Paul, p. 218; Ross, A.D., 1962, *The Hindu Family in its Urban Setting*, Toronto: University of Toronto Press, p. 10.

16 Kakar, *Inner World*, pp. 200–1.

17 Yogananda, Parmahansa, 1972, *Autobiography of a Yogi*, Los Angeles: Self-Realization Fellowship, p. 268.

18 Roopnarine, J.L. and P. Suppal, 'Kakar's Psychoanalytic Interpretation of Indian Childhood: The Need to Emphasize the Father and Multiple Caregivers in the Socialization Equation', in D. Sharma (ed.), 2003, *Childhood, Family and Sociocultural Change in India*, Delhi: Oxford University Press, pp. 115–37; see also Derne, S., 'Culture, Family Structure, and Psyche in Hindu India', in Sharma, pp. 88–114.

The Indian Mind*

IN THIS BOOK we have sought to describe the manifestations of the spirit of India in various facets of Indian life and thought. By 'spirit of India', we do not mean something elusive and ethereal, but are talking of the culturally shared part of the mind, a certain Indian-ness, that is reflected in the way the inhabitants of the subcontinent approach daily tasks as well as eternal questions of human existence. What are the building blocks of this Indian-ness? Let us begin with the Indian (here, primarily the Hindu) view of the world.

The Hindu Worldview

Every civilization has a unique way of looking at the world. This worldview, the civilization's centre of gravity, is a cluster of ideas which define the goal of human existence, the ways to reach this goal, the errors to be avoided, and the obstacles to be expected on the way. The worldview interprets central human experiences and answers perennial questions on what is good and what is evil, what is real and what is unreal, what is the essential nature of men and women and the world they live in, and what is man's connection to nature, other human beings, and the cosmos. For instance, if we look at China (and Chinese societies around the world), we can define the following elements in the dominant, Confucian worldview:

*From *The Indians: Portrait of a People,* Delhi: Viking-Penguin, 2007

There is no other world than the one we live in. The ultimate meaning of life is embedded in and not separate from ordinary practical living. The meaning of life is then realized through a personal self-cultivation within the community and through mutual aid in the family, clan, school, and work place. The glue that binds society is not law but what the Chinese call *li*, a civilized mode of conduct. A predominant feature of the Chinese worldview is a sense of duty rather than the demand for rights.

By 'worldview', we do not mean some philosophical doctrines that are relevant only for religious and intellectual elites. What we are talking of is beliefs and attitudes—many of them not conscious—of a vast number of Indians that are reflected in their lives, their songs, and their stories. Disseminated through myths and legends, proverbs and metaphors, enacted in religious rituals, conveyed through tales told to children, given a modern veneer in Bollywood films, glimpsed in the admonition of parents as also in the future vistas they hold out to their children, a worldview is absorbed from early on in life—not through the head, but through the heart.

Let us begin with three interlinked elements that comprise a major part of the Hindu worldview: *moksha*, dharma, and karma. Our interest in these concepts is not philosophical, textual, or historical, but psychological. What we want to look at closely here is the contribution of this ancient trinity in the formation of the Indian mind and its reverberations in the thoughts and actions of contemporary Indians.[1]

The Goal of Life

Moksha, which variously means self-realization, transcendence, salvation, a release from this world, has been traditionally viewed by the Hindus as the goal of human life. The idea of moksha is intimately linked with the Indian conviction in the existence of another, 'higher' level of reality beyond the shared, verifiable, empirical reality of our world, our bodies, and our emotions. A fundamental value of most schools of Hinduism (and the Sufis of Islam), the belief in the existence of an 'ultimate' reality—related to ordinary, everyday reality in the same way waking consciousness is related to the dream—is an unquestioned verity of Indian culture and the common thread in the teachings of the culture's innumerable gurus. The 'ultimate' reality, whose apprehension is considered to be the highest goal and meaning of human life, is said to be beyond conceptual thought and indeed beyond the mind. Intellectual thought, naturalistic science, and other passions of the mind seeking to grasp the empirical nature of our world, thus, have a relatively lower status in the culture as compared to meditative practices or even art, since aesthetic and spiritual experiences are supposed to be closely related. In the culture's belief system, the aesthetic power of music and verse, of a well-told tale, and a well-enacted play make them more, rather than less, real than life.

The emphasis on the spiritual underlying the practices of the various schools of 'self-realization'—those of Yoga, for instance—colors the emotional tone of the way an Indian looks at life. To most Indians, life is a combination of the tragic and the romantic. It is tragic in so far as they see human experience pervaded by ambiguities and uncertainties, where man has little choice but to bear the burden of unanswerable questions, inescapable conflicts, and incomprehensible afflictions of fate. However, superimposed on the tragic, the Indian vision of moksha offers a romantic quest. The new journey is a search and the seeker, if he withstands the perils of the road, will be rewarded by exaltation beyond normal human experience.

The belief in the existence of 'ultimate reality', this nostalgia of the Indian soul, is a beacon of 'higher feeling' in the lives of most Indians, cutting across class distinctions and caste boundaries, bridging the distance between the rural and the urban, between the illiterate and the educated, between the rich and the poor. The ironic vision of life, which brings a detached and self-deprecating perspective on the tragic, and in which gods have clay feet, is rarely found among Indians. Even among those living in enclaves of Western modernity, an ironic stance towards the spiritual is at the most an affectation of a few young people which normally disappears as they begin to age.

If spirituality has been at the centre of the Indian world image, it would be reasonable to expect that it has continued to condition the Indian mind, colouring its intellectual, artistic, and emotional responses in certain distinctive ways. In other words, there are various cultural consequences of this belief. One of these is the pervasive presence of hope, even in the most dismal of life's circumstances. For centuries, the civilization has conveyed to the growing child the almost somatic conviction that there is a hidden, even if unknown, order to our visible world. That there is a design to life that can be trusted in spite of life's sorrows, cruelties, and injustices. The Indian mind, then, tends to convert even the slightest ray of hope into a blaze of light. Consider this man from a village in Rajasthan who is living in a Delhi slum. He works a back-breaking fourteen hours a day on a construction site, lives with six other members of his family in a single room tenement and eats, if at all, stale food in a chipped enamel plate. Yet, he rejects the idea of life being better in his village with surprising astonishment. The city, with its possibilities, for example schooling for his children, has provided him with a sliver of hope. The cynic might see his aspirations for a better life as completely unrealistic, look at him as someone who clutches at the thinnest of straws and has never learnt that there is something as hoping too much, or hoping in vain. Nevertheless, what keeps this man and so many millions of others cheerful and expectant even under the most adverse economic, social and political circumstances is precisely this hope which is a sense of possession of the future, however distant that future may be.

Another consequence of the spiritual orientation, the unshakeable belief in a 'higher' reality, is the average Indian's fascination with and respect for the occult and its practitioners. Astrologers, soothsayers, clairvoyants, fakirs, and other shamanic individuals who abound in Indian society are profoundly esteemed for they are thought to be in some kind of contact with the ultimate reality. In India, it is the 'god men', the gurus, rather than political, social, or intellectual leaders who have come to incorporate our childhood yearning for omniscience and perfection in parental figures. The latter, the scholar or the scientist, may be respected but it is only the former who are revered. Their presumed contact with another reality is supposed to confer on them supernatural powers, superhuman status, and a moral excellence that is beyond the ordinary lot.

Psychologically, perhaps the most important consequence of the Hindu spiritual orientation and the widespread belief in the divinity immanent within each human being is the feeling of self-worth that comes from a pre-conscious conviction of one's metaphysical significance. However socially demeaned or economically irrelevant a person may be in day to day life, the feeling of being central to the universe and not banished to its remote extremities, of being connected equally with everyone else to the *Urgrund* of human existence, quietly nourishes the individual's self-esteem and stands as a bulwark against the despair (and rage) at life's inequities.

Right and Wrong

If moksha is the goal of life, then dharma, variously translated as law, moral duty, right action, conformity with the truth of things, is the means through which man approaches the desired goal. Today, there is a widespread bemoaning at the lack of dharma in social institutions and individual lives. Traditional and modern Indians agree that there is hardly any institution left where those in positions of power have not veered away from dharma. Whereas modern Indians will also point to the great social churning that is taking place with the advent of modern egalitarian ideologies, traditionalists see the disappearance of dharma as solely responsible for the social conflict, oppression, and unrest that characterize contemporary Indian society. And as for the dharma of individual lives, at one time, in the utopian long, long ago, every person knew that it was not what he did that was important for his spiritual progress but whether he acted in conformity with his dharma. The activity itself—whether that of a shoemaker or a priest, a housewife, or a farmer, a social worker serving others and alleviating misery or an ascetic apparently indifferent to the suffering around him—was considered equally good and equally right if it was consistent with dharma. Furthermore, since traditional Indians are inclined to tell stories whenever they wish to prove a point or convey what the world is like or ought to be like, using narrative as a way of thinking and as an inquiry into the nature of reality, they are likely to tell a story very much like this one.

There was once a king who was strolling along the banks of the river Ganges with an entourage of his ministers. It was the monsoon season and the river was in spate, its swirling waters rushing towards the sea. The broad sweep of the swollen river and its strong current filled the king with awe. Suddenly mindful of his own insignificance, he addressed his ministers: 'Is there no one on this earth who can reverse the flow of this river so that it flows from the sea to the mountains?' The ministers, shaking their heads, smiled at the king's naiveté but a prostitute who overheard his question stepped forward and addressed the river thus: 'O Mother Ganges, if I have striven to fulfil my dharma as a whore by giving my body to all comers, without distinguishing rich from poor, handsome from ugly, old from young, then reverse your flow!' The waters stood still for a moment, as if in deliberation, and then the river started flowing backwards.

Today, the conservatives will continue, the ideologies of Western modernity with their notions of egalitarianism and individual choice, their highlighting the importance of material rewards rather than the spirit of human activity, their emphasis on human aspirations rather than limits, are accountable for the widespread social envy, unbridled greed, and selfishness plaguing modern Indian society. Most would achingly agree that, of the major elements of the traditional Hindu worldview, dharma is one that is most endangered and perhaps already crumbling under the impact of modernity. Yet, there is one aspect of dharma that continues to be of vital importance in understanding the Indian mind, and not only that of the orthodox Hindu. For even if one rejects many traditional values associated with dharma, it is still pivotal in the formation of Indian ethical sensibility. The main feature of this sensibility, in which it diverges from its Judeo-Christian, and Islamic counterparts, is a pronounced ethical relativism which has become entrenched in the Hindu way of thinking. For how does any individual *know* what is right action, that he is acting in accordance with moral law and in 'conformity with the truth of things'?

The traditional answer has been that he cannot know since right action depends on the culture of his country (*desa*), the historical era in which he lives (*kala*), on the efforts required of him at his particular stage of life (*srama*) and, lastly, on the innate character (*guna*) that he has inherited from a previous life. An individual can never know the configuration of all these factors in an absolute sense, nor even significantly influence them. Nor is there a Book, or its authoritative interpreters such as the Church, which can help by removing doubts on how the individual must act in each conceivable situation. 'Right' and 'wrong', then, are relative; depending on its specific context, every action can be right ... or wrong.

In lessening the burden of an individual's responsibility for his actions, the cultural view of right action alleviates the guilt suffered in some societies by those whose actions transgress rigid 'thou-shalt' and 'thou-shalt-not' axioms. Instead, an Indian's actions are governed by a more permissive and gentle, but more ambiguous, 'thou-canst-but-try' ethos. On the one hand, this basic uncertainty makes possible the taking of unconventional and risky actions; on the other hand, actions are accompanied by a pervasive doubt as to the wisdom of individual initiative, making independent voluntary action rare for many who look for psychological security by acting as one's ancestors did in the past and as one's social group—primarily the caste—does at present. The relativism of dharma supports tradition *and* modernity, innovation *and* conformity.

The ethical relativism of dharma has been broadened by the late poet-scholar A.K. Ramanujan to embrace the very way Indians think in most situations. In his stimulating essay, 'Is There an Indian Way of Thinking?'[2] Ramanujan begins his exposition with a survey of Indian intellectuals done some thirty years ago where they were asked to describe the 'Indian Character.' As one can imagine, given the Indian talent for self-criticism, the intellectuals wrote quite sharp comments. They all seemed to agree on one thing: the Indian trait of hypocrisy. Indians don't mean what they say, and say different things at different times. Many occidental travellers in the previous centuries complain about the same thing and, in fact, in the famed Indologist Max Müeller's lectures of 1883 on India, he felt compelled to counter these accusations by writing a chapter called 'Truthful Character of Indians'.[3]

The Indian inconsistency is still regarded as puzzling. How can a reputed astronomer, working at a well-known institute of fundamental sciences, also be a practising astrologer? How can the Western educated executive of a multinational corporation consult horoscopes and holy men for family decisions? Why does an Oxford-educated cabinet minister postpone an important meeting because the hour of meeting is astrologically inauspicious?

These observed traits of inconsistency, however, Ramanujan asserts, have nothing to do with the level of a person's education or logical rigour. They are better understood if we recognize that different cultures seem to prefer either context-free or context-sensitive rules in their thought processes and that Indians operate on the basis of context-sensitivity rather than context-freedom. Let us elaborate.

There is no notion of a *universal* human nature in Indian culture and thus we cannot deduce ethical rules like 'Man shall not kill' or 'Man shall not tell an untruth' or any other unitary law for all men. What a person should or should not do depends on the context. Thus, Manu, the ancient Indian law-giver, has the following to say 'A Kshatriya (man belonging to the warrior castes), having defamed a Brahmin, shall be fined one hundred [*panas*]; a Vaishya (someone belonging to the farmer and merchant castes) one hundred and fifty or two hundred; a Shudra (man belonging to the servant castes) shall suffer corporal punishment.'[4] Even truth-telling is not an unconditional imperative. Here is a quotation from another law book: 'An untruth spoken by people under the influence of anger, excessive joy, fear, pain, or grief, by infants, by very old men, by persons labouring under a delusion being under the influence of drink, does not cause the speaker to fall (i.e. it is not a sin).'[5]

The Christian injunction against coveting 'thy neighbour's wife' is shared by Hindu law books, which proclaim that '[For] in this world there is nothing as detrimental to long life as criminal conversation with another man's wife.' In fact, Hindus are even stricter in defining adultery; talking to a woman alone in the forest, 'or at the confluence of rivers', offering her presents, touching her ornaments and dress, sitting with her on a bed, are all adulterous acts. The nature of punishment, of course, depends on the respective castes of the adulterous couple and there are also exceptions, such as the one which condones adultery with 'the wives of actors and singers.'[6] In spite of a chapter with the title 'Other Men's Wives' in the *Kamasutra*, the celebrated text shares the Hindu disapproval of adultery. However, it, too, lists exceptions to the rule: for example, if your unrequited passion makes you fall sick, and then proceeds to outline the various ways to seduce other men's wives.[7] Its position seems to be: you shouldn't do it; but if you must, then these are the ways to proceed—but, of course, you shouldn't have done it in the first place.

Virtues, too, are as dependent on the context as are transgressions. Bravery may be a virtue for the kshatriya, the warrior, but it is certainly not one for the *baniya*, the merchant. Ramanujan remarks that for a Western-Christian tradition, which is based on the premise of universalization—the golden rule of New Testament—such a view that each class of men has its own laws, its own proper ethics, which cannot be universalized, must be baffling and, ultimately, a producer of denigration.

Context-sensitivity is not just a feature of traditional moral law but extends to many areas of contemporary Indian life and thought. The cultural psychologist Richard Shweder, who has compared descriptive phrases used by Oriyas from eastern India and mid-westerners from the United States, has shown that the two describe persons very differently.[8] Americans characterize a person with abstract, generic words like 'good', 'nice', while the Oriyas use more concrete, contextual descriptions like 'he helps me', 'brings sweets' et cetera. The descriptions provided by the Indians were more situation-specific and more relational than those of Americans. Indian descriptions focus on behaviour. They describe what was done, where it was done, and to whom or with whom it was done. The Indian respondents said, 'He has no land to cultivate but likes to cultivate the land of others', or 'When a quarrel arises, he cannot resist the temptation of saying a word', or 'He behaves properly with guests but feels sorry if money is spent on them'. It is the behaviour itself that is focal and significant rather than the inner attribute that supposedly underlies it. This tendency to supply the context when providing a description characterizes the descriptions of Indians regardless of social class, education, or level of literacy. It appears, then, that the preferred Indian way of describing people is not due to a lack of skill in abstracting concrete instances to form a general proposition, but rather a consequence of the fact that global inferences about persons are typically regarded as neither meaningful nor informative.

If truth is relative, something you are never destined to know, then there is no choice but to be tolerant of the truth of others. The story of the six blind men who argued over the nature of an elephant on basis of the part of the beast each had explored with his hands is a cautionary tale that could only be Hindu in its inspiration. The roots of the vaunted Hindu tolerance, then, may well lie in this context-dependent way of thinking. Yet because of its intimate connection with matters of religious faith, to a person's deepest values, this particular civilizational heritage of ethical action being inseparable from its context does show some variation across religious communities.

We see this when we look at the moral judgements of Hindus and Muslims on their interactions with each other, both in times of peace and conflict.[9] There are many such interactions in normal times: eating with a member of the other community, working with him, punishing a member of the another community who is making fun of your religious symbols or insulting a woman of your community. And then there are the interactions during riot: killing, arson, and rape.

As compared to the Muslims, the Hindus were much more relativistic and contextual in judging a behaviour as a transgression and more easy-going in proposing punishment for actions judged as wrong. Irrespective of age and gender, 'It all depends' was an almost reflexive response. In responding to cases of interaction with the Muslims, the answers were almost always framed in terms of a context, temporal or spatial. The linkage of morality with time would be typically expressed thus: 'It was wrong (killing) when times were different but are not wrong now'. The individual can thus convincingly state that an action is wrong in right times but right in wrong times. Similarly, space is also involved in moral judgements. Hindus often said that actions such as beating up of a Muslim or arson or looting of Muslim shops during a riot were wrong if you lived in a Muslim majority area but all right if you were living in a Hindu majority neighborhood. As a consequence of this contextual stance, wrong actions by the members of the community evoked far less emotion and righteousness than the corresponding actions among the Muslims. In this particular instance Muslims were more definite and unambiguous about which actions were right and which were clearly wrong, even during a riot.

The moral relativism of the Hindu mind is not an *absence* of a moral code but only a more context-sensitive way of looking at and dealing with its violation. In many ways, Hindus are extremely strict in their definition of what constitutes a deviation from morality. Consider the following story from the Mahabharata, the epic whose centrepiece is the great war between the forces of good and evil, represented by the Pandavas and the Kaurvas. There were, of course, good men fighting on the side of the evil forces, the great archer and teacher of both the Pandava and Kaurva princes, Drona, for instance. Of course, given the Hindu penchant for relativity, good and evil are not polar opposites. Yuddhishtra, the most virtuous of the Pandava brothers, who had never told an untruth in his life, was a compulsive gambler; the mighty Bhima could not control his temper while another brother had a roving eye for women. At one point in the war, the Pandava army was being decimated by Drona's arrows. The Pandava brothers rushed to Lord Krishna who had agreed to advise them.

'There is only one way,' Lord Krishna said. 'Drona loves his son Ashwathama more than his life. If he hears that Ashwathama is no more, he will lay down his bow and die.

'But why should he believe us?'

'The only one he will believe is Yuddhishtra for every one knows that Yuddhishtra never lies,' Lord Krishna suggested.

Yuddhishtra however refused. 'I can never tell an untruth, even if it means losing this war.'

The Pandava princes again sought Krishna's counsel.

'Well,' said the god, 'You have in your forces an elephant with the same name as Drona's son. If you kill the elephant, then Yuddhishtra just has to say "Ashwathama is dead" and it will not be a lie.'

Yuddhishtra, however, was stubborn, maintaining that he would be stating a fact, not truth. After much persuasion and warnings that evil will triumph on earth if he did not help, Yuddhishtra agreed that he would shout out across enemy lines: 'Ashwathama is dead ... but the elephant', the second part of the sentence to be spoken in a normal tone of voice.

The elephant was duly killed. Yuddhishtra shouted out the news of Ashwathama's death; when he came to 'but the elephant', the Pandvas began beating the drums so that Drona only heard the first part of the sentence. The foremost of archers laid down his bow and died from grief.

Many years after the great war was over and all the protagonists were dead, their souls began the journey to the next world, dropping out one by one on the long way to heaven. Only Yuddhishtra and his dog could come right up to heaven's gates, even Lord Krishna having to spend some time in the nether world for his part in the deceit that led to Drona's death. At heaven's gates, Yuddhishtra is told that he would have to spend one day in hell before he could enter.

'But why?' the virtuousYuddhishtra protested. 'I have never told a lie in my life.'

'Perhaps,' he is informed, 'but on one occasion you did not tell the truth *loudly* enough.'

It is noteworthy that the virtuous Yuddhishtra must atone for an almost non-existent lapse because his context is that of integrity, of the 'man who never lies' while Krishna, the Lord of the Universe and thus of its moral order gets away with a slap on the wrist since his context here is not that of God but of a political and strategic adviser where deception is *de rigeur*.*

Karma, Rebirth, and the Indian Mind

The third essential idea of the Hindu worldview is karma. The popular understanding of karma is expressed by a villager thus: 'Even at the time of death man should wish to do good deeds and wish to be reborn in a place where he can do good deeds again. After many lives of good deeds (the living in dharma) a man will attain *mukti* (another word for moksha). If he does evil deeds, his form changes till he falls lower, till he becomes a *jar* (an inanimate thing).'[10] Other Hindus, when pressed for their sense of karma, are likely to express the same twin ideas: namely the cycles of birth and death in which an individual soul progresses (or regresses) through various levels of existence; and, second, the control of this movement by the karma of the individual soul, the balance of 'right' and 'wrong' actions that accompany the individual from one birth to another.

Psychologically, what interests us most in the karma theory is its idea of innate dispositions (*samskaras*), a heritage of previous life, with which a newborn is believed to come into the world and which imposes certain limits on the socialization of the child. In other words, Indians do not

*In 1976, I was travelling in the Himalayan foothills when I heard the news that the Prime Minister Indira Gandhi had declared a state of emergency and assumed dictatorial powers. I had stopped at a roadside tea shop where I overheard two middle aged men from a nearby village arguing about the step Mrs Gandhi had taken. One of the men, who had heard the Prime Minister's radio broadcast justifying the imposition of the emergency, was vehement in his opposition: 'Can't you see she is lying? Blatant lies!' The other man, a supporter, stopped the argument with the rejoinder, 'So what? In politics (*rajniti*) even Lord Krishna lied.'

consider infant nature as a *tabula rasa* which is infinitely malleable and can be moulded in any direction desired by the parents. With the cultural belief in the notion of samskaras, there is little social pressure to foster the belief that if only the caretakers were good enough, and constantly on their toes, the child's potentialities would be boundlessly fulfilled. With the Indian emphasis on man's inner limits, there is no such sense of urgency and struggle against the outside world, with prospects of sudden metamorphoses and great achievements just around the corner, that often seem to propel Western lives. Let us tell another story.

On the bank of the Ganges, there once lived a holy man called Yajnavalkya together with his wife. One day, as he was meditating, he felt something small and soft fall into the nest of his hands. He opened his eyes and saw that it was a small female mouse which must have fallen down from the claws of an eagle circling above. The holy man had pity on the mouse, and using his occult powers, transformed it into a small girl and took her home. The girl grew up as the daughter of the house, and when she reached marriageable age, Yajnavalkya's wife reproached him one day, saying, 'Don't you see your daughter is mature now and needs a husband?' Yajnavalkya answered, 'You are right. I have decided that she should have the best possible husband in all the worlds.' He then called the Sun-god and when he appeared, Yajnavalkya said, 'I have chosen you as my son-in-law.' He then turned to the girl and asked her, 'Would you like the light of three worlds as your husband?' But she answered, 'Ah father, he is much too plump and red-faced. Find me another husband.' The holy man smiled and asked the sun whether he knew of anyone who was better than him. The sun answered, 'O, holy man! The cloud is even stronger than I am, for it can cover me.' Yajnavalkya called the god of clouds, but once again when he asked his daughter's consent she replied, 'Oh, father, he looks much too morose. Find me a better husband.' Yajnavalkya asked the cloud whether there was someone in the world better than he. The cloud answered, 'The mountain is certainly better, for it can stop me.' The holy man called the mountain god, but the moment he appeared the girl cried out, 'Oh. Father, he is too massive and clumsy, find me a better husband.' Yajnavalkya's patience was nearly exhausted, but since he loved his daughter, he asked the mountain whether he knew of someone who was even better. The mountain answered, 'The mouse can bore as many holes in me as it wants to. Considering that, it must be stronger than I am.' Yajnavalkya called the mouse, and as soon as the girl saw him, she exclaimed, 'Father! This is the only husband I can be happy with. Ah, can't you change me into a mouse?' The holy man fulfilled her wish. And as the two mice disappeared into the bushes, he walked back home, smiling to himself and saying, 'Although the sun, the cloud, and the mountain stood before her as suitors, the mouse-girl needed to become a mouse again. Her innate nature could not be denied.'

The karmic balance from a previous life and, thus, the innate dispositions with which one enters the present one, serve to make a Hindu more accepting of the inevitable disappointments that afflict even the most fortunate of lives. Yet, whereas the notion of inherited dispositions can console and help to heal, it can also serve the purpose of denial of individual responsibility. Thus, a thirty-year old female patient in psychotherapy, becoming aware of her aggressive impulses towards her husband as revealed in a dream, spontaneously exclaimed, 'Ah, these are due to my bad samskaras. However hard I try to be a good wife, my bad samskaras prevent me.'[11]

I and Other—Separation and Connection

If each one of us begins life as mystic, awash in a feeling of pervasive unity where there is no distance between ourselves and the outer world, then the process of sorting out a 'me' from 'not-me is one of the primary tasks of our earliest years. The task involves the recognition—later taken for granted at least in most of our waking hours and in a state of relative sanity—that I am separate from all that is not-I, that my 'self' is not merged but detached from the 'Other.' The experience of separation has its origins in our beginnings although its echoes continue to haunt us till the end of life, its reverberations agitating the mind—at times violently—in times of psychological or spiritual crisis.

The Indian gloss on the dilemmas and pain of banishment from the original feeling of oneness, the exile from universe, has been to emphasize a person's enduring connection to nature, the Divine, and all living beings. This unitary vision, of *soma* and psyche, individual and community, self and world, is present in most forms of popular culture even today. From religious rites to folk festivals, from the pious devotion of communal singing in temples to the orgiastic excesses of *holi*, the festival of colors, there is a negation of separation and a celebration of connection.

The high cultural value placed on connection is, of course, most evident in the individual's relationships with others. The yearning for relationships, for the confirming presence of loved ones and the psychological oxygen they provide, is the dominant modality of social relations in India, especially within the extended family. Individuality and independence are not values that are cherished. It is not uncommon for family members who often accompany a patient for a first psychotherapeutic interview, to complain about the patient's *autonomy* as one of the symptoms of his disorder. Thus, the father and elder sister of a 28-years-old engineer who had a psychotic episode described their understanding of his chief problem as one of unnatural autonomy:

'He is very stubborn in pursuing what he wants without taking our wishes into account. He thinks he knows what is best for him and does not listen to us. He thinks his own life and career are more important than the concerns of the rest of the family.'[12]

The high value placed on connection does not mean that an Indian is incapable of functioning when he is by himself or that he does not have a sense of his own agency. What it does imply is his greater need for ongoing mentorship, guidance, and help from others in getting through life and a greater vulnerability to feelings of helplessness when these ties are strained.

The yearning for relationships, for the confirming presence of loved ones, and the distress aroused by their unavailability in time of need, are more hidden in Western societies where the dominant value system prizes the values of autonomy, privacy, and self-actualization, and holds that individual independence and initiative are 'better' than mutual dependence and community. However, it depends of course, on the culture's vision of a 'good society' and 'individual merit' whether a person's behaviour on the scale between fusion and isolation is nearer the pole of merger and fusion with others or the pole of complete isolation. In other words, the universal polarities of individual versus relational, nearness versus distance in human relationships are prey to culturally moulded beliefs and expectations.

The emphasis on connection is also reflected in the Indian image of the body, a core element in the development of the mind. As we saw earlier, in the traditional medical system of Ayurveda, everything in the universe, animate or inanimate is believed to be made of five forms of matter. Living beings are only a certain kind of organization of matter. Their bodies constantly absorb the five elements of environmental matter. In Ayurveda, the human body is intimately connected with nature and the cosmos and there is nothing in nature without relevance for medicine. The Indian body image, then, stresses an unremitting interchange taking place with the environment, simultaneously accompanied by a ceaseless change within the body. Moreover, in the Indian view, there is no essential difference between body and mind. The body is merely the gross form of matter (*sthulasharira*), just as the mind is a more subtle form of the same matter (*sukshmasharira*); both are different forms of the same body–mind matter, *sharira*.

In contrast, the Western image is of a clearly etched body, sharply differentiated from the rest of the objects in the universe. This vision of the body as a safe stronghold with a limited number of drawbridges that maintain a tenuous contact with the outside world has its own cultural consequences. It seems to us that in Western discourse, both scientific and artistic, there is considerable preoccupation with what is going on *within* the fortress of the individual body. Preeminently, one seeks to explain behaviour through psychologies that derive from biology—to the relative exclusion of the natural and meta-natural environment. The contemporary search for a genetic basis to all psychological phenomena, irrespective of its scientific merit, is, thus, a natural consequence of the Western body image. The natural aspects of the environment—the quality of air, the quantity of sunlight, the presence of birds and animals, the plants and the trees, are a priori viewed, when they are considered at all, as irrelevant to intellectual and emotional development. Given the Western image of the body, it is understandable that the more 'far-out' Indian beliefs regarding the effects on the sharira of planetary constellations, cosmic energies, earth's magnetic fields, seasonal and daily rhythms, precious stones and metals are summarily consigned to the realm of fantasy, where they are of interest solely to a 'lunatic fringe' of Western society.

It is not only the body but also the emotions that have come to be differently viewed by the Indian emphasis on connection. As cultural psychologists have pointed out, such emotions as sympathy, feelings of interpersonal communion, and shame, which have to do with other persons, become primary while the more individualistic emotions such as anger and guilt are secondary. The Indian mind has a harder time experiencing and expressing anger and guilt but is more comfortable than the Western individualistic psyche in dealing with feelings of sympathy and shame. If pride is overtly expressed, it is often directed to a collective of whom the self is a part. Working very hard to win a promotion at work is only secondarily connected to the individual need for achievement, the primary driving motivation in the West. The first conscious or pre-conscious thought in the Indian mind is, 'How happy and proud my family will be!' This is why Indians tend to idealize their families and ancestral background, why there is such a prevalence of family myths and of family pride, and why role models for the young are almost exclusively members of the family, very frequently a parent, rather than the movie stars, sporting heroes, or other public figures favoured by Western youth.

This greater 'dividual'[3] (in contrast to 'individual') or relational orientation is also congruent with the main thematic content of Indian art. In traditional Indian painting and especially in temple sculptures, for instance, man is not represented as a discrete presence but absorbed in his surroundings—the individual, not separate but existing in all his myriad connections. These sculptures, as Thomas Mann in his Indian novella *The Transposed Heads* remarks, are an 'all encompassing labyrinth flux of animal, human and divine ... visions of life in the flesh, all jumbled together ... suffering and enjoying in thousand shapes, teeming, devouring, turning into one another.'[14]

If one thinks of Eros not in its narrow meaning of sex but in its wider connotation of a loving 'connectedness' (where the sexual embrace is only the most intimate of all connections), then the relational cast to the Indian mind makes Indians more 'erotic' than many other peoples of the world. The relational orientation, however, also easily slips into conformity and conventional behaviour, making many Indians psychologically old even when young. On the other hand, the Western individualistic orientation has a tendency towards self-aggrandizement, 'the looking out for Number One', and the belief that the gratification of desires—most of them related to consumption—is the royal road to happiness. In a post-modern accentuation of 'fluid identities' and a transitional attitude towards relationships, of 'moving on', contemporary Western man (and the modern upper class Indian) may well embody what the Jungians call *puer aeternus*—the eternal youth, ever in pursuit of *his* dreams, full of vitality, but nourishing only to himself while draining those around him.[15]

We are, of course, not advancing any simplified dichotomy between a Western cultural image of an individual, autonomous self, and a relational, transpersonal self of Indian society. These are prototypical patterns that do not exist in their pure form in any society. Autonomy of the self, psychotherapy with patients of the Western middle class tells us, is as precarious in reality as is the notion of an Indian self that is merged in the surround of its family and community. Both visions of human experience are present in all the major cultures though a particular culture may, over a length of time, highlight and emphasize one at the expense of the other. Historically, man's connection to the universe, especially his community, has also been an important value in Western tradition, though it may have been submerged at certain periods of history, especially in the nineteenth and early twentieth centuries. This, a so-called value of counter-enlightenment, is a part of the relativist and sceptical tradition that goes back to Western antiquity. It stresses that belonging to a community is a fundamental need of man and asserts that only if a man truly belongs to such a community, naturally and unselfconsciously, can he enter the living stream and lead a full, creative, spontaneous life. Similarly, the celebration of the pleasures of individuality and of a desire-driven life, though muted, have not been completely absent in India and are, indeed, currently enjoying a resurgence among many modern Indians.

In conclusion, let us again emphasize that the Hindu worldview, the relational orientation,[16] that go into the formation of the Indian mind, are not abstractions to be more or less hazily comprehended during the adult years. They are constituents of an Indian's psyche, absorbed by the child in his relationship with his caretakers from the very beginning of life as the underlying truth of the world. Rarely summoned for conscious examination, this cultural part of mind is neither determinedly universal nor utterly idiosyncratic. The mental representation of our cultural heritage, it remains in constant conversation with the universal and individual aspects of our mind throughout life, each influencing and shaping the other two at every moment of our being.

Notes and References

1 For an elaboration of the Hindu worldview, see Kakar, Sudhir, 1978, *The Inner World: A Psychoanalytical Study of Childhood and Society in India,* Delhi and New York: Oxford University Press, ch. 2.

2 Ramanujan, A.K. 'Is there an Indian Way of Thinking?' in Marriott, M. (ed.), 1990, *India through Hindu Categories*, Newbury, CA: Sage, pp. 41–58.

3 Müeller, F. Max, 2000, *India: What Can It Teach Us*?, New Delhi: Penguin.

4 *Manu*, VIII, p. 267.

5 Gautama cited in Ramanujan, 'Is There an Indian Way of Thinking', p. 46.

6 *Manu*, VIII, pp. 352–62.

7 *Kamasutra*, Book V.

8 Shweder, R. and Bourne E.J., 'Does the Concept of the Person Vary Cross-culturally?' in R. Shweder and R. Levine (eds), 1986, *Culture Theory*, New York: Cambridge University Press, pp. 158–99.

9 Kakar, Sudhir, 1995, *The Colours of Violence*, Delhi: Viking-Penguin, ch. 5.

10 Kakar, *Inner World*, pp. 44–5.

11 Ibid., p. 49

12 Kakar, Sudhir, 1985, 'Psychoanalysis and Non-western Cultures', *International Review of Psychoanalysis*, 12, pp. 441–8.

13 The expression is by McKim Marriott; see his 'Hindu Transactions: Diversity without Duality' in Kapferer, B. (ed.), 1976, *Transactions and Meaning*, Philadelphia: Institute for the Study of Human Issues, pp. 109–42.

14 Cited in Lannoy, R., 1976, *The Speaking Tree*, London: Oxford University Press, p. 78.

15 Franz, M., 2000, *Puer Aeternus: A Psychological Study of the Adult Struggle with the Paradise of Childhood*, Toronto: Inner City Books. We owe this reference and observation to David Johnston 'A Comprehensive Approach to Psychotherapy', Unpublished MS, November 2005.

16 Elaborated in the chapter 'Clinical Work and Cultural Imagination'.

Culture and Society

A Conversation with Sudhir Kakar

MANASI KUMAR (MK): There cannot be a better time to seek a psychoanalytic perspective on Indian society and to understand the schism between the popular perception of Indian culture and the more deep-rooted psycho-historical and cultural heritage of India from an accomplished social scientist and psychoanalytic scholar like yourself. In your paper on alternative sexuality, you make a point that alternative sexualities have historically had a fraught position. While the ridicule and pathologization was always there, the persecution of those practising homosexuality is a more recent phenomenon. You also point to psychoanalysis as such being unfair to the discourse around women's psychology (and rights) and homosexuality. How do you see this debate on alternate sexuality in India shaping at this point in time? Do you feel it has greater acceptability?

SUDHIR KAKAR (SK): The most heartening point of the debate is not how it is shaping up but that it is happening at all. And this is due to the typical swing of the pendulum of Indian imagination between the ascetic and the erotic, each swing sometimes lasting for centuries. Since the last five decades, the swing has been again towards the erotic pole, which includes a willingness to engage with and acceptance of alternate sexualities. Thus, in spite of all the conservative opposition, some glaring intolerances of alternate sexualities, such as its criminalizing, are all set to disappear.

These swings between liberal and conservative, erotic and ascetic, are now getting faster because of our increasing participation in a global information structure where the global trend for a while has been towards a freeing of the erotic to a point of 'anything goes'. Of course, the conservative reaction, the reverse swing of the pendulum, taking heart from global cues, can be equally fast and what one can hope for in the near future is incremental gains.

MK: In the essay 'Is the Indian Woman a Person?', you revisit the cultural narrative of what it means to be a woman in Indian society and how the changing roles and times have not necessarily shifted the unconscious biases and layering of male dominance and ownership of woman. How do you look at the current denigration and violence targeted to women, especially modern women? What does the Indian woman need to do to be treated as a person?

SK: Until perhaps recently, the Indian male unconscious was organized to scan for signals of a woman's personhood, categorizing a woman as a person only when she appears to be a mother, a daughter, a sister, wife (or even in more distant relationships such as aunt, grandmother, or niece). The mental constructions I am talking of are deep-seated, often less than conscious, and are inculcated in early childhood by the family that is tasked with conveying the ideology of gender and gender relations of the society of which it is a part. Since modern women do not easily fit into the traditional mental categories of what constitutes a woman's personhood in their dress or deportment, these women cannot be accommodated to the relational blueprint of the woman that men have carried in their minds since childhood. Not perceived as persons, modern women encountered in the anonymity of the city are automatically, without the intervention of thought or reflection, consigned to an ambivalently despised, rest category of the *aurat* (woman) who is potentially a '*bhog ki cheez*', an object and not a subject.

Such an aurat is an accepted target for an otherwise unconscious rage many Indian men harbour against women, a rage that goes back all the way to the consciously idealized mother of childhood. In clinical psychoanalytic work with male Hindu Indian patients, I have often come across the existence of what I have called 'maternal enthralment': the wish to get away from the mother together with the dread of separation, the wish to destroy the engulfing mother who also ensures the child's survival, and, finally, incestuous desire coexisting with the terror inspired by an overwhelming female sexuality. Maternal enthralment is the largely unconscious underside of the overt and ubiquitous idealization of the mother by the Hindu son, influences unconscious attitudes towards women.

How do we approach modernity in a way that does not burden women with the responsibility of signalling their personhood or else risking violence? One way is to emphasize the individual and not the relational core of a woman's personhood. This has huge support from our Constitution, and thus the judiciary, which regards the individual and not the community as the repository of fundamental rights. However, individual lawyers and judges are still very biased by the unconscious filters I discussed earlier. The difficulty is that a recourse to the Constitution, which is based on the model of the centrality of the individual, goes against the communitarian way of thought of much of our country. Rather than dismiss the communitarian vision of life as outdated, regressive, or pathological, we need to recognize the enormous emotional valence that the community vision of life has for many Indians. In this vision of life, community sentiments and community honour take precedence over individual ones. Both women and men feel less of a sense of identification as an individual and more as part of the community, which means they affectively resonate more deeply with community sentiments than with individual rights.

Problematic, and vital to understanding violence against women, is that in the community vision, a woman, especially her sexuality, symbolizes the honour, the *izzat*, of the community. There is no price that the group is unwilling to pay to protect its honour, even if this involves the death of a daughter, sister, or wife. In so-called honour killings it is the woman who must first die or be killed for the conflict between familial love and izzat to end; any other solution, even if it be legally acceptable, simply will not do because it does not touch the affective charge of community identification.

Yet, I believe in the power of insight to alter beliefs and change behaviour. By bringing the underlying issues in honour killings and violence against women to awareness rather than simply condemning them as expressions of an outdated patriarchy, I believe there can be a change in attitudes within a generation. For we must remember, the killers of a young woman transgressing community norms are not unredeemable villains, but very often family members, charged with nurturance and protection of their wards, who are impelled by the power of group forces to betray a sacred trust. These men become convinced, at least in the moment, that loyalty to norms of the family, clan, and caste is what really makes life worth living. If we seek the kind of social change in which violence against women becomes a thing of the past, we need to think creatively about how these men may be encouraged to identify with their daughters rather than with the group of men who go on the honour killing rampage. One possibility is that mass media and grassroots organizations could be leveraged to promote the notion of fatherhood as a group phenomenon in which belonging, status, and recognition is conferred to fathers who support their daughters' individual choice, a new credo of izzat. The huge challenge of Indian modernity will be finding ways to nurture heterogeneous individual rights in ways that are harmonious with and draw upon the affective and unifying power of community structures rather than simply threaten to dismantle them.

MK: In the paper 'In Krishna's Mouth' you say that 'universality for the Hindu is the conviction that the fundamental insights of his faith also lie at the heart of all other religions'. Yet this is one thing that is forgotten by Hindu Right-wing thinkers when they question other faiths and influences in the Indian cultural psyche. At one end you bring out this beauty of the Hindu philosophy but you also allude to the infantilism in seeing every other practice or faith as being part of its own fabric. Can you elaborate on this?

SK: It is one of Hinduism's verities that all religions are different paths to the same truth: 'Ekam Sat, Viprah Bahudda Vadanti' (One truth, many ways of reaching it). For Hindu nationalist thinkers, however, universalism takes the form of a tolerance of the elite for the 'lower orders'. For them, Hindu pluralism does not exclude a hierarchy among the various faiths; there are many ways but not all of them are equal.

Although the theme of its universality is uncontested within Hinduism, the nationalist is unhappy with some of its consequences. He worries whether in placing so much emphasis on universality, on the Vedic dictum of 'Vasudhaiva Kutumbkam' (the universe is one family), Hindus have not sacrificed the development of a community feeling and the necessary unity which they have lacked in the past and which they need to face the challenge of other, more militant faiths. He is concerned whether the concept of 'Vishvabandhutva' (universal brotherhood) has not led to a weakening of 'Deshbandhutva' (national brotherhood) and 'Dharmabandhutva' (religious brotherhood). To adapt Faust's lament, in contrast to the traditional Hindu whose spirit only seeks a single quest, there are two conflicting souls, of universality and nationalism, of Hindutva militancy and Hindu dharma tolerance, that dwell in the nationalist breast, with each, if it could, gladly sundering from the other.

Finally, in perceiving other religions as all pointing towards the same truth, and thus accepting other religious traditions from the vantage point of a higher 'universal' Hindu wisdom (and not in terms of their own self-characterization), Hindu nationalists may ultimately be hindering a dialogue with other faiths. Perhaps what Yashoda saw in Krishna's mouth was the world of Hindu cosmology which the master narrative of Hinduism, with all good intentions, insists on identifying with the universe of all faiths. Given birth by the seductive power of this narrative, entranced by Yashoda's vision, the nationalist's expectation of a coming triumph of Hindu thought and belief in a globalized world is fated to be disappointed. Illusions, irrespective of their worth in mobilizing large numbers of peoples or creating utopian communities, ultimately remain just that … illusions.

MK: India is changing. The world is changing so rapidly. Politics, social media, cultural values, and traditions are evolving. Given the backdrop of this volume, there could be a number of questions in the domain of Indian culture and society in the minds of most readers, who would be keen to know your understanding of the changing dynamics, Professor Kakar. You have been a close observer, commentator, and analyst of the changing behavioural foundation of individuals, which delineate why people behave how they behave. Therefore, I would like as some questions that I feel your essays in this volume open up in the context of events today. In Indian Society, two dominant religious groups, Hindus and Muslims, have been living together at least since the early eighth century AD—harmoniously or otherwise, we do not know. But one thing we know with certainty is that Muslims are decisively in an adverse situation now than any previous point in history. So you think what has happened was inevitable?

SK: Events become inevitable only when we confuse our wishes with reality or interpret parts of reality in accordance with our wishes. Mahatma Gandhi was a realist and I cannot agree with him more. In 1924, he observed, 'I see no way of achieving anything in this afflicted country without a lasting heart unity between Hindus and Mussalmans.

... There is no question more important and more pressing than this. In my opinion, it blocks all progress."

My views on the whole issue were detailed in my 1995 book *The Colours of Violence* and in some of the papers in this volume. Briefly, I believe both the Hindu nationalist and the secularist have long engaged in wishful constructions. The Hindu nationalist believes the only way is a change in the Muslim view of the community's role, traditions, and institutions so that the Muslim can 'adapt' to the Hindu majority's culture. To ask Muslims to recognize themselves in the Hindu nationalist version of Indian history, to expect them to feel their culture confirmed in Hindu symbols, rituals, and celebrations is asking them to renounce their religious–cultural identity and to erase their collective memory so that they become indistinguishable from their Hindu neighbours. To be swamped by the surrounding Hindu culture has been the greatest fear of the Indian Muslim, an assimilation feared precisely because it is so tempting, holding the promise of a freedom from fear of violence and full participation in the majority culture. The Hindu nationalist's dilemma is that Muslims continue to decline an offer the nationalist believes they cannot refuse. The nationalist finds that the Muslim is too big to either swallow or spit out.

The 'secularist', who views the conflict as rooted in socio-economic considerations, believes the economic development of India will alter the social–structural conditions and thus assign the conflict, as the cliché would have it, 'to the dust heap of history'. Religious identities, he believes, will fade away and play less and less of a role in private and, especially, in public life. I am sceptical of the belief in the primacy of political and economic structures in the shaping of 'consciousness' (in which unconscious imagination plays a dominant role). Our consciousness is as much shaped, if not more, by cultural traditions transmitted through the family. We may have to give up Gandhi's dream of 'lasting heart unity' and content ourselves with the creation of a common public realm while regarding the other community with 'benign indifference' in private. There will be inevitable violence on the way.

MK: This question becomes important as Hindus had a sense of subjugation in the higher position in court, rulings, and so on, against Arab, Turk, Afghan, Uzbeks, and British. In documented history, Rehmat Ali and Iqbalor Jinnah could have pursued creation of a separate homeland for Indian Muslims, but in popular perception there are anecdotes and perfunctory evidence that even during late seventeenth

and early eighteenth centuries Mirasian (nomad singers) would sing that there will soon be a time where Muslim rule and Sharia law would be well established. And there will be a holy land for Muslims. You have written a lot on Indian people and their stereotypes, do you think India was tailor-made for a theocratic state and the experiment of a secular progressive state of inclusive nationalism is a failed experiment? Sitting where you are today, where do you see India thirty–fifty years from now?

SK: Given the march of exclusive nationalism all over the world in recent years, religious nationalism in Turkey, India, and much of the Islamic world, racial nationalism in the United States of America, and cultural 'sons of the soil' nationalism in most of Europe, one would be tempted to say that a secular, inclusive nationalism was a liberal dream which has few takers today. Yet, a nation where a large part of the population sees itself as victims and the majority as persecutors is sitting on a powder keg of repressed rage that can blow up at any time. I am more concerned about the next five to ten years than the long-term future, which is completely unpredictable. But what we do need to develop in the next thirty–fifty years, and preferably much sooner, is a vision of inclusive nationalism that is not of the 'secular, 'progressive' kind, which pays exaggerated homage to man's reason and conditions of material life, but a consciousness irradiated by the inclusiveness of spiritual traditions of mankind. The essence of these traditions is encapsulated in the Golden Rule, 'Do unto others what you wish others to do unto you.' In its maximal, most unconditional form, we encounter it in the Upanishads as 'he who sees all beings in his own self and his own self in all beings' and in the Christian injunction 'love thy neighbor as thyself'. In its minimal incarnation, we meet it in the Jewish Talmudic version in the words of Rabbi Hillel: 'What is hateful to yourself, do not to your fellow man. That is the whole of the Torah and the rest is but commentary.' Since the contemporary ruling deity in formation of consciousness is science and not religious–moral exhortations, we need to highlight recent developments in social psychology, socio-biology, and social neurosciences that emphasize the innate altruism of human beings, findings that demonstrate that 'doing good to others is actually doing good to yourself'. My hope, or wishful construction if you will, is that we will come to realize more and more that each one of us is deeply embedded with other human beings as also connected to animate and inanimate nature, an embeddedness demands caring for all that is not the self for our own health and happiness. Science and spirituality will combine to support St. Francis' prayer, 'Grant, that I may not so much seek to be consoled as to console; to be understood, as to understand; to be loved as to love; for it is in giving that we receive.' Or His Holiness Dalai Lama's flat statement, 'Paying attention to one's own needs is a producer of suffering; cherishing others a giver of happiness.' For me, this is a more lasting basis of an inclusive nationalism.

MK: In the paper on health and medicine in the living traditions of Hinduism, you explain how notions of health and medicine are understood in Hinduism. Do you think there have been developments in understanding health or medicine in modern Ayurveda that are worth mentioning here with regards to mental health in modern times? Do you think the understanding of manas **has changed over the period of time?**

SK: No, unfortunately not. New developments, in Ayurveda, or any other ancient system, are very difficult because of two reasons. The first is the belief that what needed to be known was known long ago. Time has just distorted that knowledge and its recovery in the original pure form is more important than any new additions. The second is the ancient Indian love of categorization: three types of this, four of that, ten of that, and so on. For instance, the three personality types—sattvik, rajas, and *tamasik*—become essentialist in the modern sense (besides being moralistic), and go against the grain of modern developments that conceive of the person in much more fluid terms rather than attributing it any fixity.

MK: In your paper on Indian love stories, you make some interesting observations that women seem to be more active as players in love stories and that in the context of what you call the 'dream of love', the woman who falls out of her marriage suffers incredibly, but this suffering also has a cultural prescription. On the one hand, you talk about the value of suffering as it brings us closer to the truth and on the other hand, you talk about suffering in love being the fate of the womankind? I keep asking you if things have changed, and if this perception has changed. Is the suffering of the woman in love inevitable?

SK: The privileging of suffering in love in our culture goes back to ancient Sanskrit poetry in which *viraha*, love in separation, was considered to be superior to *shringara*, love in union. And this is not limited to women. Majnun, the quintessential lover in many parts of north India influenced by Persian–Islamic culture, values the suffering caused by his separation from his beloved Layla more than the sexual union with her. In fact, he refuses to consummate his love when offered the opportunity to do so. And although the idea of suffering in love as somehow being superior to its satisfaction is being increasingly questioned, it still commands considerable psychic presence. The figure of Devdas, mocked and admired at the same time, testifies to the continuing hold suffering exercises on the cultural imagination of love and the ideal lover.

The questioning is greater among modern young women who refuse to see themselves as passive victims in the enterprise of love. A greater confidence in themselves as active agents and staking a claim to their own desire, the *shringara* songs of pleasure have begun to occupy more space than the suffering ones of *viraha*.

MK: Your paper on intimacy and beyond talks about sexuality, intimacy, and generativity as three interconnected themes of adulthood. Is pleasurable and satisfactory intimacy contingent on expressed mutuality in appraisal and sharing of needs? Which of these is most valuable from the psychoanalytic point of view? Do you think the Indian cultural psyche endorses one over the other?

SK: All three are closely and intimately connected parts of a whole. If asked to gauge their relative importance, I would say sexuality in early adulthood, intimacy in middle adulthood, and generativity in late adulthood. Indian culture has perhaps unduly emphasized generativity at the expense of others.

Bibliography

Books

Non-fiction

Federick Taylor: A Study in Personality and Innovation, 1970, Cambridge: MIT Press.

(co-edited with Kamla Chowdhry) *Understanding Organizational Behavior*, 1970, Delhi: Tata-McGraw Hill.

(co-authored with Kamla Cowdhry) *Conflict and Choice: Indian Youth in a Changing Society*, 1971, Bombay: Somaiya.

The Inner World: A Psychoanalytic Study of Childhood and Society in India, 1978, Delhi: Oxford University Press.

———, Second edition, 1981; Sixteen impressions.

———, Third edition, 2008.

———, French translation, 1985, Paris: Les Belles Lettres.

———, Spanish translation, 1987, Mexico: Fondo de Cultura.

———, German translation, 1988, Frankfurt: Nexus Verlag; Second edition, 2006).

———, Italian translation, 2007, Milan: Vivarium.

———, Hindi translation: 2008, Delhi: Vani Prakashan.

(edited, with a contribution and an Introduction) *Identity and Adulthood*, 1980, Delhi: Oxford University Press; Third impression, 1998).

Shamans, Mystics, and Doctors: A Psychological Inquiry into India and its Healing Traditions, 1982, New York: A. Knopf.

———, Indian edition, 1982, Delhi: Oxford University Press; Ninth impression, 2003).

———, British edition, 1984, London: Allen & Unwin.
———, Paperback edition, 1983, Boston: Beacon Press; 1991, Chicago: University of Chicago Press.
———, German translation, 1984, Munich: Biederstein Verlag; Second edition, 2006), Munich: Beck Verlag.
———, Spanish translation, 1990, Mexico: Fondo de Cultura.
———, Marathi translation, 1993, Bombay: Majestic.
———, Italian translation, 1993, Parma: Pratiche Editrice; Second edition: 1995.
———, French translation, 1997, Paris: du Seuil.
———, Hindi translation, 2005, Delhi: Rajkamal Prakashan.
———, Turkish translation, In press, Istanbul: Paradigma Yayiniari.
(co-authored with John Munder Ross) *Tales of Love, Sex, and Danger*, 1986, Delhi: Oxford University Press.
———, Second edition, 2011.
———, British edition, 1987, London: Unwin Hyman.
———, US edition, 1988, New York: Blackwell.
———, German translation, 1986, Munich: Beck Verlag.
———, French translation, 1987, Paris: PUF.
———, Italian translation, 1991, Como: Lyra Libri.
Intimate Relations: Exploring Indian Sexuality, 1990, Chicago: University of Chicago Press.
———, Indian edition, 1989, Delhi: Penguin-Viking.
———, French translation, 1990, Paris: Des Femmes, 1990.
———, Marathi translation, 1992, Pune: Raghuvanshi.
———, German translation, 1994, Munich: Verlag Waldsgut.
———, Italian translation, 1995, Parma: Pratiche Editrice.
———, Hindi translation, 2006, Delhi: Vani Prakashan.
The Analyst and the Mystic, 1992, Chicago: University of Chicago Press.
———, Indian edition, 1991, Delhi: Penguin-Viking.
(co-authored with C. Clement) *La Folle Et Le Saint*, 1993, Paris: du Seuil.
———, German translation, 1993, Munich: Beck Verlag.
———, Portuguese translation, 1997, Rio de Janeiro: Relume Dumara.
———, Italian translation, 1998, Rome: Corbaccio.
The Colours of Violence: Cultural Identities, Religion and Conflict, 1996, Chicago: University of Chicago Press.
———, Indian edition, 1995, Delhi: Viking.
———, German translation, 1997, Munich: Beck Verlag.
———, Hindi translation, In press, Delhi: Rajkamal.
Culture and Psyche: Selected Papers on Psychoanalysis and India, 1996, Delhi: Oxford University Press.
———, US edition, 1997, New York: Psyche Press.
———, German translation, In press, Giessen: Psychosozial Verlag.
The Indian Psyche, 1996, Delhi: Oxford University Press.

The Essential Writings of Sudhir Kakar, 2001, Delhi: Oxford University Press.
(co-authored with Wendy Doniger) *KAMASUTRA: A New Translation*, 2002, London: Oxford University Press.
———, US edition, 2002, New York: Oxford University Press.
———, Indian edition, 2002, Delhi: Oxford University Press.
———, German translation, 2004, Berlin:Wagenbach.
———, Italian translation, 2003, Milan: Adelphi Edizoni.
———, Latvian translation, 2004, Riga: Zvaigzne.
———, Norwegian translation, 2004, Oslo: Kagge Forlag.
———, Spanish translation, 2004, Madrid: Editorial Edaf.
———, French translation, 2006, Paris: du Seuil.
(co-authored with K. Kakar) *The Indians: Portrait of a People*, 2007, Delhi: Viking-Penguin.
———, German translation, 2006, Munich: Beck Verlag.
———, French translation, 2006, Paris: Seuil.
———, Italian translation, 2008, Milan: Neri Pozza.
———, Hindi translation, 2009, Delhi: Penguin.
———, Malyalam translation, 2010, Kottyam: DC Books.
Mad and Divine: Spirit and Psyche in the Modern World, 2008, Delhi: Viking-Penguin.
———, US edition, 2009, Chicago: University of Chicago Press.
———, German translation, 2010, Munich: Beck.
———, French translation, 2010, Paris: Seuil.
A Book of Memory: Confessions and Reflections, 2011, Delhi: Penguin-Viking.
———, German translation, In press, Munich: Beck Verlag.
———, Malyalam translation, In press, Kottyam: DC Books.
(edited) *On Dreams and Dreaming*, 2011, Delhi: Penguin-Viking.
(co-edited with J. Kripal) *Seriously Strange: Thinking Anew Psychic Phenomena*, In press, Delhi: Penguin-Viking.

Fiction

The Ascetic of Desire, 1998, Delhi: Penguin-Viking.
———, German translation, 1999, Munich: Beck Verlag.
———, Hindi translation, 1999, Delhi: Rajkamal.
———, US edition, 2000, New York: Overlook Press.
———, Brazilian edition, 2000, Rio de Janeiro: Companhia das Letras.
———, Italian translation, 2000, Milan: Neri Pozza.
———, French translation, 2001, Paris: du Seuil.
———, Portuguese edition, 2001, Lisbon: Edition Temas y Debates.
———, Hungarian translation, 2001, Budapest: Ulpius-haz.
———, Romanian translation, 2007, Bucharest: Trei.
———, Spanish translation, In press, Barcelona: Plaza y Janes.
———, Gujarati translation, In press, Ahmedabad: Image Publishing.

———, Russian translation, In press, Moscow: Ripol.
(edited) *Indian Love Stories*, 1999, Delhi: Roli Books.
———, German translation, 2006, Munich: Beck Verlag.
———, Italian translation, 2007, Milan: Neri Pozza.
Ecstasy, 2001, Delhi: Viking-Penguin.
———, German translation, 2001, Munich: Beck Verlag.
———, US edition, 2002, New York: Overlook Press.
———, Hindi translation, 2002, Delhi: Rajkamal.
———, Serbian translation, 2003, Belgrade: Stylos.
———, Italian translation, 2004, Milan: Neri Pozza.
———, French translation, 2005, Paris: du Seuil.
———, Russian translation, In press, Moscow: Sophia.
Mira and the Mahatma, 2004, Delhi: Viking-Penguin.
———, Hindi translation, 2004, Delhi: Rajkamal.
———, German translation, 2005, Munich: Beck Verlag.
———, Korean translation, 2006, Seoul: Moonhak Soochup.
———, Indonesian translation, 2006, Jakarta: Mizan Pustaka.
———, French translation, 2007, Paris: du Seuil.
———, Italian translation, 2007, Milan: Neri Pozza.
———, Brazilian edition, 2007, Rio de Janiero: Relume Dumara.
———, Marathi translation, 2007, Pune: Rajhans Prakashan.
———, US edition, 2008, Boston: Trumpeter Press.
———, Spanish translation, 2008, Barcelona: Circe.
———, Malyalam translation, 2009, Kottyam: DC Books.
———, Turkish translation, 2010, Istanbul: Kaknus.
The Crimson Throne, 2010, Delhi: Viking-Penguin.
———, Italian translation, In press, Milan: Neri Pozza.
———, Marathi translation, In press, Pune: Rajkamal.

Monographs

Indian Childhood: The R.V. Parulekar Memorial Lectures, 1979, New Delhi: Oxford University Press.

Chapters in Books

'3300 Goetter, die eine Einheit sind', in J. Ross and P. Schwartz (eds), 2008, *Was soll ich glauben—Die Weltreligionen*, Freiburg: Herder.
'Rumors and Riots', in G.A. Fine, V. Campion-Vincent, and C. Heath (eds), 2005, *Rumor Mills: The Social Impact of Rumor and Legend*, New York: Aldine.
'Myth and Psychoanalytic Concepts: Experiences from India', in Wen-shing Tseng (ed.), 2004, *Asian Culture and Psychotherapy: Implication for East and West*, Honolulu: University of Hawaii Press.

'Glaube und Begehren: Zur Psychoanalyse der spirituellen Suche', in A. Gerlach (ed.), 2004, *Psychoanalyse des Glaubens*, Giessen: Psychosozial Verlag.

'Psychoanalysis and Eastern Spiritual Healing Traditions', in J.A. Belzen and A. Geels (eds), 2003, *Mysticism: A Variety of Psychological Approaches*, Amsterdam: International Series in Psychology of Religion.

'On Domestic Violence', in F. Mayor (ed.), 1998, *Taking Action for Human Rights in the Twenty-first Century*, Paris: UNESCO.

'The Search for Middle Age in India', in R. Shweder (ed.), 1998, *Welcome to Middle Age, and Other Cultural Fictions*, Chicago: University of Chicago Press.

'Religious Conflict in the Modern World', in R. Ivekovic and N. Pagon (eds), 1998, *Otherhood and Nation*, Ljublijana: Institutum Studiorum Humanitatis.

'The Construction of a New Hindu Identity', in K. Basu and S. Subramanyan (eds), 1996, *Unravelling the Nation*, Delhi: Penguin.

'Klinische Arbeit und Kulturelle Imagination', in P. Mohring and R. Apsel (eds), 1995, *Interkulturelle Psychoanalytische Therapie*, Frankfurt: Brandes & Apsel.

'Gandhi et le fantasme de l'erotisme', in L. Lapierre (ed.),1992, *Imaginaire et leadership*, Montreal: Presses HEC.

'Some Unconscious Aspects of Ethnic Violence in India', in V. Das(ed.), 1990, *Mirrors of Violence*, Delhi: Oxford University Press.

'Psychoanalysis in India: Text and Context', in J. Stigler, R. Shweder, et. al (eds), 1989, *Cultural Psychology*, New York: Cambridge University Press.

'Health and Medicine in the Living Traditions of Hinduism', in L. Sullivan (ed.), 19989, *Health in World Religious Traditions*, New York: Macmillan.

'Das Hindustische Weltbild' and 'Der Mensch in Ayurveda', in D. Reimenschneider (ed.), 1986, *Shiva tanzt: Das Indien Lesebuch*, Zurich: Union Verlag.

'Psychotherapy and Culture: Healing in the Indian Tradition', in S. Pollack and M. White (eds), 1986, *The Cultural Transition*, New York: Basic Books.

'The Child in India', in *Aditi* Catalogue, 1985, Washington: Smithsonian Press; also in A. Cohn and L. Leach (eds), 1987, *Generations*, New York: Pantheon.

'Fathers & Sons: The Indian Experience', in S. Cath, A. Gurwit, and J. Ross (eds), 1982, *Father & Child: Developmental and Clinical Perspectives*, Boston: Atlantic Little Brown.

Six Chapters on the Healthy Personality, in 1982, *Encyclopedia of Health*, vol.3, Lausanne: Editions Grammont; (in Spanish) *La Personalidad Sana*, Barcelona: Salvat Editores.

(with Ashis Nandy) 'Culture and Personality in India', in U. Pareek (ed.), *Review of Research in Psychology*, New Delhi: Indian Council of Social Science Research.

'Images of the Life Cycle and Adulthood in Hindu India', in E. James Anthony and C. Chiland (eds), 1978, *The Child in his Family*: Children and their Parents in a Changing World, New York: John Wiley.

Papers in Professional Journals

'The Resurgence of Imagination', 2009, *Harvard Divinity Bulletin*, 37(1).

'Culture and Psychoanalysis', 2006, *Social Analysis*, 50(2).

'Hindoe-moslimgeweld', 2004, *Groepspsychotherapie*, 38(2).
'Psychoanalysis and Eastern Spiritual Healing Traditions', 2003, *Journal of Analytical Psychology*, 48(5).
'Kali's Zeit, Gewalt zwischen Religionsgruppen in Indien', 2003, *Internationales Asienforum*, 34(3-4).
'Seduction and the Saint: Desire and the Spiritual Quest', 2002, *Annual of Psychoanalysis*, 30.
'Psychoanalyse und oestliche Traditionen des Heilens', 2002, *Zeitschrift fuer psychoanalytische Theorie und Praxis*, 17(3).
'Leadership in Indian Organizations in a Comparative Perspective', 2002, *International Journal of Cross-Cultural Management*, 2(2).
'The Time of Kali: Violence between Religious Groups in India', 2000, *Social Research*, 67:3.
'La Double Quete: La Vie des Femmes dans e'Inde Moderne', 1998), *Bulletin d'Information des Cadres*, 37.
'Gesundheit und Kultur. Heilung in oestlicher und westlicher Perspektive', 1998), *Jahrbuch fuer Komplexitaet in den Natur-, Sozial- und Geisteswisseschaften*, Bd. 7
'Clinical Work and Cultural Imagination', 1995, *Psychoanalytic Quarterly*, 64, 2); Spanish translation in 2001 in *Los Caminos de Eros*, Buenos Aires: Psicoanalisis.
'Encounters of the Psychological Kind: Freud, Jung and India', 1994, *The Psychoanalytical Study of Society*, 19.
'Ramakrishna and the Mystical Experience', 1992, *Annual of Psychoanalysis*, 20.
'The Maternal Feminine in Indian Psychoanalysis', 1989, *International Review of Psychoanalysis*, 16(3).
'Notes on the History and Development of Indian Psycho-analysis', 1989, *Revue Internationale d'histoire de la Psychanalyse*, 2; also in P. Kutter, ed., 1995, *Psychoanalysis International*, 2, Stuttgart: Frommann.
'Doctors and Patients in the Hindu Tradition', 1995, *Indian Horizons*, 37.
'Psychoanalytic Reflections on Religion and Mysticism', 1988, *Zen Buddhism Today*, 6.
'Psychoanalysis and Anthropology: A Renewed Alliance', 1987, *Contributions to Indian Sociology*, 21(1).
'Male and Female in India: Identity Formation and its Effects on Cultural Adaptation', 1986, *Studies in Third World Societies*, 38.
'Psychoanalysis and Non-Western Cultures', 1985, *International Review of Psychoanalysis*, 12(4).
'Psychotherapie et Culture: La guerison dans la traditon', 1985, *Confronations*, 13.
'Les meres et leurs fils en Inde', 1985, *Frayages*.
'Erotic Fantasy: The Secret Passion of Radha and Krishna', 1985, *Contributions to Indian Sociology*, 19(1).
'Psychoanalysis and Religious Healing: Siblings or Strangers?', 1985, *Journal of American Academy of Religion*, 53(3); also in R. Hart, ed., 1982, *Trajectories in the Study of Religion*, Atlanta: Scholars Press.

'Reflections on Psychoanalysis, Indian Culture and Mysticism, A Review Essay', 1982, *Journal of Indian Philosophy*,, 10).

'The Person in Tantra and Psychoanalysis', 1981, *Samiksa, Journal of Indian Psychoanalytic Society*, 35(4); also published in *International Journal of Asian Studies*.

'Observations on the "Oedipal Alliance" in a Patient with a Narcissistic Personality Disorder', 1980, *Samiksa*, 32(4).

'A Case of Depression', 1979, *Samiksa*, 33(3).

'Childhood in India: Traditional Ideals and Contemporary Reality', 1979, *International Social Science Journal*, 31(3); German translation: 'Kindheit in Indien', *Kindheit*, 1.

'Relative Realities: Images of Adulthood in Psychoanalysis and the Yogas', 1977, *Samiksa*, 31(2).

'Authority in Work Organizations', 1977, *Vikalpa*, 2(4).

'Leaders, Power and Personality', 1977), *Vikalpa*, 2(2).

'Curiosity in Children and Adults: A Review Essay', 1976, *Indian Journal of Psychology*, 51(2).

'Leadership Training in Industry and Administration: A Critical Review', 1976, *Management in Government*.

'Neurosis in India: An Overview and Some Observations', 1975, *Indian Journal of Psychology*, 50(2).

'Indische Kultur und Psychoanalyse, Indian Culture and Psychoanalysis)', 1974, *Psyche*, 28(7).

'Aggression in Indian Society: An Analysis of Folk Tales', 1974, *Indian Journal of Psychology*, vol. 49, Pt.2; (a shorter version appeared in *Journal of Social Psychology*, 87).

'Authority Relations in Indian Organization', 1972, *Management International Review*, 1.

'Rationality and Irrationality in Business Leadership', 1971, *Journal of Business Policy*, 2(2).

'Authority Patterns and Subordinate Behavior in Indian Organizations', 1971, *Administrative Science Quarterly*, 16(5).

'The Theme of Authority in Social Relations in India', 1971, *Journal of Social Psychology*, 84.

'The Logic of Psychohistory', 1970, *Journal of Interdisciplinary History*, 1(1).

(co-authored) 'Time and Content of Significant Life Experience', 1968, *Perceptual and Motor Skills*, 27. 'The Human Life Cycle: The Traditional Hindu View and the Psychology of Erik Erikson', 1968, *Philosophy East and West*, 18(5).

About the Author

Psychoanalyst, scholar, and writer Sudhir Kakar has been a lecturer at Harvard University, Boston, USA; research fellow at the Harvard Business School, professor at the Indian Institute of Management, Ahmedabad; head of the Department of Humanities and Social Sciences at the Indian Institute of Technology, Delhi; and adjunct professor of leadership at INSEAD in Fontainebleau, France. He was senior fellow at the Centre for Study of World Religions at Harvard as also visiting professor at the universities of Chicago, Harvard, McGill, Melbourne, Hawaii, and Vienna. He has also been a fellow at the Institutes of Advanced Study at Princeton and Berlin, and at the Centre for Advanced Study, University of Cologne, Germany.

Dr Kakar is a member of the New York Academy of Sciences; the International Psychoanalytic Association; the Board of Sigmund Freud Archives at the Library of Congress, Washington; and the Academie Universelle des Culture, France. He serves on the editorial boards of several professional journals.

His many honors include the Kardiner Award from Columbia University; the Boyer Prize for psychological anthropology from the American Anthropological Association; Germany's Goethe Medal; the Rockefeller Residency; the McArthur Fellowship; the Distinguished Service Award from the Indo-American Psychiatric Association; the Merck-Tagore Award; Fellow of the National Academy of Psychology; and the Bhabha, Nehru, and ICSSR National Fellowships in India. In

February 2012, he was conferred with the Order of Merit of the Federal Republic of Germany, the country's highest civilian order.

A leading figure in the fields of cultural psychology and the psychology of religion, as well as a novelist, Dr Kakar's person and work have been profiled in *The New York Times*, *Le Monde*, *Frankfurter Allgemeine*, *Neue Zuricher Zeitung*, *Die Zeit*, *Le Nouvel Observateur* (which listed him as one of the world's twenty-five major thinkers), and German weekly *Die Zeit* (which included him among the twenty-one important thinkers of the twenty-first century).

Kakar is the author/editor of twenty-three books of non-fiction. These include: *The Inner World*; *Shamans, Mystics and Doctors*; *Tales of Love, Sex and Danger*; *Intimate Relations*; *The Analyst and the Mystic*; *The Colors of Violence*; *Culture and Psyche*; *The Indians: Portrait of a People*; a new translation of the *Kamasutra* for Oxford World Classics (with Wendy Doniger); *Mad and Divine: Spirit and Psyche in the Modern World*; and *Young Tagore*. He is also the author of the novels *The Ascetic of Desire*; *Ecstasy*; *Mira and the Mahatma*; *The Crimson Throne* (shortlisted for the Crossword Vodaphone Prize); *The Devil Take Love*; *The Kipling File* (shortlisted for the Valley of Words Prize); and the editor of *Indian Love Stories*. His books have been translated into twenty-two languages around the world.

